T0340937

Emerging
Non-Clinical
Biostatistics in
Biopharmaceutical
Development and
Manufacturing

Chapman & Hall/CRC Biostatistics Series

Published Titles

Published Titles

Published Titles

Emerging Non-Clinical Biostatistics in Biopharmaceutical Development and Manufacturing
Harry Yang

Empirical Likelihood Method in Survival Analysis
Mai Zhou

Essentials of a Successful Biostatistical Collaboration
Arul Earnest

Exposure–Response Modeling: Methods and Practical Implementation
Jixian Wang

Frailty Models in Survival Analysis
Andreas Wienke

Fundamental Concepts for New Clinical Trialists
Scott Evans and Naitee Ting

Generalized Linear Models: A Bayesian Perspective
Dipak K. Dey, Sujit K. Ghosh, and Bani K. Mallick

Handbook of Regression and Modeling: Applications for the Clinical and Pharmaceutical Industries
Daryl S. Paulson

Inference Principles for Biostatisticians
Ian C. Marschner

Interval-Censored Time-to-Event Data: Methods and Applications
Ding-Geng (Din) Chen, Jianguo Sun, and Karl E. Peace

Introductory Adaptive Trial Designs: A Practical Guide with R
Mark Chang

Joint Models for Longitudinal and Time-to-Event Data: With Applications in R
Dimitris Rizopoulos

Measures of Interobserver Agreement and Reliability, Second Edition
Mohamed M. Shoukri

Medical Biostatistics, Third Edition
A. Indrayan

Meta-Analysis in Medicine and Health Policy
Dalene Stangl and Donald A. Berry

Mixed Effects Models for the Population Approach: Models, Tasks, Methods and Tools
Marc Lavielle

Modeling to Inform Infectious Disease Control
Niels G. Becker

Modern Adaptive Randomized Clinical Trials: Statistical and Practical Aspects
Oleksandr Sverdlov

Monte Carlo Simulation for the Pharmaceutical Industry: Concepts, Algorithms, and Case Studies
Mark Chang

Multiregional Clinical Trials for Simultaneous Global New Drug Development
Joshua Chen and Hui Quan

Multiple Testing Problems in Pharmaceutical Statistics
Alex Dmitrienko, Ajit C. Tamhane, and Frank Bretz

Noninferiority Testing in Clinical Trials: Issues and Challenges
Tie-Hua Ng

Optimal Design for Nonlinear Response Models
Valerii V. Fedorov and Sergei L. Leonov

Patient-Reported Outcomes: Measurement, Implementation and Interpretation
Joseph C. Cappelleri, Kelly H. Zou, Andrew G. Bushmakin, Jose Ma. J. Alvir, Demissie Alemayehu, and Tara Symonds

Quantitative Evaluation of Safety in Drug Development: Design, Analysis and Reporting
Qi Jiang and H. Amy Xia

Quantitative Methods for Traditional Chinese Medicine Development
Shein-Chung Chow

Randomized Clinical Trials of Nonpharmacological Treatments
Isabelle Boutron, Philippe Ravaud, and David Moher

Chapman & Hall/CRC Biostatistics Series

Emerging Non-Clinical Biostatistics in Biopharmaceutical Development and Manufacturing

Harry Yang

MedImmune, LLC

Gaithersburg, Maryland, USA

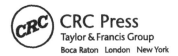

CRC Press

Taylor & Francis Group

Boca Raton London New York

CRC Press is an imprint of the
Taylor & Francis Group, an **informa** business

A CHAPMAN & HALL BOOK

CRC Press
Taylor & Francis Group
6000 Broken Sound Parkway NW, Suite 300
Boca Raton, FL 33487-2742

Printed on acid-free paper
Version Date: 20160923

International Standard Book Number-13: 978-1-4987-0415-1 (Hardback)

Visit the Taylor & Francis Web site at
http://www.taylorandfrancis.com

and the CRC Press Web site at
http://www.crcpress.com

Printed and bound in the United States of America by
Edwards Brothers Malloy on sustainably sourced paper

Contents

Section III Process Development

Section IV   Manufacturing

Preface

In August 2002, the Food and Drug Administration (FDA) launched a significant initiative, "Pharmaceutical Current Good Manufacturing Practices (cGMPs) for the 21st Century." This initiative, coupled with other subsequent regulatory publications, including ICH Q8–Q11, ushered in a risk-based and life cycle approach to process and product development. The initiative encourages manufacturers to capitalize on new technological advances and adopt risk-based approaches and quality system techniques. An increased emphasis has been placed on product and process understanding. This includes understanding the mechanism of action of the product, its safety profile, variability of raw materials, bulk and finished products, analytical method variations, relationships between process parameters and the product's critical quality attributes (CQAs), and the impact of CQAs on clinical responses and product quality. This enhanced product and process knowledge not only enables product quality to be built by design but also provides a basis for the development of robust control strategies.

A holistic approach, QbD begins in development and continues throughout the manufacturing life cycle. It involves defining desired clinical performance, identifying CQAs that have an impact on clinical outcomes, determining necessary raw material attributes and manufacturing process parameters to achieve the desired product attributes, and designing manufacturing controls to ensure consistent manufacturing. Furthermore, QbD enhances development capability, shortens development speed, and enables robust manufacturing. It also helps proactively prevent manufacturing failures. An additional benefit of QbD is that, in certain instances, it enables a manufacturer to make postapproval changes and scale-up operations without prior approval from regulatory authorities.

However, despite the plethora of opportunities to reduce manufacturing costs while ensuring product quality, implementation of QbD is often very challenging because of the large number of variables to consider, interactions among the variables, uncertainties in measurements, and missing data involved in product and process development. Such intrinsic complexities argue for advanced statistical methods in both study design and analysis. In fact, the preceding guidelines specifically call for use of such statistical tools. For example, ICH Q8 recommends the use of design of experiments (DOE) to aid the development of a design space, which is defined as the "multidimensional combination and interaction of input variables (e.g., material attributes) and process parameters that have been demonstrated to provide assurance of quality." The successful determination of a design space makes continued process improvements within the design space possible, without overly regulatory oversight. Furthermore, the FDA guidance on Process Analytical

Technology specifically cites the use of multivariate tools for study design, data acquisition, and data analysis to aid quality assessment. In addition, the 2011 FDA process validation guidance recommends the use of a broad array of statistical tools, including DOE, acceptance sampling, multivariate modeling, and statistical process control. It has been widely recognized by both pharmaceutical manufacturers and regulators that novel statistical methods are key to delivering on the promise of the new pharmaceutical development paradigm.

In recent years, statistical science has made significant inroads in advancing the new product and process development paradigm and quality initiatives. As the entire pharmaceutical industry is adopting a QbD approach, statistics is likely to continue to play a central role in realizing the full benefits of QbD. However, no book so far has been written to discuss the QbD-related statistical advances. As such, a single book covering important biopharmaceutical development issues, relevant regulatory requirements, and associated statistical solutions would provide an invaluable resource for practitioners in biopharmaceutical development and manufacturing.

Drawing from the author's extensive drug research and development experience and published statistical works, this book is intended to provide a single source of information on emerging statistical approaches to QbD and risk-based pharmaceutical development. It combines in-depth explanations of advanced statistical methods with real-life case studies that illustrate practical applications of these methods in QbD implementation. The book is divided into four sections, consisting of a total of 12 chapters. Each chapter begins with a summary of the scientific issues, related regulatory requirements, and pitfalls of statistical methods either currently in use or recommended in regulatory guidance, followed by an introduction to and discussion of the advantages of the emerging statistical techniques used to address the scientific questions. The use of the statistical methods in practice is further illustrated through case studies. Each chapter concludes with a summary of key points and directions for possible extension and new applications of the statistical methods in future research. A brief description of each chapter follows:

Section I (Chapter 1) provides a background about the evolution of regulatory thinking and industry practice from "testing into compliance" to QbD. The chapter highlights challenges associated with the implementation of QbD and related statistical opportunities.

Section II (Chapters 2 through 4) is devoted to discussions of various statistical advances in analytical method development and validation, notably with focus on the validation of accuracy and precision, parallelism testing for bioassay, and validation of assay linearity.

Chapter 2 discusses a formal statistical framework for the validation of analytical methods, using QbD principles. The use of total error to control the risk of incorrect decision-making is summarized, including a new statistical method based on the total error concept; the performance of the new method is compared with other statistical methods conventionally used.

Chapter 3 is concerned with an important issue of bioassay, namely, parallelism testing. Parallelism is a prerequisite for the estimation of relative potency in many bioassays. Implicit in parallelism is that the test sample is a dilution of the reference standard. In this chapter, various parallelism test methods are evaluated through simulation and receiver operating characteristic analysis. A new Bayesian test method, which overcomes the shortcomings of the current statistical approaches, is also discussed.

In Chapter 4, we focus on current statistical practices and emerging statistical methods in the validation of linearity, a key characteristic of analytical methods. Central to the discussion is a new equivalence test that compares the quality of a linear fit to that of a higher-order polynomial. By using orthogonal polynomial regression and generalized pivotal quantity analysis, the method allows for estimation of the probability of equivalence in either the assay response space or the dose concentration space. In addition, a simpler and more practical but theoretically rigorous alternative is also presented.

Section III (Chapters 5 through 8) concentrates on four major scientific issues related to biopharmaceutical process development, validation, and verification.

Chapter 5 concerns the assessment of oncogenicity and infectivity risk. It is well known that biological products manufactured in cells contain residual DNA derived from host cell substrates. Therefore, it is theoretically possible that the residual DNA could transmit activated oncogenes or latent infectious viral genomes to subjects receiving the product and induce oncogenic or infective events. A probabilistic model to estimate the risks due to residual DNA is discussed. The model takes into account the enzyme inactivation process and allows for more accurate risk assessment when compared to statistical methods currently in use. An application of the method to determine the safety factor for a vaccine product is provided as a case study. The model is further applied to establish acceptable limits of residual DNA that may differ from the current regulatory specifications. An extension of the proposed statistical method based on Bayesian inference is also discussed.

Chapter 6 discusses novel statistical methods in evaluating results of viral clearance studies. Statistical methods robust to both missing data and zero viral counts post process are presented along with results of simulation studies conducted to compare the performance of the current and new methods. These results provide practical guidance on the selection of statistical methods for assessing purification process capability.

In Chapter 7, we introduce a risk-based statistical approach to establishing prefiltration bioburden acceptance limits and alternative test volumes. The relationship between bioburden risk, prefiltration bioburden test limits, and sterile filtration process parameters, such as filtration volume, filter surface area, and microbial retention capacity of the sterilizing filter, is established through statistical modeling. The method provides a sound rationale for justifying prefiltration bioburden test volumes and acceptance limits, as an alternative to the regulatory limit (10 colony-forming units/100 mL), without compromising sterility assurance.

Chapter 8 is dedicated to the latest statistical developments in adopting QbD principles in the life cycle approach to process validation. Various multivariate statistical methods to model relationships between process parameters and CQAs, to link CQAs to clinical responses, and to define a design space and set specifications are introduced and illustrated through examples. Also included in this chapter are methods for addressing key issues such as the number of lots used for process performance quantification and monitoring strategies for large dimensional data, with interdependent responses.

Section IV (Chapters 9 through 12) is devoted to quality control and assurance in manufacturing, in order to fulfill the requirements of the FDA's cGMPs. These chapters cover a wide range of important GMP topics, including specifications, environmental monitoring, stability study design and analysis, and the investigation of out-of-specification results.

Chapter 9 focuses on setting specifications for drug products, which are quality standards providing assurance that the product is fit for its intended use. While quality attributes may be correlated, specifications are often determined without taking into account any such interdependencies. Such practice may result in specifications that are narrower than the actual acceptable ranges of product performance, thus causing unnecessary out-of-specification investigations. Through multiple case studies, the chapter discusses how this issue can be avoided using multivariate statistical modeling and other advanced statistical techniques such as generalized pivotal quantity analysis.

Chapter 10 discusses statistical methods for trending environmental data of classified rooms. By modeling the excess of zeroes and overdispersion, caused by sampling population heterogeneity, the proposed statistical methods provide a clear improvement over the traditional approaches. Additionally, a new approach to constructing multivariate control charts for cleanroom environmental monitoring is presented.

Chapter 11 introduces a statistical framework for the evaluation of various commonly used shelf life estimation methods. In addition, through several case studies, it describes how novel statistical methodologies such as Arrhenius modeling, simulation, and Bayesian analysis can be effectively used in stability testing to achieve both quality assurance and cost reduction objectives.

Finally, Chapter 12 discusses current and new statistical methods for out-of-specification (OOS) result investigations and out-of-trend (OOT) result identification. Despite improved regulatory clarity on OOS investigations, how OOS results are evaluated and batches disposed continues to be a leading cause of warning letters issued by the FDA. Numerous working practices and various degrees of understanding of current expectations in this area have led to many different statistical approaches to investigating OOS results. In this chapter, statistical methods for OOS investigation that represent good science and conform to current regulatory guidelines are presented. In addition, various statistical methods for identifying OOT results are also included in the chapter.

I am extremely grateful to John Kimmel, executive editor, Chapman & Hall/ CRC Press, for the opportunity to work on this book. I would like to express my deepest gratitude to Katherine Giacoletti, Kicab Castaneda-Mendez, Lorin Roskos, Brad Evans, Liang Zhao, and three anonymous reviewers for their expertly review of the book/book proposal and constructive comments that have greatly helped improve both the content and the presentation of the book. I would also like to thank Steve Novick, Rick Burdick, Jianchun Zhang, Na Li, Wei Zhao, Binbing Yu, Lanju Zhang, Lingmin Zeng, Terry O'Day, Percerval Sondag, John Peterson, David LeBlond, Charles Tan, Tim Schofield, and Stan Altan for collaborative statistical research on various statistical subjects pertinent to biopharmaceutical development and manufacturing. I also wish to thank Athula Herath, David Christopher, Tony Lonardo, Don Bennett, Meiyu Shen, Xiaoyu Dong, and Yi Tsong for many inspiring discussions on statistical issues of interest to the biopharmaceutical industry and regulatory agencies, and my colleagues, Robert Singer, Bruno Boulanger, Tony Okinczyc, and Dennis Sandell, on the USP Statistics Expert Committee for helpful discussions on important topics such as analytical method validation and analysis, treatment, and interpretation of analytical data. I am deeply indebted to my wife, Hongji Liu, and daughters, Katarina Yang and Kelsey Yang, for their strong support during the writing of this book.

Last, the views expressed in this book are those of the author and not necessarily those of MedImmune.

Harry Yang
Gaithersburg, Maryland

Section I

Background

1

Quality by Design in Biopharmaceuticals

1.1 Introduction

A biopharmaceutical is a drug product that is produced from living sources such as cells or tissues. Also known as biologics, biopharmaceutical products include not only recombinant therapeutic proteins but also naturally sourced proteins, live virus vaccines, and blood components. The discovery of penicillin in 1920 led to the first biopharmaceutical product. However, it was not until the creation of recombinant technology that production of therapeutic proteins in a laboratory setting became possible. The first boom in the discovery and production of biopharmaceuticals took place in the 1980s, as evidenced by the approval and marketing of recombinant human insulin, human growth hormone, interferon gamma, and other important therapeutic molecules. Leveraging the advances in cellular and molecular sciences and technologies, biopharmaceutical firms have been able to develop targeted therapies for treating diseases ranging from cancers to rare genetic disorders. As of 2014, more than 300 biopharmaceuticals have been approved for marketing. The biopharmaceutical industry clearly has become one of the fastest-growing sectors. At present, there are more than 900 biopharmaceutical molecules in various stages of development for the treatment and prevention of a wide range of diseases. With some older biologics coming off patent, biosimilar product development has emerged as a nascent and rapid growing area as well. However, chemistry, manufacturing, and control (CMC) issues present a host of unique challenges in the development of biopharmaceutical products.

In this chapter, we discuss the impact of the evolving regulatory environment on biopharmaceutical development and manufacturing, challenges of biopharmaceutical CMC development, implications of quality by design (QbD), and statistical innovations that can help advance successful CMC development of biopharmaceuticals.

1.2 Evolving Regulatory Environment

The pharmaceutical industry is strictly regulated. Before marketing approval of a new drug is granted by regulatory agencies such as the US Food and Drug Administration (FDA) and European Medicines Agency, the drug must be shown to be both safe and efficacious (Peltzman 1973). For this reason, a large body of clinical, nonclinical, and analytical CMC data are generated in support of the premarketing approval. Furthermore, manufacturing regulations, such as the US current good manufacturing practices (cGMPs), also stipulate that modern standards and technologies be adopted in the design, monitoring, and control of manufacturing processes and facilities to ensure consistent supply of high-quality drug products to the patient. In fact, manufacturing practices that deviate from the cGMPs constitute violations of law. Specifically, under the Federal Food, Drug, and Cosmetic Act, a drug is adulterated if "the methods used in, or the facilities or controls used for, its manufacture, processing, packing or holding do not conform to or are not operated or administered in conformity with cGMP to assure that such drug meets the quality and purity characteristics, which it purports or is represented to possess" (21 U.S.C. § 351(a) (2) (B)). Violations of GMP may result in costly recalls and lost sales. In some cases, they may lead to closure of manufacturing facilities and denial of access to the US market. Thus, noncompliance findings may also lead to severe shortage of drug supplies, causing serious public health concerns. In the United States, the FDA has the authority to inspect drug manufacturing facilities and to examine, investigate, and collect samples to ensure conformance to cGMPs. The FDA has control over virtually every aspect of manufacturing processes. Therefore, adherence to government regulations, including cGMPs, is essential to ensuring consistent supply of high-quality drug products to patients.

Traditionally, quality of a drug product was ensured through various testing. The testing was carried out not only on the finished product but also on raw materials including drug substance and excipients. Since only a small sample out of potentially millions of units in a batch is tested, extensive in-process tests were expected by the regulatory agencies (Yu 2008). In addition, any change to the manufacturing process required a postapproval filing. This made manufacturers wary of improving their processes, for example, by utilizing new technologies. Such concern spilled over to the biopharmaceutical sectors in the 1990s when the FDA shifted its attention from individual products to the biotechnology industry as a whole (Elliott et al. 2013). The enactment of the 1997 FDA Modernization Act, which was intended to minimize the differences in the regulation of drug and biologic applications, reinforced the FDA oversight of biopharmaceutical manufacturing.

However, despite frequent regulatory inspections and intense oversight, there was a series of serious manufacturing failures in the United States in the mid to late 1990s that led to plant closures and massive product recalls, as well as FDA injunctions and consent decrees. By the early 2000s, the FDA had uncovered a number of widespread issues, including uneven quality and substandard practices in pharmaceutical manufacturing, insufficient understanding of manufacturing breakdowns, low manufacturing efficiencies, and slow uptake of new technologies. It became apparent to the FDA that manufacturing processes needed to be modernized in order to improve manufacturing efficacy and reliability. Also clear was that the FDA's extensive control over virtually every aspect of the manufacturing process had caused pharmaceutical manufacturers to be reluctant to improve their manufacturing processes, thus impeding innovation (Woodcock 2012). As a result, in August 2012, the FDA launched a significant initiative entitled "Pharmaceutical cGMPs for the 21st Century: A Risk-Based Approach" (FDA 2004a). It was intended to encourage pharmaceutical companies to invest in and commit to modern production systems able to meet established regulatory standards. In addition, through this initiative, the FDA was committed to developing risk-based review, compliance, and inspection policies so that CMC reviews would be focused on high-risk issues. As discussed by Dr. Woodcock (2012), the initiative was driven by a vision to achieve a desired state of the pharmaceutical industry as "a maximally efficient, agile, flexible manufacturing sector that reliably produces high-quality drug products without extensive regulatory oversight." The initiative brought about several important regulatory changes. Among these changes, most noticeable were publications of several ICH guidance documents [ICH Q8 (R2), 9, 10, and 11] related to pharmaceutical development, quality risk management, and pharmaceutical quality systems (ICH 2006, 2007a,b, 2011, respectively). These guidance documents stress the importance of manufacturing process development based on systematic product and process understanding, control of risk, and implementation of quality management systems. They represented a significant shift from the traditional "testing into compliance" to "quality by design." The culmination of these regulatory activities was the publication in 2011 of the long-awaited guidance *FDA Guidance for Industry on Process Validation: General Principles and Practices* (FDA 2011). This guidance document aligns process validation activities with a risk-based product life cycle approach, as well as other existing ICH guidelines Q8–Q10.

Over the past decade, there has also been growing interest in utilization of process analytical technology (PAT) to optimize products and processes and provide assurance of quality. In ICH Q8 (R2) (ICH 2006), PAT is defined as "A system for designing, analyzing, and controlling manufacturing through timely measurements (i.e., during processing) of critical quality and performance attributes of raw and in-process materials and processes with the goal of ensuring final product quality." Within the PAT framework, there are several important tools that can be used to effectively acquire information for process understanding, continuous improvement, development of risk-mitigation strategies, and knowledge management. As PAT advances, application of PAT in process development has gained rapid regulatory and industry support as evidenced by the 2004 publication of an FDA guidance document on PAT (FDA 2004b).

As pointed out by Kozlowski and Swann (2009), manufacturing processes may still be improved, based on QbD principles, even if PAT tools are not readily available for real-time analysis of material attributes (MAs) and linkage to process control. QbD is a more general and systematic approach to development "that begins with predefined objectives and emphasizes product and process understanding and process control, based on sound science and quality risk management" [ICH Q8 (R2)]. Under QbD, product quality is built into the product through understanding manufacturing risks and developing control strategies to mitigate these risks. Successful implementation of QbD will ultimately lead to more efficient and reliable manufacturing processes that produce drug products with desired clinical performance. Over the past decade, substantial progress has been made in implementing QbD in product and process development. In 2008, a working group, consisting of representatives from seven pharmaceutical companies, was formed to create a case study that would support application of QbD in monoclonal antibody development. This was followed by another case study on vaccine development. Various other examples of successful applications of QbD in improving recombinant expression systems, cell culture, virus clearance, and formulation development have been reported (Rathore and Mhatre 2009). More recently, QbD principles have been applied to analytical method development (Borman et al. 2007; Martin et al. 2013; Nethercote and Ermer 2012; Nethercote et al. 2010).

1.3 Bioprocess Development

Process development for a biopharmaceutical is generally more labor intensive and time consuming when compared to chemically synthesized small-molecule pharmaceuticals, owing to the large number of unit operations, variability in both input materials and processes, and control of organism-mediated production (Gronemeyer et al. 2014). To reduce cost and improve manufacturing efficiency and consistency, it is critical to have a fundamental understanding of the processes and effective controls. Employment of modern technologies such as PAT and application of novel statistical methods can help gain deep insights about factors that affect process performance, speed up development, and ensure regulatory compliance. The processes by which biologic products are manufactured are often referred to as bioprocesses. In broad terms, a bioprocess can be divided into the upstream process (USP) and downstream process (DSP), each having well-defined objectives. Figure 1.1 displays a typical manufacturing process for monoclonal antibodies.

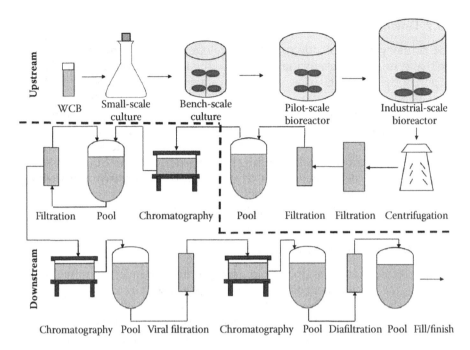

FIGURE 1.1
Manufacturing process of monoclonal antibody.

1.3.1 Upstream Process

USP development is concerned with selection of host cell line, development of culture medium, and design of the bioreactor and its operating conditions. Upstream processing may also include cell harvesting, process control, and corresponding analytics (Gronemeyer et al. 2014). Consider the manufacture of a monoclonal antibody based on recombinant-DNA technologies. A cell line is selected based on its ability to meet high productivity and other quality criteria. Special consideration should be given to the cell growth behavior, stability, and posttranslational properties including level of expression of the desired product. Development of the growth medium usually commences at a small scale using shake flasks of 250-mL to 1-L capacity. Experiments are carried out to determine the optimum culture environment. After the optimal culture conditions are identified, scale-up efforts take place first in a benchtop bioreactor (1–2 L) and then in a pilot-scale reactor (100–1000 L). These systems are capable of monitoring or adjusting environmental and process parameters (PPs) such as temperature, pH, and dissolved-oxygen concentration. Data collected from this stage of development provide critical information to allow for optimizing culture medium and the process for commercialization. When the culture medium and process are deemed to be viable, design and development of the commercial-scale bioreactor along with aseptic manufacturing facilities begin.

1.3.2 Downstream Process

The primary focus of downstream development is to maximize product yield and minimize impurities. Typically, the DSP involves a series of steps to purify the product, using various chromatographic separation methods such as affinity, size-exclusion, ion-exchange, and reversed-phase chromatography. To ensure the sterility of the product, DNA and virus inactivation processes are employed. Also needed are a filtration step and a final diafiltration operation, which are followed by final polishing steps, yielding the final drug bulk substance. Depending on the product, either filling or lyophilization may be performed on the drug substance. Downstream processing is a critical component of the overall manufacturing process as exceptional purity of biopharmaceutical products is expected.

1.3.3 Challenges of Bioprocessing

While biological drug products hold great promise for meeting unmet medical needs, the development of manufacturing processes for biologicals presents a host of challenges. To begin with, there are many variables (such as media composition, aeration, metabolites, sheer forces, and cell density) that may affect the performance of the cell substrate used for manufacturing (Kozlowski and Swann 2009). Subtle variations in these variables may result in significant changes in quality attributes such as glycosylation and oxidation. Most formidable is that translational modifications of the protein may have a negative impact on drug safety, efficacy, PK, or immunogenicity. In addition to these upstream challenges, the quality of raw materials varies significantly and is difficult to control. Furthermore, since downstream processing usually consists of many complex unit operations, it is challenging to optimize DSPs from a holistic perspective. To reduce cost and improve efficiency and consistency, a fundamental understanding of the processes and controls are essential. Employment of modern tools such as PAT and the application of statistical techniques can provide deep insights into these complex process steps, increase process knowledge, and speed the development of robust manufacturing processes.

1.4 Quality by Design

As previously discussed, the traditional product and process development is concentrated on the assurance of product quality through extensive testing. This testing includes the inspection of raw materials, in-process material testing, and final drug substance and product release testing. The lack of product and process understanding and limited knowledge of variability lead to stringent specifications that prohibit the release of products that otherwise may have acceptance clinical performance (Yu et al. 2014). As changes to the process and test methods required postapproval submissions, there were no incentives for the manufacturers to improve their manufacturing processes. Pharmaceutical QbD provides a framework for both the industry and FDA to adopt a scientific, risk-based, holistic, and proactive approach to pharmaceutical development. Under QbD, product and process development begins with predefined quality objectives, followed by the identification of critical quality attributes (CQAs) that have significant impact on the drug product. Experiments are carried out to understand process variability and establish the relationships between process performance and input materials and PPs. This knowledge serves as the basis for developing effective controls centered on parameters or areas of high risk. It also lends the manufacturer the ability to develop a manufacturing process that is flexible and consistent in delivering high-quality product.

As outlined in ICH Q8 (R2), key steps to implementing QbD include the following: (1) define quality target product profile (QTPP), (2) determine CQAs through risk assessment, (3) link raw MAs and PPs to CQAs, (4) develop design space for key MAs and PPs, (5) develop and implement effective control strategies, and (6) manage product life cycle through continued process improvement. The overall QbD approach is illustrated in Figure 1.2.

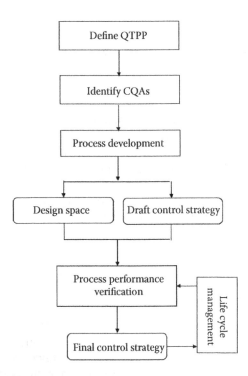

FIGURE 1.2

QbD process development paradigm. (Adapted from CMC Biotech Working Group (2009). A-Mab: A Case Study in Bioprocess Development. www.casss.org/associations/9165/.../A -Mab_Case_Study_Version_2-1.pdf (accessed on April 15, 2016).)

Successful implementation of QbD requires significant efforts in each of the above steps.

1.4.1 Quality Target Product Profile

The QTPP defines a new drug product in terms of its desired clinical benefits and quality standard. The QTPP is the foundation for the drug product development. A drug product designed, developed, and manufactured according to its QTPP can consistently provide the desired clinical performance. According to ICH Q8 (R2) (2006), a QTPP is a "prospective and dynamic summary of the quality characteristics of a drug product that ideally will be achieved to ensure that the desired quality, thus the safety and efficacy, of a drug product is realized." When developing a QTPP, the following considerations should be given:

- Intended use in clinical setting, route of administration, dosage form, and delivery systems
- Dosage strength(s)
- Container closure system
- Therapeutic moiety release or delivery and attributes affecting pharmacokinetic characteristics (e.g., dissolution, aerodynamic performance) appropriate to the drug product dosage form being developed
- Drug product quality criteria (e.g., sterility, purity, stability, and drug release) appropriate for the intended marketed product

Depending on the complexity of the product, more attention may be paid to some of these considerations than others (Kozlowski and Swann 2009). How to develop a robust QTPP has been extensively discussed in two case studies (CMC Biotech Working Group 2009; CMC Vaccine Working Group 2012). As the QTPP is the guiding principle for product development, its importance can never be overstated.

1.4.2 Product and Process Design

1.4.2.1 Critical Quality Attributes

Identification of CQAs follows immediately after the QTPP is developed. This allows for evaluation and control of product characteristics that have impact on quality, safety, and efficacy. A CQA is defined as a physical, chemical, biological, or microbiological property or characteristic that should be within an appropriate limit, range, or distribution to ensure the desired product quality [ICH Q8 (R2)]. The identification of CQAs is usually accomplished through a criticality assessment that evaluates the risk for each attribute, which includes severity (consequences to the patient) and probability (likelihood of occurrence) of nonconformance with acceptable limits. Both prior product knowledge and process capability are useful sources of information for such evaluation. The former includes cumulative laboratory, nonclinical, and clinical experience related to the quality attribute under evaluation, as well as data from molecules in the same class and publications in literature. The latter consist of data from process development studies and manufacturing experience. Both product knowledge and process capability serve as the basis for establishing the acceptable range for a CQA. Since changes in CQAs might have a significant impact on product safety and efficacy, it is critical to establish the relationships between CQAs and clinical performance and define acceptable ranges for CQAs. This knowledge provides a foundation for developing robust control strategies for the product and constructing a design space for the manufacturing process. However, it can be difficult to link a particular quality attribute to clinical performance (safety and efficacy) in a qualitative or quantitative manner.

1.4.2.2 Process Development

After the CQAs are defined, the focus is shifted to the development of a manufacturing process that produces a product with the desired quality. At this stage of development, studies are carried out, using multivariate design of experiment (DOE) strategies, to evaluate the effects of process variables and their interactions on process performance. Knowledge gleaned from the results of these studies, perhaps combined with platform knowledge and data from other molecules in the same class, will be used to define critical process parameters (CPPs) through a risk assessment. The next step is to optimize the process based on the CPPs identified from the risk assessment. This experimentation also gives rise to the design space. The above sequence of activities is repeated for each unit operation, establishing design space for each set of input PPs.

1.4.3 Process Control

Implementation of control strategies enables a manufacturing process to consistently deliver product that meets established quality attribute ranges that in turn ensure drug safety and efficacy. QbD principles call for using a risk-based approach to develop control strategies. Knowledge of CQAs and the impact of PPs and other input materials on these CQAs enable manufacturers to avoid unnecessary testing for maintaining product quality. In essence, the level of control of each quality attribute should reflect the criticality of the attribute. Effective control strategies integrate a number of elements including input material controls, procedural controls, PP controls, in-process testing, specification testing, characterization/comparability testing, and process monitoring applied as appropriate.

TABLE 1.1

Contrasts between Minimal and QbD Approaches

Aspect	Minimal Approaches	Enhanced QbD Approaches
Overall pharmaceutical development	• Mainly empirical • Development research often conducted one variable at a time	• Systematic, relating mechanistic understanding of material attributes and process parameters to drug product CQAs • Multivariate experiments to understand product and process • Establishment of design space • PAT utilized
Manufacturing process	• Fixed • Validation primarily based on initial full-scale batches • Focus on optimization and reproducibility	• Adjustable within design space • Life cycle approach to validation and ideally continuous process verification • Focus on control strategy and robustness • Use of statistical process control methods
Process controls	• In-process test primarily for go/no-go decisions • Off-line analysis	• PAT tools utilized with appropriate feed forward and feedback controls • Process operations tracked and trended to support continual improvement efforts post-approval
Product specifications	• Primary means of control • Based on batch data available at time of registration	• Part of overall control strategy • Based on desired product performance with relevant supportive data
Control strategy	• Drug product quality controlled primarily by intermediates (in-process materials) and end product testing	• Drug product quality ensured by risk-based control strategy for well-understood product and process • Quality control shifted upstream, with the possibility of real-time release testing or reduced end-product testing
Life cycle management	• Reactive (i.e., problem solving and corrective action)	• Preventative action • Continual improvement facilitated

Source: ICH (2006). Q8 (R2) Pharmaceutical Development. http://www.fda.gov/downloads /Drugs/.../Guidances/ucm073507.pdf

1.4.4 Contrast between Minimal Approaches and QbD

The QbD approach distinguishes itself from the traditional practice in many aspects of pharmaceutical development, thanks to the adoption of modern technologies such as PAT and utilization of advanced quality system techniques and multivariate statistical methods. Table 1.1 lists potential contrasts between a minimal approach and an enhanced QbD approach for different aspects of pharmaceutical development and life cycle management, which are presented in ICH Q8 (R2) (2006). The intent is to illustrate the tools that can help fully realize the benefits of QbD. Note that these tools are by no means all-encompassing, and for a particular product and process development, not all of the listed methods are always expected to be used in the enhanced QbD approach. However, there is a common thread in QbD approaches. That is, to fully capitalize the benefits of QbD, it is necessary to gain understanding of the product and process, in terms of relationships between process and input material parameters and CQAs.

1.5 Statistical Opportunities

Statistics has been applied to virtually all aspects of biopharmaceutical development. This is in part because, for most processes, there are no theoretical or mechanistic models that can be used to fully describe the process performance (Haaland 1989). As a result, successful development of robust CMC processes relies on trial and error through well-thought-out DOEs. Scientific questions are addressed using the data collected from various experiments. As data are usually multifactorial, inherently variable and random, and oftentimes incomplete, parsing information and knowledge from one experiment and using it to guide the next study can be challenging. Statistics concerns itself with "learning from data" or "translating data into knowledge"; thus, it is an effective tool for pharmaceutical development. The recent advances in regulatory policies have brought statistics to the forefront of CMC development. For example, in the FDA PAT guidance (2004b), it is reiterated how important it is to use multivariate tools for design, data acquisition, and analyses. The use of statistical methods is also recommended in the FDA process validation guidance (2011). Statistics is a critical enabler that allows for understanding of pharmaceutical development and confirms product quality.

While the recent regulatory initiatives have brought about many opportunities for the industry to modernize manufacturing process development, a wide range of new challenges have emerged. For example, the adoption of PAT tools allows companies to generate large amounts of complex data in a short period. The data tend to be noisy. There may be missing data and outliers. In many cases, collinearity may exist. As a result, extracting useful information from these data may pose significant challenges. These challenges have spurred statistical innovations, not only in terms statistical methodology development but also in terms of the ways in which statisticians are working with other stakeholders in biopharmaceutical development. An excellent overview of statistical applications in the CMC areas was provided by Peterson et al. (2009b). In commenting on the article by Peterson et al., Hofer (2009) discussed future opportunities for statistics in the rapidly changing pharmaceutical industry. In the following sections, areas within a QbD development paradigm in which statistics may play a significant role are discussed.

1.5.1 Analytical Method QbD

Analytical methods are critical components in bioprocess development as data collected through analytical testing are used to optimize the manufacturing process and ensure quality standards (identity, quality, safety, purity, and potency). The inclusion of descriptions of analytical methods used for process development in a biological licensure application is required by regulatory guidelines. Therefore, analytical methods are an integral part of drug research and development. Apart from applications in early drug discovery and preclinical development, analytical methods are also widely used in formulation, process development and optimization, and quality control of marketed products. Since the quality of analytical methods has a direct and significant impact on the quality, safety, and efficacy of the product, analytical methods must be developed and validated for their intended use. Statistical techniques that have been conventionally used in analytical method development include DOE, development of acceptance criteria, and monitoring and control of method performance. In recent years, there has been a growing interest in applying the QbD concept to enhance the understanding, control, and performance of analytical methods. Parallel to QTTP in process development, an analytical target profile (ATP) needs to be developed to guide method development. The ATP should include "fit for purpose" criteria that directly link performance of analytical methods to product safety, efficacy, and quality. The application of science- and risk-based approaches and the concept of continued validation and verification make it possible to concentrate method development efforts in areas that have a significant impact on the method performance. These advances in analytical method development ask for closer collaboration between scientists and statisticians to use multivariate study design and analysis to gain understanding of the analytical method, define testable fit-for-purpose hypothesis so that quality data can be generated to assess analytical method performance, construct an analytical method design space to facilitate continued method improvement and validation, and develop effective control strategies to ensure consistent performance of the method.

Along these lines, several examples were given by researchers (Ermer and Nethercote 2015). The publication of USP Chapter <1210> Statistical Tools for Analytical Procedure Validation (USP 2013) is also a step forward toward applying rigorous statistical modeling approaches to method validation. The concept of total error (see Chapter 2) has the potential to be used to formulate the ATP in terms of quantifiable objectives.

1.5.2 CQAs and Clinical Performance

As previously pointed out, one of the challenges in implementing QbD is to link quality attributes to clinical performance related to bioactivity, safety, PK/PD, and immunogenicity in a qualitative or quantitative manner. Such links make it possible to develop acceptable ranges of CQAs, which are essential for developing both a design space and control strategies. However, to date, little research has been done in this area. This in part is attributed to there being few mechanistic models available to describe the relationships between CQAs and clinical performance and that only limited clinical data are available at the early stage of drug development. One potential solution is to use PK/PD parameters as surrogate markers for clinical endpoints and assess the effect of CQAs on those PK/PD markers. As shown in an example in Chapter 10, such a method may provide an effective means for establishing the relationship between CQAs and clinical endpoints. Furthermore, a joint acceptable range can be constructed for multiple CQAs, taking into account the interdependency among those attributes (Yang 2013a).

1.5.3 Design Space

After the CQAs are identified, process characterization studies are carried out. These studies are based on multifactorial experiments, in which the effects of PPs and input MAs on the CQAs are evaluated. The aim of these experiments is to design manufacturing processes that produce a product with the desired CQAs. Typically statistical DOEs are used to gain experimental efficiency. Note that not all the PPs and MAs have a significant impact on CQAs. Before the characterization studies, a risk analysis is performed to select experimental factors that are deemed to be of high or medium impact on CQAs. Knowledge gained from these studies, coupled with other historical data and manufacturing experience, serves as the basis for establishing a design space, product specifications, and manufacturing control strategies. Per ICH Q8 (R2) (2006), a design space is "[t]he multidimensional combination and interaction of input variables (e.g., material attributes) and process parameters that have been demonstrated to provide assurance of quality." For example, a design space for a cell culture system may have ranges for temperature, pH, feed volume, and culture duration that provide quality product. Design space is a key concept intimately tied with quality system risk management principles. By linking manufacturing variations with the variability of CQAs, it sets the stage for developing effective manufacturing controls. A design space also has regulatory implications for postapproval changes as "working within the design space is not considered as a change. Movement out of the design space is considered to be a change and would normally initiate a regulatory post-approval change process" [ICH Q8 (R2)]. A well-developed design space enables the manufacturer to continuously improve the manufacturing process by adapting to novel technologies without incurring additional risk and creating more regulatory hurdles.

There is a misconception that the design space is a direct product of the traditional multifactorial DOE. As pointed out by Peterson (2009), the design space is more related to process capability. It is an operating region under which the process produces products with high assurance of quality. Therefore, the traditional "overlapping mean response surfaces" method suggested in ICH Q8 is inadequate. An appropriately constructed design space needs to account not only for measurement uncertainties but also for variations in the parameters of statistical models, as well as intercorrelations among the measurements. In the past years, a significant advance has been made in developing design space using Bayesian multivariate analysis (Peterson 2004, 2008, and 2009; Peterson and Lief 2010; Peterson and Yahyah 2009; Peterson et al. 2009a,b; Stockdale and Cheng 2009). Further statistical opportunities for design space development also exist. For example, thus far, the concept of design space is, by and large, applied to input materials and PPs. The same statistical principles and methodologies can be borrowed or further developed for establishing design space of CQAs. In addition, design space is usually developed based on experiments and data from small-scale processes. How to update such design spaces, based on pilot- and full-scale data, remains to be further researched. It is also of great benefit to bring these statistical methods into common practice through software development (Hofer 2009). Equally beneficial is to implement these methods in analytical method development.

1.5.4 Control Strategy

In the risk-based framework, pharmaceutical control strategies are multi-tiered. Future opportunities for statistical applications lie in each of the above areas. For instance, as noted by Peterson et al. (2009b) and Hofer (2009), most acceptance criteria including product specifications are established based on process capability as opposed to impact on drug safety and efficacy. This presents an opportunity for setting fit-for-purpose acceptance ranges, using statistical modeling. Furthermore, both consumer and producer risks can be minimized by setting joint acceptance range of CQAs that accounts for interdependence among the CQAs. Advanced multivariate modeling approaches such as principal component analysis and partial least squares models can be used for the purposes of OOS (out-of-specification) investigation and process control. Bayesian analysis can be used to establish risk-based release limits.

1.5.5 Continued Improvement

Harnessing the advances in technologies, pharmaceutical companies often strive to improve their manufacturing processes, after product approval, to increase product yield while minimizing costs and ensuring quality. Therefore, continued improvement in analytical methods and manufacturing process is a norm. This affords additional statistical opportunities for the generation of design spaces that allow for continued improvement for both assays and manufacturing processes.

1.5.6 Predictive Modeling of Bioprocesses

Predictive modeling is another area where statistical treatment is advantageous. Over the past several years, numerous predictive models have been developed to assess risk associated with residual host cell DNA (Yang 2013a; Yang and Zhang 2016; Yang et al. 2010), evaluate the efficiency of viral purification processes (Li and Yang 2012), and develop risk-based prefiltration bioburden testing schemes (Yang et al. 2013a). These modeling approaches bring about greater insights about process performance by linking the outcomes of the process to PPs. The knowledge gained can be further used to devise effective control strategies. Predictive modeling can also be used to determine release limits to ensure a high probability for the product to remain within specification during its shelf life. Modeling approaches are also critical in developing acceptance sampling plans and in understanding process variability.

1.5.7 Statistical Computing Tools

Never before have we seen such an explosion of data as now in the new QbD era. Since data generated from process development are usually massive, incomplete, noisy, and random, parsing information and knowledge from various sources has become increasingly challenging. A key to successful delivery on the promise of the science- and risk-based approach to product and process development is an ability to integrate, analyze, and understand the deluge of biological and clinical data generated from various sources. Several authors discussed the impact of statistical software and information technology in facilitating the synthesis of information and knowledge management (Hofer 2009; Peterson et al. 2009b; Zhao and Yang 2015). Statistical computational tools, coupled with product- and process-specific knowledge and expertise, can substantially enable risk assessment, CQA identification, development of design space, and control strategies. Bringing these methodologies into common practice allows a manufacturer to attain efficiency and ensure regulatory compliance. Deployment of these tools through web-based applications can further enable scientists to fully capitalize on the utility of novel statistical methods for product and process development.

1.5.8 Regulatory Science

Advances in science and technology have a profound impact on regulatory policies. For example, although initially viewed with much caution, PAT technologies have emerged as important resources for successful implementation of QbD. The latest QbD approach has helped shift the assurance of product quality from regulatory oversight more toward the manufacturers. By adopting a science- and risk-based approach, quality assurance effort can be focused on high-risk areas. Likewise, statistical innovation may greatly influence regulatory thinking and facilitate implementation of regulatory initiatives.

As described by Woodcock (2012), CMC reviews are typically conducted during the initial stage of licensure application and for certain manufacturing changes. In those reviews, the FDA reviewers try to address two questions: (1) Is the product performance acceptable? (2) If so, does the manufacturer have a control strategy to ensure that the product continues to have acceptable performance? Statisticians who have been intimately involved in study design and analysis in analytical, product, and process development, or across multiple products using the same technology platform, are uniquely positioned in helping to put together a robust CMC submission package and ensure successful registration.

Statisticians can also influence regulatory thinking by working with peers on industry consortia, working groups, or USP expert committees. The active participation of statisticians in the two case studies (CMC Biotech Working Group 2009; CMC Vaccine Working Group 2012) greatly helped demonstrate the utility of using multivariate statistical models such as principal component analysis for material qualification, design space, and risk assessment. Joint efforts by statisticians and validation scientists lead to the development risk-based approach to process validation. Various novel statistical methods including use of equivalence test for parallelism testing and assay linearity validation were developed to support fit-for-purpose method validation and the concept of continued method validation and verification (Burdick et al. 2013; LeBlond et al. 2013). Some of these methods have been recommended in USP chapters (USP 2013). On an annual basis, industry and FDA statisticians jointly organize CMC sessions for the FDA/Industry Statistics Workshop to promote communication between industry and the FDA on the topic of statistical methods to address CMC issues. All of these contribute to statistical advancements in the pharmaceutical industry.

1.6 New Role of Statisticians

As discussed above, statistics is clearly a critical enabler in product and process development. In the areas of process development, statisticians are known to be subject-matter experts in quantitative analysis. Their technical contributions are also well recognized. However, as the entire pharmaceutical industry and regulatory bodies move toward adopting a science- and risk-based paradigm for process development, statisticians needs to grow out of their traditional roles as technical consultants to take more leadership responsibilities (Peterson et al. 2009b). Central to the fulfillment of the new leadership role that statisticians assume are business acumen, regulatory knowledge, process and systems thinking, and communication and interpersonal skills (Peterson et al. 2009b). To be able to interact at an executive level, the statisticians need to understand how business is run, how to define objectives, and develop strategies and implementation plans to achieve those goals. The individuals should keep abreast of regulatory trends, in addition to technical know-how.

1.7 Concluding Remarks

Since the launch of the FDA initiative "Pharmaceutical cGMPs for the 21st Century" in 2002, significant progress has been made in implementing QbD principles for product and process development to boost manufacturing efficiency and reliability. The new regulatory and industry trends have also brought about many unique challenges, particularly in the area of synthesis of information from many sources, quantifying manufacturing variability and risk and devising effective control strategies. The changing environment opens windows of opportunity for statisticians to take on more of a leadership role in the fulfillment of QbD. Drug product development is a complex, costly, and lengthy process. Only through collaborations among statisticians, pharmaceutical scientists, and engineers can QbD bear fruit.

Section II

Analytical Method

2

Analytical Method Validation

2.1 Introduction

Analytical methods are measurement systems that are used to determine the identity, strength, quality, purity, and potency of the drug substance and drug product. As such, they are an integral part of drug research and development, allowing for process understanding and conformance to quality standards. Many key decisions in biopharmaceutical development and manufacturing are made based on results from analytical methods. In early drug discovery, analytical results concerning the properties of candidate drugs are used to guide the selection of the lead drug candidates. In both preclinical and clinical development, analytical methods aid optimal dose selection and assess study endpoints. Analytical methods are also widely used in formulation and process development and optimization, and in quality control of marketed products. Since the quality of analytical methods has a direct and significant impact on successful development of a new drug, analytical methods must be developed and validated for their intended use.

As previously discussed, through the "Pharmaceutical Quality for the 21st Century" initiative of the US Food and Drug Administration (FDA), many deficiencies in pharmaceutical manufacturing processes were uncovered (FDA 2004a). They included uneven quality and substandard manufacturing practices, insufficient understanding of manufacturing breakdowns, low manufacturing efficiencies, and slow uptake of new technologies. In general, these problems also exist for analytical methods. The quality by design (QbD), risk-based, life cycle development paradigm for the development of manufacturing processes described in ICH Q8, Q9, and Q10 is adaptable to analytical methods as they can be viewed as processes as well. Enhanced understanding of sources of variability that affect an analytical method's performance can lead to better design, control, and reliability of the method.

In this chapter, we provide an overview of statistical approaches used for analytical method development and validation with an emphasis on the latest innovations. The concept of total error as an analytical method validation characteristic is described and the utility of using β-expectation tolerance intervals, β-content tolerance intervals, and generalized pivotal quantities

(GPQs) is discussed. On the basis of both empirical evaluation and theoretical argument, it is demonstrated that the β-content tolerance interval and GPQ approaches have the potential to be adopted for validating analytical methods for their intended use.

2.2 Regulatory Requirements

Analytical method validation consists of a series of experiments intended to demonstrate that an analytical method is fit for its intended use. It is a regulatory requirement. In the past two decades, several regulatory guidelines have been published to provide guidance on method validation (FDA 2000, 2001b, 2015; ICH 1995a, 1996; USP 1989). The first guidance was developed by the United States Pharmacopeia (USP) and published as a general chapter in USP <1225> Validation of Compendial Methods in 1989. For the pharmaceutical industry, the FDA has issued several guidelines on analytical method validation, stipulating specific requirements for the demonstration of fitness for use of analytical methods. However, there exist discrepancies among these documents. Consequently, an effort was led by the International Conference of Harmonization (ICH) to harmonize validation requirements. In 1995, the ICH guideline Q2 (R1) Validation of Analytical Procedures: Text and Methodology was published (EMA 1995). According to ICH Q2 (R1), there are typically four types of analytical procedures:

- Identification tests for active product ingredients (APIs)
- Quantitative tests for APIs
- Quantitative tests for impurities
- Qualitative or limit tests for impurity content

Although these regulatory documents provide general concepts for method validation as well as specific requirements of performance characteristics to be validated (see Table 2.1), they appear to focus on a one-time evaluation of an analytical procedure (Borman et al. 2007). Even if an analytical procedure meets the acceptance criteria for the specified performance characteristics, this does not provide a high degree of assurance that the analytical procedure will perform well after it is transferred from the analytical laboratory to the quality control department. In addition, the traditional validation approaches do not provide means for understanding sources of variations, nor do they provide control strategies. Without such knowledge, the transferred method may fail to perform in the receiving laboratory, incurring costly root cause analyses intended to identify variables that caused the performance issues (Ermer and Nethercote 2015).

TABLE 2.1

Validation Characteristics for Different Types of Analytical Methods

		Impurity		
Validation Characteristics	**Identity**	**Quantitative**	**Limit**	**Assay**
Accuracy	No	Yes	No	Yes
Precision				
Repeatability	No	Yes	No	Yes
Intermediate precision[a]	No	Yes	No	Yes
Specificity[b]	Yes	Yes	Yes	Yes
Detection limit	No	No[c]	Yes	No
Quantitation limit	No	Yes	No	No
Linearity	No	Yes	No	Yes
Range	No	Yes	No	Yes

Source: ICH Q2A (1995).

Note: Yes, normally evaluated; no, not evaluated.

[a] In cases where reproducibility is performed, intermediate precision is not needed.

[b] Lack of specificity of one analytical method could be compensated by other supporting analytical method(s).

[c] May be needed.

2.3 Life Cycle Approach

In recent years, there has been a growing interest in applying the QbD concept to analytical procedure development and validation. The efforts were motivated by the latest shift in regulatory thinking in pharmaceutical development, evidenced by ICH 8, 9, 10, and 11, and the *FDA Guidance for Industry on Process Validation: General Principles and Practices*, in January 2011 (FDA 2011). The ICH documents describe how robust manufacturing processes can be developed, based on systematic understanding of the processes and control of sources of variations. The new process validation guideline encourages the use of modern pharmaceutical development concepts, quality risk management, and quality systems at all stages of the manufacturing process life cycle.

Applying the same principles, Borman et al. (2007) suggest using a QbD approach for analytical methods that includes risk assessment, robustness and ruggedness testing, and assessment of method variability compared with the specification limits to determine whether the method is fit for its intended purpose. Viewing an analytical procedure as a process and data as its product, Nethercote et al. (2010) argue that QbD concepts for manufacturing process development can be applied to analytical methods, including the concepts of life cycle validation. The idea of using QbD and life cycle approaches to gaining enhanced understanding of sources of variability and better controls of analytical procedures is further described in several publications (Borman et al. 2007; Martin et al. 2013; Nethercote and Ermer 2012).

These authors propose a holistic approach to analytical method development and validation that aligns understanding of analytical method variability with its intended use. The culmination of these efforts is the proposal that the three stages of process validation be applied to analytical method validation (Martin et al. 2013; Nethercote and Ermer 2012) as depicted in Figure 2.1.

The starting point of this approach is to define an analytical target profile (ATP) that describes the quality of the data that the method is required to produce. The concept of ATP was first proposed by the EFPIA/PhRMa working group (2010) and adopted by the USP Validation and Verification Expert Panel (Martin et al. 2013). The ATP is constructed based on measurement uncertainty, and the required level of assurance regarding the reportable results. Several considerations need to be taken into account when defining the ATP (Colgan et al. 2014). They include (1) the range over which the analytical method is expected to reliably quantify the amount or potency of analyte; (2) the total uncertainty or error that measures the closeness between the reportable value and the true value, which is expressed as the sum of systematic and random errors; and (3) a description of the analyte to be tested, including the sample or matrix in which it will be tested. The ATP is used to guide method development, performance qualification, and continued verification throughout the life cycle of the method. It is critical to link the traditional assay characteristics such as accuracy and precision to the ATP. Such a link enables the definition of acceptance criteria for these performance parameters in the method performance qualification study.

After the ATP is defined, the analyst proceeds to Stage 1 Method Design, in which the analyst selects an appropriate technique and develops a draft method that may meet the requirements defined in the ATP. As understanding sources of variability is one of the primary focuses at this stage, risk assessment tools, such as Ishikawa or fishbone diagrams, failure modes and

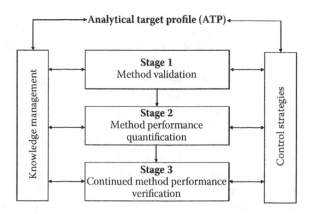

FIGURE 2.1
Life cycle approach to analytical procedure validation.

effects analysis, and so on, can be used to gain understanding of variables that may have an impact on the method performance and help prioritize experimentation (Martin et al. 2013). Designs of experiment are carried out to determine ranges of key variables in which the ATP may be met. Stage 2 Method Qualification is intended to confirm that the method is fit for its purpose through formal studies. This stage involves the collection of data from performing the analytical procedure under routine operating conditions and demonstration that the data meet acceptance criteria in the ATP. In addition, knowledge of the analytical procedure gleaned from the method quantification studies can be used to refine control strategies. The objective of Stage 3 Continued Procedure Performance Verification is to provide assurance that the method remains in a state of control during routine use. This involves routine monitoring to confirm the analytical procedure performance as well as performance verification after any changes made to the method. Statistical process control charts can be used to capture any special-cause variation.

2.4 Validation Study Design

An important consideration in method validation is to design experiments so that statistical inference can be made regarding validation parameters. If designed properly, the studies use a minimum number of experimental runs while generating the maximum amount of information. Experimental efficiency can be obtained if assay performance parameters can be validated simultaneously. As discussed previously, typical validation characteristics include accuracy, precision, specificity, detection limit, quantitation limit, linearity, and range. However, in this chapter, we primarily concern ourselves with validation of accuracy and precision, as they are two key measures of analytical method performance. A comprehensive discussion of statistical methods for linearity validation is provided in Chapter 4.

2.4.1 Accuracy and Precision

For quantitative methods, accuracy and precision are often considered to be the primary performance characteristics. Accuracy measures the closeness of test results obtained by the analytical method to the true value of the sample. The closeness (or lack thereof), also termed bias, can be expressed either as the absolute difference between the measured result and the true value or as the relative difference, which is the ratio of the absolute difference to the true value. As per regulatory requirements, accuracy should be validated across the range of analyte concentrations to which the analytical method is intended to apply.

Precision is the degree of agreement among individual test results of the analytical method. There are various sources of variations such as analyst, day, and instrument that may contribute to the overall variability of a test. Intra-instrument variation is also referred to as repeatability of the test. Precision is usually expressed as the standard deviation or relative standard deviation (coefficient of variation) (USP 2005).

2.4.2 Experimental Design

As stated above, validation of analytical method accuracy and precision requires well-designed studies. These experiments should mimic the process by which the method is routinely applied after validation. Factors that may affect method accuracy and precision need to be considered in designing the validation experiment so that their effects can be properly estimated. For example, analyst, high-performance liquid chromatography (HPLC) instrument, and column are typical experimental factors for a relative purity assay. Depending on the population from which a factor is chosen, it may be viewed as either fixed or random. In the above example, HPLC instrument can be considered fixed if the laboratory only has a limited number of instruments that are routinely used for the test. However, if the number of available instruments is large, and only a few instruments are used in the validation study, it is more appropriate to deem the factor as random. As a rule of thumb, the larger the population, the more reasonable to assume that the factor is random. However, in the following discussion, we consider a common design in which all factors are treated as random variables. The measurements of the analytical method are described through a statistical model. Consider that there are p factors. Let $X_{i_1,i_2,\dots,i_p}$ ($i_k = 1, 2,\dots,I_k$; $k = 1, 2,\dots, p$) be the test results from the runs where the random conditions are $i_1, i_2,\dots,i_p$. $X_{i_1,i_2,\dots,i_p}$ can be described as follows:

$$X_{i_1,i_2,\dots,i_p} = \mu + \alpha_{1,i_1} + \alpha_{2,i_2} + \cdots + \alpha_{p-1,i_{p-1}} + \varepsilon_{i_1,i_2,\dots,i_p} \quad (i_k = 1,2,\dots,I_k;\ k = 1,2,\dots,p)$$

where each α_{k,i_k} (for $k = 1, 2,\dots, p - 1$) is independently normally distributed with mean 0 and variance σ_k^2; the within-run replication error terms $\varepsilon_{i_1,i_2,\dots,i_p}$ are within-run measurement errors and are independently normally distributed with mean 0 and variance σ_p^2. The α_{k,i_k} and $\varepsilon_{i_1,i_2,\dots,i_p}$ are also assumed to be independent of each other.

The quantity $\sigma_{IP}^2 = \sum_{k=1}^{p-1} \sigma_k^2$ is often referred to as intermediate precision (IP), and σ_p^2 is called repeatability. The total variance is $\sigma^2 = \sigma_{IP}^2 + \sigma_p^2$. Treating the random conditions in the experiment as a randomly selected sample from the population of all possible conditions, the above model is simplifed to a one-way random effect model that contains two random components (Burdick et al. 2013):

$$X_{ij} = \mu + A_i + \varepsilon_{ij}, \tag{2.1}$$

where A_i is the effect associated with the random condition i and ε_{ij} is the measurement error of the jth sample tested under condition i.

To estimate the effects of the random conditions, it is necessary to assume that the A_i are independent. In theory, there is mutual dependence among some of the conditions as they may have a common component such as analyst. However, such dependence lessens as the time between two experimental conditions increases; therefore, it is reasonable to assume independence. Without loss of generality, we assume that each A_i follows a normal distribution $N\left(0, \sigma_a^2\right)$ and that ε_{ij} is distributed $N\left(0, \sigma_e^2\right)$. As noted by Burdick et al. (2013), consideration should be given to the relative contribution of the IP σ_a^2 and repeatability σ_e^2 to the total error $\sigma^2 = \sigma_a^2 + \sigma_e^2$ for a particular application. In general, the larger the ratio σ_a^2 / σ^2, the larger the number of treatment conditions needed to provide adequate power for a validation test (for details, see Burdick et al. 2013). On the other hand, if prior knowledge suggests σ_a^2 is relatively small with respect to σ^2, Model 2.1 can be further reduced to

$$X_j = \mu + \varepsilon_j, \tag{2.2}$$

which only involves random measurement errors ε_j. In such cases, statistical tests for validation performance characteristics can be more easily constructed.

After the experiment is conducted and the results are collected, the effects of the random components in Model 2.1 are estimated and assessed through analysis of variance (ANOVA) using the statistics in Table 2.2. Taken together, these estimates allow us to construct statistical tests to evaluate if the validation performance characteristics such as accuracy and precision meet preselected acceptance criteria.

TABLE 2.2

ANOVA of One-Way Random Effect Model

Source	df[a]	Sum of Squares[b]	Mean Square	Expected Mean Square
Between-run	$n_a - 1$	$SSA = n_w \sum_{i=1}^{na}(\bar{X}_i - \bar{\bar{X}})^2$	$MSA = \dfrac{SSA}{n_a - 1}$	$n_w \sigma_a^2 + \sigma_e^2$
Within-run	$n_a(n_w - 1)$	$SSE = \sum_i \sum_j (X_{ij} - \bar{X}_i)^2$	$MSE = \dfrac{SSE}{n_a(n_w - 1)}$	σ_e^2
Total	$n_a n_w - 1$	$SST = \sum_i \sum_j (X_{ij} - \bar{\bar{X}})^2$		

[a] *df*, degree of freedom.

[b] $\bar{\bar{X}} = \dfrac{1}{n_a n_w} \sum_i \sum_j X_{ij}$ and $\bar{X}_i = \dfrac{1}{n_w} \sum_{j=1}^{n_w} X_{ij}$; n_a = number of runs; n_w = number of replicates.

Let μ_T be the true value of the analytical method. We assume that μ_T is either known or can be well estimated. Thus $\delta = \mu - \mu_T$ represents the bias of the analytical method. From Table 2.1, estimates of the parameters δ, σ_a^2, σ_e^2, and σ^2 are given by

$$\hat{\delta} = \bar{\bar{X}} - \mu_T$$

$$\hat{\sigma}_a^2 = (\text{MSA} - \text{MSE})/n_w$$

$$\hat{\sigma}_e^2 = \text{MSE}$$

$$\hat{\sigma}^2 = \hat{\sigma}_a^2 + \hat{\sigma}_e^2 = \text{MSA}/n_w + (1 - 1/n_w)\text{MSE}. \tag{2.3}$$

For a balanced design, these estimators are the same as those obtained using the method of restricted maximum likelihood estimation (RMLE). RMLE gives unbiased estimates and is thus preferred to maximum likelihood estimation (MLE).

2.5 Current Validation Methods

2.5.1 Point Estimate

Validation of analytical method accuracy and precision is traditionally based on whether or not the point estimates in Model 2.1 meet certain threshold criteria. For example, accuracy and precision are considered as validated if the estimate of bias falls within ±15% of the true value and the estimates of variabilty (typically quantified as the coefficient of variation) do not exceed 15% (FDA 2001b). However, because this approach does not take into account uncertainties in those point estimates, even if the acceptance criteria are met, there is no adequate assurance that the method is accurate and precise. Likewise, failing the acceptance criteria does not necessarily imply that the method is inaccurate or imprecise for its intended use.

2.5.2 Confidence Interval Approach

To address the above issues, an alternative approach has been proposed (Burdick et al. 2013; USP 2013). This method calculates confidence intervals for accuracy and precision measures and compares them against prespecified acceptance criteria. An approximate two-sided $(1 - 2\alpha) \times 100\%$ confidence interval for δ is given by

$$\hat{\delta} \pm t_{n_a-1,1-\alpha}\sqrt{\hat{\sigma}_b^2/n_a n_w} \, , \tag{2.4}$$

where $t_{n_a-1,1-\alpha}$ is the $100(1 - \alpha)$th percentile of the t-distribution with $n_a - 1$ degrees of freedom and $\sigma_b^2 = \text{MSA}$ is the between-run mean square given in Table 2.1. The bias is deemed acceptable if the above interval is contained entirely within prespecified limits.

For the IP, Burdick et al. (2013) applied a method by Graybill and Wang (1980) to construct a one-sided upper $(1 - \alpha) \times 100\%$ confidence interval. This method, called the modified large-sample confidence interval, was also used by Nijhuis and Van den Heuvel (2007) to assess precision. The one-sided upper $(1 - \alpha) \times 100\%$ confidence interval for σ_a is obtained as

$$\sqrt{\hat{\sigma}_a^2 + \sqrt{H_1^2\left(\frac{1}{n_e}\right)^2 \hat{\sigma}_b^4 + H_2^2\left(1-\frac{1}{n_e}\right)^2 \hat{\sigma}_e^4}} \, , \tag{2.5}$$

where

$$H_1 = \frac{n_a - 1}{\chi^2_{\alpha,n_a-1}} - 1 \text{ and}$$

$$H_2 = \frac{n_a(n_w - 1)}{\chi^2_{\alpha,n_a(n_w-1)}} - 1 \, ,$$

with χ^2_{α,n_a-1} and $\chi^2_{\alpha,n_a(n_w-1)}$ being 100αth percentiles of chi-square distributions with degrees of freedom $n_a - 1$ and $n_a (n_w - 1)$, respectively. The IP considers meeting the acceptance criterion if the one-sided confidence limit in Equation 2.5 is bounded by a preselected limit.

An alternative method based on the Satterthwaite (1946) approximation was also suggested by Burdick et al. (2013). A one-sided upper $(1 - \alpha) \times 100\%$ confidence interval for σ_a^2 is

$$\hat{\sigma}_a^2 \times df / \chi^2_{\alpha,df}$$

where

$$df = \frac{\hat{\sigma}_{IP}^2}{\dfrac{\hat{\sigma}_b^4}{(n_a-1)n_w^2} + \dfrac{(n_w-1)\hat{\sigma}_e^4}{n_a n_w^2}} \, . \tag{2.6}$$

A challenging aspect of method validation is to establish numerical acceptance criteria. Ideally, the acceptance critieria should be set based on the impact on product quality, safety, and efficacy. However, in practice, it is difficult to acquire such information. Factors that may be helpful in setting the acceptance criteria include (1) process knowledge; (2) performance of similar analytical methods and historical practice; (3) data generated in the life cycle of the method, including development and prevalidation work; (4) the desired state of control of the method in routine use; and (5) most importantly, the intended use of the method.

Example

Burdick et al. (2013) considered a method validation design with five concentration levels (40, 60, 100, 200, and 300). At each concentration level, three analysts and three pieces of equipment were utilized. Three replicates were taken for each combination of analyst and equipment. Assuming that the nine combinations of analyst and equipment are a random sample from the population of all combinations, the data collected at each combination can be described through Model 2.1. An example data set is provided in Table 2.3. The response values are the differences between each measured value and the true target value of 100.

It is further assumed that the bias and precision of the method are deemed to be acceptable if their confidence interval estimates are within ±5% and less than 3%, respectively. Fitting the data in Table 2.3 to Model 2.1 results in Table 2.4.

From Tables 2.3 and 2.4, $\hat{\mu} = 0.374$, $\hat{\sigma}_b^2 = 4.672$, and $\hat{\sigma}_e^2 = 1.299$. The two-sided 90% confidence interval for the bias is $(-5\%, 5\%)$, which is enclosed

TABLE 2.3

Measured Responses Expressed as Change from the Target Value 100

Combination	Analyst	Equipment	Replicate 1	Replicate 2	Replicate 3
1	1	A	1.4	−1.4	2
2	2	B	1.2	−1.8	0.6
3	3	C	1.8	−0.8	−0.9
4	1	B	0.6	−0.3	−0.4
5	2	C	−0.6	−0.8	−1.8
6	3	A	2.5	2.5	2.8
7	1	C	−1.3	0.7	−0.9
8	2	A	3.1	1.8	1.7
9	3	B	0.6	−1.4	−0.8

Source: Burdick, R., LeBlond, D., Sandell, D., and Yang, H. (2013). Acceptance criteria for method validation of accuracy and precision. *Pharmacopeial Forum*, May–June Issue, 39(3).

TABLE 2.4

ANOVA Table of Example Data

Source	df	Sum of Squares	Mean Square	F Value	Pr > F
Model	8	37.379	4.672	3.60	0.012
Error	18	23.3739	1.299		
Corrected total	26	60.752			

in (−5%, 5%); hence, the bias of analytical method has passed its acceptance criterion. From Equation 2.5, the one-sided upper 95% confidence limit on the IP is 2.4%. Since this is smaller than 3%, the method meets the acceptance criterion for intermediate precision as well.

2.5.3 Total Error Approach

The methods described in Section 2.5.2 validate analytical method accuracy and precision separately. In particular, the method is acceptable if the point or interval estimates for bias and precision are within prespecified limits (USP 2013). However, these methods have a serious drawback. That is, they are not directly related to the method's intended purpose as recognized by various authors (Hoffman and Kringle 2007; Yang and Zhang 2015). Specifically, an analytical method may pass the validation of accuracy and precision, but it is not demonstrated that, with high assurance, test results of future samples will be close to their true values. Furthermore, they are incompatible with acceptance criteria when the analytical method is in routine use in the quality control laboratory for in-process and product release testing (Hoffman and Kringle 2007). The in-study criteria are required by regulatory guidance to be expressed as the percentage of test results being within acceptance limits (FDA 2001a). In addition, accuracy and precision affect the usefulness of an analytical procedure in a joint manner. That is, a relatively precise method can tolerate a larger bias than a less precise one, and vice versa.

For these reasons, several alternative methods have been proposed, with the focus on the total error of an analytical method, which incorporates both systematic bias and random variation (Boulanger et al. 2003; DeSilva et al. 2003; Findlay et al. 2000; Hubert et al. 2004, 2007a,b; Kringle and Khan-Malek 1994; Lee et al. 2006; Miller et al. 2001). The total error is the difference between the observed value and the true value of a test sample. Since an analytical method is usually intended to be used to give results close to the true value, setting acceptance criteria based on the concept of total error is consistent with the true purpose of method validation.

2.5.3.1 "Fit for Purpose" Hypothesis

Validation is a confirmatory process to demonstrate that an analytical method is fit for its intended purpose. One way to define "fit for purpose" is to warrant high assurance that the absolute difference between any future result of the analytical method and the true value of the analyte is bounded by a prespecified acceptable limit. Let X and μ_T be the measured value and true value of a future sample, respectively. Let $\pi = P(|X - \mu_T| < \lambda)$, where λ is a prespecified acceptable limit on $|X - \mu_T|$ consistent with the analytical procedure's intended purpose. The quantity π is the probability that the error of a future measurement is bounded by λ. Validation of the method can be achieved through testing the following fit-for-purpose hypotheses:

$$H_0: \pi < \beta \text{ versus } H_1: \pi \geq \beta, \tag{2.7}$$

where β is the desired level of assurance that the total error of any future test result does not exceed λ.

Under the normality assumption, the probability π can be expressed as

$$\pi = \Phi\left(\frac{\lambda + \mu_T - \mu}{\sigma}\right) - \Phi\left(\frac{-\lambda + \mu_T - \mu}{\sigma}\right), \tag{2.8}$$

where Φ is the cumulative probability function of the standard normal distribution.

The inequality $\pi \geq \beta$ can be used to define a joint acceptance region for bias and precision. For example, Figure 2.2 depicts the acceptance region when $\lambda = 15\%$ and $\beta = 80\%$, 90%, and 95%.

The plot in Figure 2.2 depicts the interdependence between the bias and precision. That is, the larger the bias is, the smaller the precision or variability needs to be in order to maintain the same level of quality assurance.

Methods for testing the hypotheses in Equation 2.7 have been explored by several authors (Boulanger et al. 2003; DeSilva et al. 2003; Findlay et al. 2000; Hoffman and Kringle 2005; Hubert et al. 2004; Kringle and Khan-Malek 1994; Lee et al. 2006; Miller et al. 2001). However, there has been no consensus as to which method is most appropriate for testing the fit-for-purpose hypotheses (Equation 2.7). More recently Yang and Zhang (2015) investigated this issue, using a series of simulation studies, and concluded that the approaches based on a β-content tolerance interval (Hoffman and Kringle 2005) and GPQ analysis (Yang and Zhang 2016) provide adequate protection of Type I error (consumer risk), whereas the β-expectation tolerance interval (Hubert et al. 2004) approach has inflated Type I error, thus affording inadequate protection of Type I error. In Section 2.8, based on Model 2.2, we quantify the degree of inflated Type I error of the β-expectation tolerance interval.

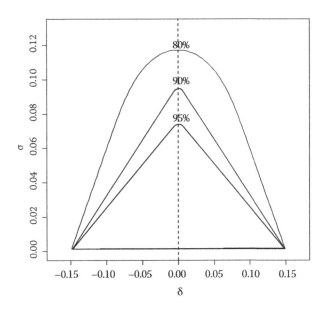

FIGURE 2.2
Joint acceptance region for bias and precision with $\lambda = 15\%$ and $\beta = 80\%$, 90%, or 95%. (From Yang, H. and Zhang, J. (2015). A generalized pivotal quantity approach to analytical method validation based on total error. *PDA J. Pharm. Sci. Technol.*, 69, 725–735.)

2.5.3.2 Maximum Likelihood

The testing strategy proposed by Boulanger et al. (2007b) and Govaerts et al. (2008) is based on comparing the one-sided lower confidence limit for π to the acceptable level β. The null hypothesis (Equation 2.7) is rejected if the one-sided lower confidence limit for π is no less than β. Two approaches were considered for the construction of the lower confidence limit. The first (Govaerts et al. 2008) utilizes the Taylor expansion to estimate the variance of the maximum likelihood estimator (MLE) of π:

$$\hat{\pi} = \Phi\left(\frac{\lambda - \hat{\delta}}{\hat{\sigma}}\right) - \Phi\left(\frac{-\lambda - \hat{\delta}}{\hat{\sigma}}\right),$$

where $\hat{\mu}$ and $\hat{\sigma}$ are the MLEs of μ and σ, respectively, and $\hat{\delta} = \hat{\mu} - \mu_T$. The variance of $\hat{\pi}$ is approximated using the Taylor expansion as follows (Govaerts et al. 2008):

$$\mathrm{Var}(\hat{\pi}) \cong \left(\frac{\partial \hat{\pi}}{\partial \hat{\delta}}\right)^2 \mathrm{Var}(\hat{\delta}) + \left(\frac{\partial \hat{\pi}}{\partial \hat{\sigma}^2}\right)^2 \mathrm{Var}(\hat{\sigma}^2),$$

where, for a balanced design,

$$\text{Var}(\hat{\delta}) = \frac{\text{MSA}}{n_a n_w},$$

$$\text{Var}(\hat{\sigma}^2) = 2\left(\frac{\text{MSA}^2}{n_a - 1} + \frac{(n_w - 1)\text{MSE}^2}{n_a}\right)\bigg/ n_w^2,$$

$$\frac{\partial \hat{\pi}}{\partial \hat{\delta}} = \frac{1}{\hat{\sigma}^2}\left[\phi\left(\frac{-\lambda - \hat{\delta}}{\hat{\sigma}}\right) - \phi\left(\frac{\lambda - \hat{\delta}}{\hat{\sigma}}\right)\right], \text{ and}$$

$$\frac{\partial \hat{\pi}}{\partial \hat{\sigma}^2} = \frac{1}{2\hat{\sigma}^3}\left[(\lambda + \hat{\delta})\phi\left(\frac{-\lambda - \hat{\delta}}{\hat{\sigma}}\right) + (\lambda - \hat{\delta})\phi\left(\frac{\lambda - \hat{\delta}}{\hat{\sigma}}\right)\right].$$

The one-sided $(1 - \alpha) \times 100\%$ lower confidence bound for π is obtained as

$$\pi_L^\alpha = \hat{\pi} - z_{1-\alpha}\sqrt{\widehat{\text{Var}}(\hat{\pi})}, \tag{2.9}$$

where $\widehat{\text{Var}}(\hat{\pi})$ is the estimator of $\text{Var}(\hat{\pi})$ by replacing unknowns δ and σ with $\hat{\delta}$ and $\hat{\sigma}$, respectively; $z_{1-\alpha}$ is the $100(1 - \alpha)$th quantile of a standard normal random variable. This approach is referred to as the MLE method.

2.5.3.3 Modified MLE

Based on the work by Mee (1988), Govaerts et al. (2008) proposed a modified version of the MLE method. An approximate one-sided $(1 - \alpha) \times 100\%$ lower confidence bound for π is provided as follows:

$$\pi_{\text{Mee}}^\alpha = \frac{n'}{n' + z_{1-\alpha}^2}\left(\left(\hat{\pi} + \frac{z_{1-\alpha}^2}{2n'}\right) - z_{1-\alpha}\sqrt{\frac{z_{1-\alpha}^2}{4n'^2} + \widehat{\text{Var}}(\hat{\pi})}\right), \tag{2.10}$$

with $n' = \dfrac{\hat{\pi}(1 - \hat{\pi})}{\widehat{\text{Var}}(\hat{\pi})}$. We refer to this method as Mee's modified MLE method.

2.5.3.4 β-Expectation Tolerance Interval

An approach based on the β-expectation tolerance interval was also proposed for testing the hypotheses in Equation 2.7 (Boulanger et al. 2007b; Govaerts et al. 2008; Hoffman and Kringle 2005; Hubert et al. 2004). The β-expectation tolerance interval for X is defined as

$$E_{\hat{\delta},\hat{\sigma}}\left\{P_X\left(\hat{\delta} - k\hat{\sigma} < X - \mu_T < \hat{\delta} + k\hat{\sigma}\right) \big| \hat{\delta}, \hat{\sigma}\right\} = \beta. \qquad (2.11)$$

That is, the expected probability for the interval to cover the future observations is equal to a prespecified number β. The analytical method is considered validated if the β-expectation tolerance interval falls within the acceptance limits $[-\lambda, \lambda]$.

When X comes from Model 2.2, that is, $X - \mu_T \sim N(\delta, \sigma^2)$, the $100(1 - \beta)\%$ prediction interval for the future observation $X - \mu_T$ based on sample mean $\hat{\delta}$ and standard deviation $\hat{\sigma}$ of the observed values $X_1 - \mu_T, \ldots, X_n - \mu_T$ is given by

$$\hat{\delta} \pm t_{n-1,1-\beta/2}\hat{\sigma}\sqrt{1 + \frac{1}{n}}\ .$$

Because $\dfrac{X - \mu_T - \hat{\delta}}{\hat{\sigma}\sqrt{1 + \dfrac{1}{n}}} \sim t_{n-1}$,

$$E_{\hat{\delta},\hat{\sigma}}\left[P_X\left(X - \mu_T \in \hat{\delta} \pm t_{n-1,1-\beta/2}\,\hat{\sigma}\sqrt{1 + \frac{1}{n}}\right)\big| \hat{\delta}, \hat{\sigma}\right]$$

$$= E_{\hat{\delta},\hat{\sigma}}\left[P_X\left(-t_{n-1,1-\beta/2} \leq \frac{X - \mu_T - \hat{\delta}}{\hat{\sigma}\sqrt{1 + \dfrac{1}{n}}} \leq t_{n-1,1-\beta/2}\right)\big| \hat{\delta}, \hat{\sigma}\right]$$

$$= E_{X,\hat{\delta},\hat{\sigma}}\left[I_{\left\{-t_{n-1,1-\beta/2} \leq \frac{X - \mu_T - \hat{\delta}}{\hat{\sigma}\sqrt{1 + \frac{1}{n}}} \leq t_{n-1,1-\beta/2}\right\}}(X, \hat{\delta}, \hat{\sigma})\right]$$

$$= P_{X,\hat{\delta},T}\left[-t_{n-1,1-\beta/2} \leq \frac{X - \mu_T - \hat{\delta}}{\hat{\sigma}\sqrt{1 + \dfrac{1}{n}}} \leq t_{n-1,1-\beta/2}\right]$$

$$= \beta,$$

where $I_{\left\{-t_{n-1,1-\beta/2} \leq \frac{X - \mu_T - \hat{\delta}}{\hat{\sigma}\sqrt{1 + \frac{1}{n}}} \leq t_{n-1,1-\beta/2}\right\}}(X, \hat{\delta}, \hat{\sigma})$ is an indicator function that assumes either 1 or 0 depending on whether the condition in the bracket is met or not.

The above derivations show that the β-expectation tolerance interval in Equation 2.11 is a prediction interval when the observations can be described through Model 2.2. It is also well known that for a balanced one-way random effect model, the β-expectation tolerance interval is a prediction interval. Various methods have been developed for the construction of tolerance intervals for variance component models (Govaerts et al. 2008; Hoffman and Kringle 2007). From Mee (1984), it can be shown that the coefficient in Equation 2.11 is given by

$$k = t_{f,(1+\beta)/2}\sqrt{1+1/N_E},$$

where N_E is the effective sample size that accounts for the uncertainty in the mean μ and is estimated as $\hat{N}_E = \dfrac{n_a(\text{MSA} + (n_w - 1)\text{MSE})}{\text{MSA}}$, f is the degrees of freedom for the estimator of total variance and is estimated as $\hat{f} = \dfrac{(\text{MSA} + \text{MSE})^2}{\dfrac{\text{MSA}^2}{n_a - 1} + (n_w - 1)\text{MSE}^2/n_a}$ using the Satterthwaite method, and $t_{f,(1+\beta)/2}$ is the $\dfrac{100(1+\beta)}{2}$% quantile of a t-distribution with degrees of freedom f.

2.5.3.5 β-Content Tolerance Interval

Alternatively, a β-content, γ-confidence tolerance interval was proposed based on similar probabilistic considerations (Govaerts et al. 2008; Hoffman and Kringle 2007). The β-content, γ-confidence tolerance interval of a future test result X is defined as

$$P_{\hat{\delta},\hat{\sigma}}\left\{P_X(\hat{\delta} - h\hat{\sigma} < X - \mu_T < \hat{\delta} + h\hat{\sigma}) > \beta|\hat{\delta},\hat{\sigma}\right\} = \gamma. \tag{2.12}$$

To apply this approach to method validation, the confidence level γ needs to be prespecified. Various suggestions have been made in literature. For example, Boulanger et al. (2007b) and Govaerts et al. (2008) proposed to set γ at 50% to make it comparable to the β-expectation method, whereas Hoffman and Kringle (2007) independently proposed to use 90% confidence. To facilitate the comparison of the statistical approaches in Section 2.5, we refer to them as β-expectation, β-content(0.5), and β-content(0.9), respectively.

As noted by Burdick et al. (2013) and Yang and Zhang (2015), the use of a β-content tolerance interval has an intuitive interpretation when the acceptance limit is one sided. In this case, the hypotheses in Equation 2.7 can be restated as

$$H_0: \pi = P(X - \mu_T < \lambda) < \beta \text{ versus } H_1: \pi = P(X - \mu_T < \lambda) \geq \beta, \tag{2.13}$$

which are obviously equivalent to the following hypotheses by inverting the probability:

$$H_0: q_X(\beta) > \lambda + \mu_T \text{ versus } H_1: q_X(\beta) \leq \lambda + \mu_T,$$

where $q_X(\beta)$ is the 100βth quantile of X.

A test of the above hypotheses (Equation 2.13) can be constructed based on the fact that the one-sided upper β-content tolerance bound for a future test result X is essentially the one-sided upper γ-confidence bound for $q_X(\beta)$. Specifically, the test rejects the null hypothesis in Equation 2.13 if the one-sided upper β-content, γ-confidence tolerance bound for $q_X(\beta)$ is less than or equal to $\lambda + \mu_T$. An advantage of this test is that it controls the Type I error. However, for the hypotheses with two-sided acceptance limits in Equation 2.12, that is, $-\lambda < X - \mu_T < \lambda$, there is no intuitive interpretation of the test procedure based on a two-sided β-content, γ-confidence tolerance interval. The size of the test for a test with two-sided acceptance limits can only be examined through statistical simulation.

A β-content, γ-confidence tolerance interval can be constructed using the method by Hoffman and Kringle (2005), in which the coefficient h in Equation 2.12 is determined to be

$$h = z_{(1+\beta)/2} C_\sigma \sqrt{1 + 1/N_E},$$

where $\hat{\sigma}^2 C_\sigma^2$ is the one-sided upper γ-confidence bound for σ^2. For a balanced one-way random effect model, C_σ is obtained as

$$C_\sigma = \sqrt{1 + \frac{1}{\hat{\sigma}^2} \sqrt{\frac{H_1^2 \text{MSA}^2}{n_w^2} + H_2^2 \left(1 - \frac{1}{n_w}\right)^2 \text{MSE}^2}},$$

where $H_j = \left(\dfrac{1}{F_{1-\gamma;r_j;\infty}}\right) - 1$ for $(j = 1,2)$ with $r_1 = n_a - 1$; $r_2 = n_a(n_w - 1)$.

2.6 Generalized Pivotal Quantity Method

Although the above methods are intended to test the "fit for use" hypothesis, it is unclear how the risk of accepting unsuitable methods (i.e., Type I error) is controlled. Since an exact test statistic of the null hypothesis in Equation 2.7 is hard to construct, Yang and Zhang (2015) proposed an alternative approach based on GPQ inference. The GPQ was first developed by Weerahandi (1993, 2004) and has been applied to a wide range of statistical estimation and inference problems (Krishnamoorthy and Mathew 2004). The method is particularly useful for problems where exact test statistics do not exist. A GPQ is a function of both the observed values of random variables and the unknown parameters of their distributions. Although a GPQ may involve the unknown parameters, its distribution is free of the unknown parameters. Specifically, let $R(X, x, \theta)$ be a test statistic of the parameter θ. It is a GPQ of θ if it satisfies the following two conditions (Weerahandi 2004):

(A1) The distribution of R does not depend on θ.

(A2) The observed value of R, $r = R(x, x, \theta)$ is equal to θ.

These properties allow for making inference about θ based on the distribution of R, as is illustrated below.

2.6.1 GPQ of Quality Level

To test the null hypothesis in Equation 2.7, we assume that x_{ij} is the observed value of X_{ij} and is a random test result that may be collected from a validation experiment that has a one-way ANOVA design. We also let $\bar{\bar{x}}$, ssa, and sse be the observed values of $\bar{X}$, SSA, and SSE, respectively. Since the quality level π in Equation 2.7 is a function of the parameters $\theta \equiv \left(\mu, \sigma_a^2, \sigma_e^2\right)$, a GPQ of π can be constructed by substituting GPQs for μ, σ_a^2, and σ_e^2 into Equation 2.7. For the one-way random effect model (Model 2.1), the GPQs for μ, σ_a^2, and σ_e^2 are given by

$$\bar{\bar{x}} - \frac{\sqrt{n_a n_w}\left(\bar{\bar{X}} - \mu\right)}{\sqrt{SSA}}\sqrt{\frac{ssa}{n_a n_w}},$$

$$\frac{n_w \sigma_a^2 + \sigma_e^2}{n_w SSA}ssa - \frac{\sigma_e^2}{n_w SSE}sse, \text{ and}$$

$$\frac{\sigma_e^2}{n_w SSE}sse, \text{ respectively.} \tag{2.14}$$

Note that $\bar{\bar{X}}$, SSA, and SSE are independently distributed according to

$$Z = \sqrt{n_a n_w}\frac{\left(\bar{\bar{X}} - \mu\right)}{\sqrt{n_w \sigma_a^2 + \sigma_e^2}} \sim N(0,1),$$

$$U_a^2 = \frac{SSA}{n_w \sigma_a^2 + \sigma_e^2} \sim \chi_{n_a-1}^2, \text{ and } U_e^2 = \frac{SSE}{\sigma_e^2} \sim \chi_{n_a(n_w-1)}^2, \tag{2.15}$$

where χ_d^2 is the chi-squared distribution with degree of freedom d. Let

$$R(X,x,\theta) = \Phi\left(\frac{(\lambda+\mu_T)-\left(\bar{\bar{x}}-\dfrac{Z}{U_a}\sqrt{\dfrac{\mathrm{ssa}}{n_a n_w}}\right)}{\dfrac{\sqrt{\dfrac{\mathrm{ssa}}{U_a^2}+(n_w-1)\dfrac{\mathrm{sse}}{U_e^2}}}{\sqrt{n_w}}}\right) - \Phi\left(\frac{(-\lambda+\mu_T)-\left(\bar{\bar{x}}-\dfrac{Z}{U_a}\sqrt{\dfrac{\mathrm{ssa}}{n_a n_w}}\right)}{\dfrac{\sqrt{\dfrac{\mathrm{ssa}}{U_a^2}+(n_w-1)\dfrac{\mathrm{sse}}{U_e^2}}}{\sqrt{n_w}}}\right).$$

It can be easily verified that $R(X, x, \theta)$ satisfies Conditions A1 and A2. Therefore, $R(X, x, \theta)$ is a GPQ of π. A one-sided lower $100(1 - \alpha)\%$ generalized confidence interval (GCI) for π can be constructed through simulation, using the following procedures (Weerahandi 1993):

Step 1. For $i = 1, \ldots, m$, simulate $\left(Z^i, U_a^{2i}, U_e^{2i}\right)$ as distributed in Equation 2.15.

Step 2. Calculate $R(X^i, x, \theta)$.

Step 3. Let $R^{(\alpha)}$ be the 100αth percentile of $\{R(X^i, x, \theta), i = 1,\ldots m\}$. $R^{(\alpha)}$ is an estimate of the one-sided lower $(1 - \alpha \times 100)\%$ GCI of π.

2.6.2 GPQ Test

Let $R^{(0.05)}$ be the 5th percentile of the simulated random sample described above. It is the one-sided lower 95% GCI for π. A test of the hypothesis in Equation 2.7 is constructed such that the null hypothesis is rejected if $R^{(0.05)}$ is greater than β. This method is called the GPQ test. It is of interest to know how well the test performs when compared to the existing tests described in Section 2.5.

2.7 Statistical Test Comparisons

Yang and Zhang (2015) conducted a simulation study to compare the performance of the GPQ test with the five existing approaches. The acceptance limit λ and acceptance level β were chosen to be the same as used in Govaerts et al. (2008), namely, 0.15 and 80%, respectively. The corresponding acceptable region for bias and precision is depicted in Figure 2.3, with the combinations of bias and precision under the curve corresponding to valid assays and those above the curve corresponding to invalid assays.

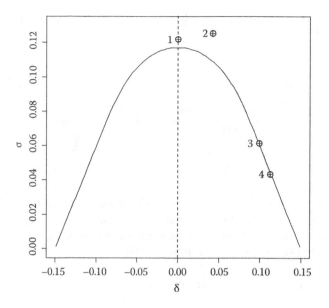

FIGURE 2.3

Acceptance region for bias and precision and the combinations used in simulation study, with $\lambda = 0.15$ and $\beta = 80\%$. (From Yang, H. and Zhang, J. (2015). A generalized pivotal quantity approach to analytical method validation based on total error. *PDA J. Pharm. Sci. Technol.*, 69, 725–735.)

Several experimental designs were evaluated with combinations of numbers of runs × replicates being 3 × 3, 4 × 4, 4 × 8, 8 × 8, and 20 × 20. As the intraclass coefficient (ICC) $\rho = \dfrac{\sigma_a^2}{\sigma_a^2 + \sigma_\varepsilon^2}$ also has an impact on assay performance, two levels of ρ, 0.25 and 0.75, were explored. In total, four scenarios listed in Table 2.5 were simulated. They all represent invalid assays as their corresponding quality levels are all below 80%.

Methods 1 and 2 represent analytical methods with 0 or small bias and high variability, whereas methods 3 and 4 have large bias and small to

TABLE 2.5

Four Analytical Methods with Unacceptable Quality Levels

Method	Bias	Precision	Quality Level (π)
1	0	0.12	0.789
2	0.05	0.12	0.750
3	0.1	0.06	0.798
4	0.13	0.03	0.748

Source: Yang, H. and Zhang, J. (2015). A generalized pivotal quantity approach to analytical method validation based on total error. *PDA J. Pharm. Sci. Technol.*, 69, 725–735.

moderate variability. These four methods are also shown in Figure 2.3. For each of the eight scenarios (combinations of bias and precision in Table 2.5 for each ICC level), 10,000 samples were generated from the one-way random effect model, with normally distributed random errors, for each of the five designs, 3×3, 4×4, 4×8, 8×8, and 20×20. Type I error, which is the probability of incorrectly accepting unsuitable analytical methods, is estimated by the proportion of times the null hypothesis in Equation 2.7 is rejected. The results are summarized in Tables 2.6 through 2.9.

The simulation results indicate that regardless of the sample size, both the GPQ method and the β-content(0.9) approach control Type I error at <0.05, thus protecting consumer risk, while the other four methods provide less control of Type I error. The contrast is more pronounced when either the sample size is not large ($N \leq 32$) or interrun variability is high (ICC = 0.75). In addition, the magnitude of bias of the analytical method has an impact on how the GPQ and β-content(0.9) methods compare to each other. Specifically, when the analytical method bias is greater than 0.1, the Type I error of the GPQ method is closer to the nominal level of 5% when compared to the β-content(0.9) method, for almost all sample sizes and ICCs. This suggests that the former is less conservative than the latter. As a result, the GPQ method potentially has greater power in accepting the methods when they have large biases. Where little or no method bias exists, the Type I error of the GPQ method is farther from the nominal level of 5% than the β-content method. In other words, it is more conservative than the β-content(0.9) method. In light of these findings, it is preferable to use the GPQ test for

TABLE 2.6

Estimated Type I Error for Method 1 (Bias = 0 and Precision = 0.12)

ICC ρ	Test Method	Sample Size ($N = n_a \times n_w$)				
		3×3	4×4	4×8	8×8	20×20
0.25	MLE	0.104	0.074	0.064	0.044	0.027
	Mee's modified MLE	0.035	0.031	0.034	0.026	0.022
	β-Expectation	0.141	0.125	0.117	0.104	0.067
	β-Content(0.5)	0.154	0.132	0.116	0.104	0.066
	β-Content(0.9)	0.010	0.011	0.011	0.010	0.005
	GPQ	0.003	0.005	0.006	0.008	0.008
0.75	MLE	0.167	0.134	0.139	0.094	0.061
	Mee's modified MLE	0.079	0.069	0.083	0.051	0.041
	β-Expectation	0.166	0.149	0.157	0.139	0.131
	β-Content(0.5)	0.181	0.162	0.163	0.150	0.138
	β-Content(0.9)	0.026	0.027	0.030	0.022	0.017
	GPQ	0.013	0.016	0.019	0.016	0.018

Source: Yang, H. and Zhang, J. (2015). A generalized pivotal quantity approach to analytical method validation based on total error. *PDA J. Pharm. Sci. Technol.*, 69, 725–735.

TABLE 2.7

Estimated Type I Error for Method 2 (Bias = 0.05 and Precision = 0.12)

ICC ρ	Test Method	Sample Size ($N = n_a \times n_w$)				
		3×3	4×4	4×8	8×8	20×20
0.25	MLE	0.070	0.047	0.033	0.015	0.001
	Mee's modified MLE	0.022	0.018	0.017	0.009	0.001
	β-Expectation	0.089	0.072	0.050	0.021	0.000
	β-Content(0.5)	0.099	0.077	0.050	0.021	0.000
	β-Content(0.9)	0.006	0.005	0.004	0.002	0.000
	GPQ	0.002	0.003	0.003	0.002	0.000
0.75	MLE	0.131	0.103	0.099	0.052	0.019
	Mee's modified MLE	0.062	0.052	0.059	0.029	0.012
	β-Expectation	0.129	0.114	0.109	0.067	0.023
	β-Content(0.5)	0.144	0.122	0.113	0.073	0.025
	β-Content(0.9)	0.020	0.018	0.020	0.012	0.002
	GPQ	0.009	0.012	0.015	0.011	0.005

Source: Yang, H. and Zhang, J. (2015). A generalized pivotal quantity approach to analytical method validation based on total error. *PDA J. Pharm. Sci. Technol.*, 69, 725–735.

TABLE 2.8

Estimated Type I Error for Method 3 (Bias = 0.1 and Precision = 0.06)

ICC ρ	Test Method	Sample Size ($N = n_a \times n_w$)				
		3×3	4×4	4×8	8×8	20×20
0.25	MLE	0.165	0.144	0.140	0.107	0.075
	Mee's modified MLE	0.076	0.080	0.090	0.071	0.056
	β-Expectation	0.134	0.109	0.078	0.029	0.000
	β-Content(0.5)	0.146	0.114	0.077	0.028	0.000
	β-Content(0.9)	0.016	0.014	0.012	0.003	0.000
	GPQ	0.016	0.028	0.035	0.041	0.040
0.75	MLE	0.230	0.196	0.187	0.135	0.089
	Mee's modified MLE	0.122	0.105	0.104	0.067	0.055
	β-Expectation	0.190	0.170	0.163	0.097	0.028
	β-Content(0.5)	0.215	0.184	0.172	0.104	0.030
	β-Content(0.9)	0.041	0.036	0.038	0.021	0.004
	GPQ	0.033	0.039	0.040	0.043	0.047

Source: Yang, H. and Zhang, J. (2015). A generalized pivotal quantity approach to analytical method validation based on total error. *PDA J. Pharm. Sci. Technol.*, 69, 725–735.

TABLE 2.9

Estimated Type I Error for Method 4 (Bias = 0.13 and Precision = 0.03)

ICC ρ	Method	Sample Size ($N = n_a \times n_w$)				
		3×3	4×4	4×8	8×8	20×20
0.25	MLE	0.099	0.076	0.063	0.028	0.004
	Mee's modified MLE	0.044	0.038	0.039	0.017	0.002
	β-Expectation	0.079	0.052	0.031	0.004	0.000
	β-Content(0.5)	0.088	0.055	0.031	0.004	0.000
	β-Content(0.9)	0.001	0.005	0.004	0.001	0.000
	GPQ	0.012	0.015	0.016	0.009	0.002
0.75	MLE	0.167	0.132	0.126	0.066	0.023
	Mee's modified MLE	0.088	0.068	0.068	0.032	0.011
	β-Expectation	0.137	0.113	0.107	0.043	0.004
	β-Content(0.5)	0.154	0.124	0.111	0.046	0.004
	β-Content(0.9)	0.027	0.022	0.024	0.008	0.001
	GPQ	0.028	0.027	0.030	0.020	0.009

Source: Yang, H. and Zhang, J. (2015). A generalized pivotal quantity approach to analytical method validation based on total error. *PDA J. Pharm. Sci. Technol.*, 69, 725–735.

method validation if development or prevalidation data indicate an appreciable bias of the method; otherwise, it is advantageous to use β-content(0.9). It is also worth pointing out that with a large sample size, the Type I error of the GPQ method is closer to the nominal level than all of the five current methods. This implies that the GPQ test has a better asymptotic property and improved power in accepting analytical methods fit for its intended purpose.

Also of interest is to compare the power of the tests described above. For this purpose, Yang and Zhang (2016) conducted additional simulations using combinations of acceptable bias and precision: (0.0, 0.03), (0.05, 0.04), and (0.1, 0.04); ICC 0.25, 0.75; and runs × replicates of 3 × 3, 4 × 4, 4 × 8, 8 × 8, and 20 × 20. Two key findings are as follows: (1) the power of the MLE, modified MLE, β-expectation, and β-content(0.5) is larger than that of β-content(0.9) and GPQ tests; (2) the GPQ test is more powerful than the β-content(0.9) test when the method is more biased. In addition, the overall power of the latter is low regardless of the sample size, which implies a poor asymptotic property of the β-content(0.9) test. By contrast, when the analytical method has little or no bias, the two tests are comparable to each other, with β-content(0.9) having slightly higher power than the GPQ test.

However, it should be noted that the power comparison between the group of MLE, modified MLE, β-expectation, and β-content(0.5) and that of GPQ and β-content(0.9) should be interpreted with caution, as the four tests in the first group have inflated Type I errors. It is also worth bearing in mind that because of practical limitations, the sample size for method validation cannot be too large. Therefore, improvement in method bias and precision rather than increased sample size is the preferred way to ensure sufficient power. In addition, when the design is unbalanced, several alternative methods can be used to construct a GPQ for the probability π (Krishnamoorthy and Mathew 2004; Liao et al. 2005). Last, the β-content(0.9) method often has a test size significantly less than the nominal level of 0.05. One potential remedy is to construct a table that contains, for various pratical sample sizes, β-content intervals with content less than 0.9 but having test size close to 0.05. This can be achieved through simulations. The same remark can be made for the GPQ method. By fine-tuning the confidence level, potentially for each choice of design, a GPQ with an appropriately chosen confidence level can be used to ensure a test size close to 0.05.

2.8 Other Alternate Methods

2.8.1 Method Based on Capability

The performance of an analytical method can be characterized through a capability measure defined as (Burdick et al. 2013)

$$C = \min\left[\frac{\lambda - \delta}{3\sigma}, \frac{\delta + \lambda}{3\sigma}\right], \tag{2.16}$$

which is estimated by

$$\hat{C} = \min\left[\frac{\lambda - \hat{\delta}}{3\hat{\sigma}}, \frac{\hat{\delta} + \lambda}{3\hat{\sigma}}\right].$$

When the acceptance limits $\pm\lambda$ are equal to the lower and upper specification limits LSL and USL, respectively, the measure C is the traditional capability index, often denoted as C_{pk}. In either case, C measures the analytical method's ability to produce results within acceptance range or specifications. Let P_{OOR} denote the probability for a test result to be out of the range (OOR) of $\pm\lambda$. Thus, $P_{OOR} = P(|X - \mu_T| \geq \lambda) = 1 - \pi$. It can be easily verified that

$$P_{OOR} \leq 2[1 - \Phi(3C)], \tag{2.17}$$

where $\Phi(\cdot)$ is the cumulative probability function of the standard normal distribution.

Therefore, the larger is the value of C, the smaller is the OOR probability. For example, for $C = 1, 1.5$, and 2, the corresponding upper bounds of P_{OOR} are $2.70 \times 10^{-3}, 6.70 \times 10^{-5}$, and 1.97×10^{-9}, respectively. Because of this monotonic relationship, one may validate the analytical method through testing the following hypotheses:

$$H_0: C < C_0 \text{ versus } H_1: C \geq C_0, \tag{2.18}$$

where C_0 is chosen such that

$$1 - \beta = 2[1 - \Phi(3C_0)]. \tag{2.19}$$

Solving Equation 2.19 for C_0, we obtain

$$C_0 = \frac{1}{3}z_{(1+\beta)/2}. \tag{2.20}$$

For example, when $\beta = 0.95$, $C_0 = \frac{1}{3}z_{(1+0.95)/2} = 0.653$. A statistical test can be constructed such that it rejects the null hypothesis in Equation 2.18 at a significance level of α if the lower limit of the one-sided $100(1 - \alpha)\%$ confidence interval of C exceeds C_0. Based on the method by Kushler and Hurley (1992), an approximate $100(1 - \alpha)\%$ lower confidence limit of C is obtained as (Burdick et al. 2013)

$$\hat{C} - z_{1-\alpha}\sqrt{\frac{1}{9n_a n_w} + \frac{\hat{C}^2}{2df_{\text{Approx}}}}, \tag{2.21}$$

where the degree of freedom df_{Approx} is estimated from Equation 2.6.

From Equation 2.17, the following can be derived:

$$\pi \geq 2\Phi(3C) - 1. \tag{2.22}$$

By Equations 2.19 and 2.22, $\pi < \beta$ implies $C < C_0$. Therefore, a statistical test that rejects the null hypothesis in Equation 2.18 would also reject the null hypothesis in Equation 2.7. Consequently, the analytical method can be considered validated if the null hypothesis in Equation 2.18 is rejected.

Using the data in Tables 2.2 and 2.3, the following can be calculated from Equation 2.3:

$$\hat{\sigma}^2 = MSA/n_w + (1 - 1/n_w)MSE = 4.672/3 + (1 - 1/3) \times 1.299 = 2.423,$$

$$\hat{\delta} = 0.372,$$

$$\hat{C} = \min\left[\frac{15 - 0.372}{3\sqrt{2.432}}, \frac{15 + 0.372}{3\sqrt{2.432}}\right] = 3.132.$$

By Equation 2.21, the 95% lower confidence limit is given as 2.242, which is greater than $C_0 = 0.653$. Hence, the null hypothesis in Equation 2.18 is rejected and the analytical method is validated for its intended use.

2.8.2 Bayesian Approach

Another alternative is to use a Bayesian tolerance interval to test the hypotheses (Equation 2.7). In general, Bayesian analysis makes inference about either the future observations or the model parameters, based on predictive and posterior distributions, which can be derived by combining the current data with prior distributions of the model parameters. When the closed-form representations of these distributions are unobtainable, Markov chain Monte Carlo sampling can be performed, using software packages such as Winbugs (MCR Biostatistics Unit 2016). For the balanced random effects model (Model 2.1), the Bayesian intervals can be obtained, using the simulation-based approach by Wolfinger (1998). This simulation-based approach for Bayesian tolerance intervals is also discussed by Krishnamoorthy and Mathew (2009). Applications of Bayesian analysis for method validation was demonstrated by several researchers (Burdick et al. 2013; Rozet et al. 2011; Saffaj and Ihssane 2012). After Krishnamoorthy and Mathew (2009), Saffaj and Ihssane (2012) described an algorithm for constructing β-expectation tolerance interval, based on simulation. The method is briefly described below.

Assume that the data from the validation study X_{ij} were generated from the one-way random effect model (Model 2.1). Under the model assumptions, the sufficient statistics $\bar{\bar{X}}$, SSA, and SSE, defined in Table 2.2, are independently distributed such that

$$\bar{\bar{X}} \sim N\left(\mu, \frac{n_w \sigma_a^2 + \sigma_e^2}{n_a n_w}\right)$$

$$\frac{SSA}{n_w \sigma_a^2 + \sigma_e^2} \sim \chi_{n_a}^2$$

$$\frac{SSE}{\sigma_e^2} \sim \chi_{n_a(n_w-1)}^2.$$

Therefore, the likelihood of the observed data is the product of the joint distributions of the three sufficient statistics of Model 2.1. Under Jeffrey's noninformative prior of $\left(\mu, \sigma_a^2, \sigma_e^2\right)$,

$$p\left(\mu, \sigma_a^2, \sigma_e^2\right) \propto \frac{1}{\sigma_e^2 \left(n_w \sigma_a^2 + \sigma_e^2\right)},$$

it can be shown that the posterior distributions of $\sigma_A^2 \left(\equiv n_w \sigma_a^2 + \sigma_e^2\right)$, σ_e^2, and the conditional posterior distribution of μ are given by (Krishnamoorthy and Mathew 2009)

$$\sigma_A^2 \mid \bar{\bar{X}}, \text{SSA}, \text{SSE} \propto \text{IG}\left(\frac{n_a - 1}{2}, \frac{\text{SSA}}{2}\right), \qquad (2.23)$$

$$\sigma_e^2 \mid \bar{\bar{X}}, \text{SSA}, \text{SSE} \propto \text{IG}\left(\frac{n_a(n_w - 1)}{2}, \frac{\text{SSE}}{2}\right), \qquad (2.24)$$

$$\mu \mid \bar{\bar{X}}, \text{SSA}, \text{SSE}, \sigma_A^2, \sigma_e^2 \propto N\left(\bar{\bar{X}}, \frac{\sigma_A^2}{n_a n_w}\right), \qquad (2.25)$$

where IG(u, v) is an inverse-gamma distribution with parameters (u, v).

To simulate a sample from the predictive density $p(X_f \mid \bar{X}, \text{SSA}, \text{SSE})$, where X_f is a future observation, one may generate an observation from $p\left(X_f \mid \left(\mu, \sigma_a^2, \sigma_e^2\right)^*, \bar{\bar{X}}, \text{SSA}, \text{SSE}\right)$ for each observation $\left(\mu, \sigma_a^2, \sigma_e^2\right)^*$ from $p\left(\mu, \sigma_a^2, \sigma_e^2 \mid \bar{\bar{X}}, \text{SSA}, \text{SSE}\right)$. This is a valid approach because under the one-way random effect model (Model 2.1),

$$X_f \mid \left(\mu, \sigma_a^2, \sigma_e^2, \bar{\bar{X}}, \text{SSA}, \text{SSE}\right) \sim N\left(\mu, \sigma_a^2 + \sigma_e^2\right). \qquad (2.26)$$

Using the distributions in Equations 2.23 through 2.26, the following procedure can be used to construct a Bayesian β-expectation tolerance interval:

1. Simulate $\left(\sigma_A^2\right)^*$ and $\left(\sigma_e^2\right)^*$ from Equations 2.23 and 2.24, for m_0 times. Retain the sample only if $\left(\sigma_A^2\right)^* \geq \left(\sigma_e^2\right)^*$. Let m denote the number of times for the above condition to hold.
2. Generate μ^* from the distribution in Equation 2.25.
3. Simulate X_f from Equation 2.26 for each observation of $\left(\mu^*, \left(\sigma_A^2\right)^*, \left(\sigma_e^2\right)^*\right)$ out of a total of m.
4. The lower β_1th and upper β_2th percentiles of the above sample $(\beta_2 - \beta_1 = \beta)$ provide a Bayesian β-expectation tolerance interval for future observation.

The null hypothesis in Equation 2.7 is rejected if the (β_1, β_2) is contained within $(-\lambda, \lambda)$. Similarly a β-content, γ-confidence tolerance interval of the future observations can be constructed (see Krishnamoorthy and Mathew 2009 for details).

2.9 Concluding Remarks

The objective of an analytical method is to generate accurate and reliable data to aid decision-making related to product quality. Method validation through systematic experimentation and rigorous statistical evaluation plays an important role in achieving this objective. Good manufacturing practice and other regulatory guidance also requires that analytical test methods used in assessing compliance of pharmaceutical products should meet proper standards for accuracy, sensitivity, specificity, precision, and so on, and be shown to be suitable for their intended purpose. Traditionally, method validation was viewed as a one-time checklist exercise to demonstrate and document the performance of the analytical method with a focus on validation of individual performance characteristics. Application of the QbD and life cycle approach to process validation concepts to analytical methods presents an opportunity to gain enhanced understanding of the analytical method and ensure continual validation and verification of the method. However, implementation of the life cycle approach to analytical methods may pose some statistical challenges. For example, it is necessary to develop statistical tests that can be used to evaluate the performance of the analytical method against the ATP that is directly related to the intended purpose of the method. Validation based on the concept of total error is a step forward in testing fit-for-purpose hypotheses. Although some advancement has been made in statistical tests based on total error, more research is needed, particularly when designs are unbalanced and missing data occur. While protection of Type I error is of primary concern in selecting a statistical test for analytical method validation, it is also important to consider the power of the statistical test. Factors affecting the power and Type I error include true bias and precision of the assay, numbers of runs and replicates, and intraclass correlation. For a detailed discussion, see Burdick et al. (2013).

3

Parallelism Testing of Bioassay

3.1 Introduction

Although the advances in chemical characterization have greatly reduced the dependence on bioassays to characterize drug products in recent years, bioassays continue to play a significant role in drug development, particularly in the determination of potency and bioactivity of biological and biotechnological products. A typical bioassay involves the use of biological substrates such as live animals, living tissues, or cells. The inherently large variability of the assay often makes an absolute measure impractical. A practical remedy is to utilize a relative test method. The method determines the potency or bioactivity of a test sample relative to a reference standard, tested in the same run. The result is reported as "relative potency," for example, the ratio of EC_{50} values. However, for the relative potency to be meaningful, the test sample must behave like a dilution or concentration of the reference standard. In other words, the dose–response curve of the test sample must be a horizontal shift of that of the reference standard along the logarithmic dose axis. This idea of this similarity between the test sample and reference standard was first introduced by Wood (1946) and was mathematically formulated by Finney (1978).

In bioassay literature, similarity between two dose–response curves is often referred to as parallelism. Although parallelism has nothing to do with method validation, it is necessary to ensure the validity of relative potency. In fact, testing for parallelism in relative potency assays is recommended by both the United States Pharmacopeia (USP) (USP 2010a,b) and European Pharmacopeia (EP) (European Directorate for the Quality of Medicines 2004).

To date, various statistical tests for parallelism have been proposed (Callahan and Sajjadi 2003; Gottschalk and Dunn 2005; Hauck et al. 2005; Jonkman and Sidik 2009). In a broad sense, the current statistical approaches can be classified into two categories: significance tests and equivalence tests. Significance tests proposed for parallelism include the t test for a parallel line model (USP <111>) (USP 2000) and the F test based on a four-parameter logistic (4PL) model and extra sum of squares (Gottschalk and Dunn 2005), whereas equivalence tests for parallelism include interval tests (Callahan and Sajjadi 2003; Hauck et al. 2005), the intersection–union test (IUT) (Jonkman and Sidik 2009) for comparison of model parameters, and a Bayesian approach that directly tests the hypothesis that the test sample is a dilution or concentration of the reference standard (Novick et al. 2012).

Historically, there has been much debate regarding whether significance or equivalence tests are more appropriate for demonstrating parallelism. Using a receiver operating characteristic (ROC) analysis, Yang and Zhang (2012) compared the overall performance of the two classes of methods. It was demonstrated that the equivalence tests outperform the significance tests when the equivalence limits are selected based on some optimality criteria such as area under the ROC curve (AUC). However, as with equivalence tests applied in other settings, the selection of equivalence limits for parallelism remains challenging. Although several methods were proposed (Hauck et al. 2005; Liao et al. 2011; Yang and Zhang 2012a), it is evident that more research along this line is needed.

The primary focus of this chapter is advances in statistical tests for parallelism. Key points of interest include dose–response models, advantages and disadvantages of various parallelism test methods, parallelism test comparisons, and the selection of equivalence limits.

3.2 Dose–Response Models

Determination of the relative potency of a bioassay relies on characterization of the assay response across a range of doses (concentrations). The dose–response relationship usually can be described through a mathematical function. For bioassays, both linear and nonlinear functions have been used to describe dose–response data. Let $f(\theta, x)$ denote a dose–response function, with x being the concentration on either the raw or the transformed scale and θ being the parameters describing the dose–response function. The expected dose–response curves of the test sample and reference standard preparations are described through $f(\theta_T, x)$ and $f(\theta_R, x)$, respectively. Under the similarity definition by Wood (1946), there exists a constant ρ such that $f(\theta_T, x) = f(\theta_R, \rho x)$ if x is the raw concentration or $f(\theta_T, x) = f(\theta_R, x + \rho)$ if x is the logarithmic concentration. The calibration constant ρ is commonly known as the relative or log-relative potency of the test sample. It is often estimated after the similarity in dose–response curve between the test sample and reference standard is established. Although $f(\theta, x)$ can take many different forms, most common are linear and 4PL functions. Including measurement error ε_{ij}, a linear model takes the form of

$$y_{ij} = \alpha_i + \beta_i x_j + \varepsilon_{ij}. \tag{3.1}$$

A 4PL model (Gottschalk and Dunn 2005; Jonkman and Sidik 2009) of a dose–response relationship is described through a nonlinear function, with ε_{ij} measurement errors, such that

$$y_{ij} = a_i + \frac{d_i - a_i}{1 + \exp[b_i(x_j - \log(c_i))]} + \varepsilon_{ij}, \tag{3.2}$$

where y_{ij} is the assay response at log dose (or concentration) x_j of a test or reference preparation and ε_{ij} are the measurement errors following $N(0, \sigma^2)$, with $i = 1$ and 2 corresponding to the test sample and reference standard preparations, respectively, $j = 1, ..., n$, and σ is the assay variability. Under the parameterization of Model 3.2, the model parameters have intuitive interpretations. Specifically, a_i and d_i are the upper and lower asymptotes, respectively, b_i is the Hill slope, and c_i is the inflection point where curvature changes direction. The parameter c_i, often referred to as EC_{50}, is the dose corresponding to a response midway between the lower and upper asymptotes. Through re-parameterization, the above 4PL may take different forms.

It is conceivable that the model selected to describe the dose–response relationship has a significant impact on parallelism testing. For instance, an inadequate model may incur large variability in model parameter estimation, thus decreasing the performance of the test for parallelism. However, despite the importance of model selection, it is not the primary focus of this chapter. Statistical considerations and appropriateness of using these models to fit dose–response curves have been discussed in the literature (Callahan and Sajjadi 2003). Interested readers may also refer to work by O'Connell et al. (1993) and Boulanger et al. (2007a) for a detailed discussion.

3.3 Parallelism Testing

3.3.1 Measure of Parallelism

An essential part of parallelism testing is the quantification of parallelism, that is, the metric that describes the similarity of two dose–response curves. Existing metrics are based on either model parameters or dose–response curves. For example, metrics by Callahan and Sajjadi (2003), Gottschalk and Dunn (2005), Hauck et al. (2005), and Jonkman and Sidik (2009) are related to the difference in model parameters. For many bioassays, the dose–response curves can be adequately described through the 4PL model in Equation 3.2. Figure 3.1 displays two 4PL dose–responses curves. They typically are either monotonically increasing or decreasing with plateaus at both extremes of the dose concentration range.

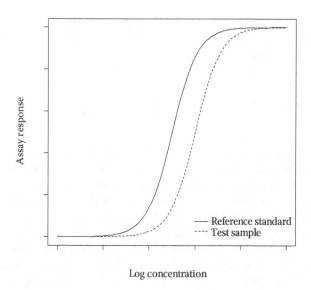

FIGURE 3.1
Example of a 4PL model used to describe dose–response curves of a test sample and a reference standard.

There are several ways in which the measure of parallelism can be defined. For example, it can be described as differences in the parameters, $a_1 - a_2$, $b_1 - b_2$, and $d_1 - d_2$. As c_i are used to estimate relative potency, they are not expected to be identical and therefore are not part of the parallelism test. Alternatively, one may define the metric for parallelism as the ratios of parameters: a_1/a_2, b_1/b_2, and d_1/d_2.

Yang et al. (2012) proposed to re-parameterize (a_i, b_i, d_i) as (a_i, f_i, s_i), with $f_i = d_i - a_i$ and $s_i = -(d_i - a_i)b_i/4$, respectively. They argued that such re-parameterization has two advantages. First of all, it offsets potentially large variability in the ratio estimate of lower asymptotes between the test sample and reference standard because the lower asymptotes tend to be close to zero. Second, s_i represents the slope of the dose–response curve at EC_{50}. It makes both intuitive and practical sense to test equivalence in slope between the two response curves, as opposed to b_i, which is a factor of slope. In practice, f_i, the difference between the lower and upper asymptotes, is often referred to as the effective window. Yang et al. (2012) also suggested a test for parallelism using $r_1 = a_1/a_2$, $r_2 = f_1/f_2$, and $r_3 = s_1/s_2$, which represent the ratios of upper asymptote, effective window, and slope at EC_{50}, respectively. However, as noted by Novick et al. (2012), the metrics based on model parameters have a serious drawback; namely, the closeness between two sets of model parameters does not readily translate into the similarity of the two dose–response curves.

As a remedy, Novick et al. (2012) proposed a metric that measures the maximum difference between the two dose–response curves after properly shifting the dose–response curve of the reference standard. Specifically, it is defined as

$$\min_{\rho} \max_{x \in [x_L, x_U]} |f(\theta_1, x) - f(\theta_2, x + \rho)| < \delta, \tag{3.3}$$

where $[x_L, x_U]$ is a range of dose concentration.

Interestingly, when the dose–response curves are linear as shown in Figure 3.2, the above metric is equivalent to that based on the difference in model parameters.

It is clear that the two lines are parallel if they have the same slope; thus, the parallelism metric can be defined as $\beta_1 - \beta_2$. Novick et al. (2012) showed that the value of ρ that minimizes Equation 3.3 for the linear dose–response model is given by

$$\rho = [(b_1 - b_2)(x_L + x_U)/2 + (a_1 - a_2)]/b_2. \tag{3.4}$$

Substituting this in Equation 3.3 gives rise to

$$(\beta_1 - \beta_2)(x_U - x_L)/2, \tag{3.5}$$

which is proportional to the metric $\beta_1 - \beta_2$. Therefore, the two metrics are essentially the same. However, in general, there does not exist a direct

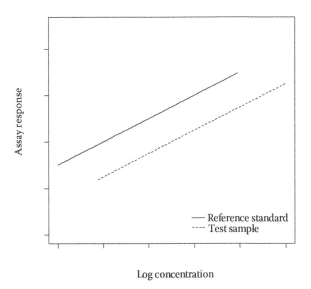

Log concentration

FIGURE 3.2
Parallel-line model used to describe dose–response curves of a test sample and a reference standard.

relationship between the two metrics when the dose–response curves are nonlinear. An important advantage of the metric in Equation 3.3 is that it is consistent with Wood's definition of similarity between the dose–response curves of the test sample and reference standard. As is shown in Section 3.4, the properties of statistical tests for parallelism based on these two types of metrics greatly differ from each other.

3.3.2 Statistical Parallelism Tests

As previously mentioned, there are two categories of parallelism test methods, namely, significance tests and equivalence tests. In this section, we present a detailed discussion of how the tests are constructed and the advantages and disadvantages associated with these types of tests.

3.3.2.1 Significance Tests

What differentiates significance and equivalence approaches for parallelism testing is how the associated hypotheses of each test are formulated. For a significance test, the hypotheses are stated as

H_0: Parameters of the two dose–response curves are identical

versus

H_1: The parameters are not identical.

For Model 3.1, the corresponding hypotheses of parallelism are

$$H_0: \beta_1 = \beta_2 \text{ versus } H_1: \beta_1 \neq \beta_2. \tag{3.6}$$

Let

$$T = \frac{\hat{\beta}_1 - \hat{\beta}_2}{\hat{\sigma}\sqrt{2/S_x}}, \tag{3.7}$$

where $\hat{\beta}_1, \hat{\beta}_2,$ and $\hat{\sigma}$ are least square estimators of the two slopes and common assay variability, respectively, and $S_x = \sqrt{\sum_{i=1}^{n}(x_i - \bar{x})^2}$ with $\bar{x} = \frac{1}{n}\left(\sum_{i=1}^{n} x_i\right)$. Under the assumptions of Model 3.1 and the null hypothesis H_0, the test statistic T follows a t distribution with $(2n - 4)$ degrees of freedom. The parallelism claim H_0 is rejected if the test statistic results in a P value less than or equal to α (typically chosen to be 0.05). In other words, the parallelism claim is rejected if $|T| \geq t_{1-\alpha/2, 2n-4}$, where $t_{1-\alpha/2, 2n-4}$ is the upper $(1 - \alpha/2) \times 100\%$ critical value of a central t distribution with $(2n - 4)$ degrees of freedom.

Similarly for Model 3.2, we may formulate the parallelism hypotheses as

H_0: $a_1 = a_2$ and $b_1 = b_2$ and $d_1 = d_2$ versus H_1: $a_1 \neq a_2$ or $b_1 \neq b_2$ or $d_1 \neq d_2$.

Define

$$\hat{F} = \frac{|\text{SSE(Reduced)} - \text{SSE(Full)}|/3}{\text{SSE(Full)}/(2n - 8)}, \tag{3.8}$$

where SSE(Reduced) and SSE(Full) are sum of squared errors from fitting Model 3.2 under H_0 and H_1, respectively (Gottschalk and Dunn 2005; Jonkman and Sidik 2009). Under H_0, $\hat{F}$ follows an F distribution with $(3, 2n - 8)$ degrees of freedom. The null hypothesis is rejected if $\hat{F}$ exceeds its upper $(1 - \alpha) \times 100\%$ critical value $F_{3,2n-8}(1 - \alpha)$, where α is typically chosen to be 0.05. An alternative test statistic based on the same 4PL model was proposed by Gottschalk and Dunn (2005). It is given by

$$\hat{H} = \text{SSE(Reduced)} - \text{SSE(Full)}, \tag{3.9}$$

which follows a χ^2 distribution with $2n - 8$ degrees of freedom under the null hypothesis. Although lacking in an apparent theoretic basis, it was empirically shown that this χ^2 statistic is more reliable than the F test (Gottschalk and Dunn 2005).

3.3.2.2 Equivalence Tests

All of the above P value–based tests in Section 3.3.2.1 are referred to as significance tests. As noted by several researchers (Callahan and Sajjadi 2003; Hauck et al. 2005; Jonkman and Sidik 2009), these significant tests may be fundamentally flawed in two ways, as they rely on lack of statistical significance to declare parallelism. The issue stems from how the parallelism hypotheses are formulated. Specifically, parallelism is claimed if the null hypothesis is *not* rejected. Since a small sample size and large variability of the assay would render a larger P value, the smaller the experiment or the larger the variability, the less likely one will reject the null hypothesis of parallelism. This obviously does not make any scientific sense as it rewards insufficient experimentation and imprecise assays. On the other hand, when the assay is precise, statistical significance may be achieved even if the differences in model parameters are trivial. This results in untoward rejection of parallelism, thus penalizing precise assays (Callahan and Sajjadi 2003; Hauck et al. 2005).

To overcome the shortcomings of the significance tests, several authors suggested that parallelism testing be reformulated as testing the hypothesis of equivalence.

3.3.2.2.1 Frequentist Solutions

For the linear case, in the context of equivalence testing, the hypotheses of interest are

$$H_0: |\beta_1 - \beta_2| \geq d \text{ versus } H_1: |\beta_1 - \beta_2| < d. \tag{3.10}$$

The intent of an equivalence test for parallelism, for a linear model, is to disprove that the slopes of test sample and reference standard differ by greater than or equal to an amount d, which is deemed a practically important difference and referred to as the equivalence limit. As the burden of disproving the null hypothesis is on the experimenter, it lends him or her more incentives to properly design the study. A test for the hypotheses in Equation 3.10 can be constructed using two one-sided t tests (TOST) (Chow and Liu 1992). It is well known that the TOST is operationally equivalent to declaring parallelism if the two-sided $(1 - \alpha) \times 100\%$ confidence interval (CI) for the mean slope difference $(\beta_1 - \beta_2)$ falls within the interval $(-d, d)$ (Schuirmann 1987):

$$\hat{\beta}_1 - \hat{\beta}_2 \pm t_{1-\alpha, 2n-4} \, \hat{\sigma} \sqrt{2/S_x} \in (-d, d). \tag{3.11}$$

The above interval approach makes testing the hypotheses in Equation 3.10 straightforward.

Jonkman and Sidik (2009) extended the equivalence test for parallelism to a nonlinear model based on a 4PL function. Parallelism is assessed through testing the following hypotheses:

$$H_0: \frac{a_1}{a_2} \leq D_L \text{ or } \frac{a_1}{a_2} \geq D_U \text{ or } \frac{b_1}{b_2} \leq D_L \text{ or } \frac{b_1}{b_2} \geq D_U \text{ or } \frac{d_1}{d_2} \leq D_L \text{ or } \frac{d_1}{d_2} \geq D_U$$

$$\text{versus } H_1: D_L < \frac{a_1}{a_2} < D_U \text{ and } D_L < \frac{b_1}{b_2} < D_U \text{ and } D_L < \frac{d_1}{d_2} < D_U, \tag{3.12}$$

where D_L and D_U are equivalence limits. The parameters $c_i (i = 1, 2)$ are not part of the hypotheses as they are related to relative potency and are therefore not expected to be the same. Depending on the bioassay, different equivalence limits may be appropriate for each parameter. Under the assumption that the parameters (a_2, b_2, c_2) are positive, the hypotheses in Equation 3.12 can be rewritten as (Jonkman and Sidik 2009)

$$H_0 : \begin{array}{lclcl} a_1 - D_L a_2 \le 0 & \text{or} & a_1 - D_L a_2 > 0 & \text{or} \\ b_1 - D_L b_2 \le 0 & \text{or} & b_1 - D_L b_2 > 0 & \text{or} \\ c_1 - D_L c_2 \le 0 & \text{or} & c_1 - D_L c_2 > 0 & \text{or} \end{array}$$

versus

$$H_1 : \begin{array}{lclcl} a_1 - D_L a_2 > 0 & \text{and} & a_1 - D_L a_2 > 0 & \text{and} \\ b_1 - D_L b_2 \le 0 & \text{and} & b_1 - D_L b_2 > 0 & \text{and} \\ c_1 - D_L c_2 \le 0 & \text{and} & c_1 - D_L c_2 > 0 & \text{and.} \end{array} \quad (3.13)$$

Jonkman and Sidik (2009) argued that it is reasonable to assume that the lower and upper asymptotes a_i and d_i are positive, as assay responses are typically positive. As for the parameters b_i, they may be positive or negative depending on whether the assay is intended to measure activity of an agonist or an antagonist. However, since each b_i would assume the same sign, the above hypotheses can be re-expressed with b_i being replaced by $-b_i$ when they are known to be negative. In this way, the reformulated hypotheses would take exactly the same form as in Equation 3.13.

3.3.2.2.2 Intersection–Union Test

The null hypothesis in Equation 3.13 is a union of six subhypotheses concerning ratios of three parameters of the 4PL model, and the alternative is an intersection of six hypotheses. An IUT test was constructed by Jonkman and Sidik (2009) using six one-sided tests, each testing a component set of hypotheses in Equation 3.13. Take the first component hypothesis as an example:

$$H_{01}: a_1 - D_L a_2 \le 0 \text{ versus } H_{11}: a_1 - D_L a_2 > 0. \quad (3.14)$$

Let $\theta = (a_1, b_1, c_1, d_1, a_2, b_2, c_2, d_2)$. We let $\hat{\theta} = (\hat{a}_1, \hat{b}_1, \hat{c}_1, \hat{d}_1, \hat{a}_2, \hat{b}_2, \hat{c}_2, \hat{d}_2)$ denote the estimate of θ from fitting Model 3.2, and let $\hat{\Sigma}(\theta)$ be the estimated associated variance–covariance matrix of θ. Further, let $K = (1, 0, 0, 0, -D_L, 0, 0, 0)$. A t statistic for testing the hypotheses in Equation 3.14 is given by

$$T_1 = \frac{K\hat{\theta}}{K'\hat{\Sigma}(\theta)K},$$

which has a t distribution with $n - 8$ degrees of freedom. The null hypothesis in Equation 3.14 is rejected if $T_1 > t_{1-\alpha, n-8}$. Similarly, we could construct five additional tests for the other five subhypotheses. Combined, these tests form an IUT that has a size of α (Berger 1982; Berger and Hsu 1996; Casella and Berger 1990). The IUT protects the consumer risk and is desirable from a compliance point of view.

More recently, Yang et al. (2012) developed an IUT based on re-parameterization of the model parameters (a_i, b_i, d_i), namely, using (a_i, f_i, s_i), which were previously described, in lieu of (a_i, b_i, d_i). Hence, the corresponding hypotheses are obtained as follows:

$$H_0: \frac{a_1}{a_2} \le D_{L1} \text{ or } \frac{a_1}{a_2} \ge D_{U1} \text{ or } \frac{f_1}{f_2} \le D_{L2} \text{ or } \frac{f_1}{f_2} \ge D_{U2} \text{ or } \frac{s_1}{s_2} \le D_{L3} \text{ or } \frac{s_1}{s_2} \ge D_{U3}$$

$$\text{versus } H_1: D_{L1} < \frac{a_1}{a_2} < D_{U1} \text{ and } D_{L2} < \frac{f_1}{f_2} < D_{U2} \text{ and } D_{L3} < \frac{s_1}{s_2} < D_{U3}, \qquad (3.15)$$

where D_{Lk} and D_{Uk} are equivalence limits ($k = 1, 2, 3$). Similar to the linear case, testing one of these hypotheses approach is operationally equivalent to the $(1 - 2\alpha) \times 100\%$ CIs for the parameter ratios being fully contained within the intervals (D_{Lk}, D_{Uk}), $k = 1, 2, 3$. For simplicity, we use r_k, $k = 1, 2, 3$ to denote the ratios $\frac{a_1}{a_2}$, $\frac{f_1}{f_2}$, and $\frac{s_1}{s_2}$, respectively. As functions of θ, they can be denoted as $r_k = g_k(\theta)$. Let $g'_k(\theta) = \partial g_k(\theta)/\partial \theta$ be the partial derivative of r_k with respect to the model parameters θ. Then, $\hat{r}_k = g_k(\hat{\theta})$ is an estimate of r_k with the variance of $\hat{r}_k$ being estimated by $\hat{\text{var}}[\hat{r}_k] = [g'_k(\hat{\theta})]^T \hat{\Sigma}(\theta)[g'_k(\hat{\theta})]$. An approximate $(1 - 2\alpha) \times 100\%$ CI of r_k is given by

$$\left(\hat{r}_k - z_{1-\alpha}\sqrt{\hat{\text{var}}[\hat{r}_k]}, \ \hat{r}_k + z_{1-\alpha}\sqrt{\hat{\text{var}}[\hat{r}_k]} \right),$$

where $z_{1-\alpha}$ is the upper $(100\alpha)\%$ critical value of the standard normal distribution. The null hypothesis in Equation 3.15 is rejected if the above interval is contained in (D_{Lk}, D_{Uk}) for $k = 1, 2, 3$. As an illustration, we demonstrate how to construct the $(1 - 2\alpha) \times 100\%$ CI for r_1. The partial derivative of r_1 is

$$g'_1(\theta) = \left(\frac{1}{a_2}, 0, 0, 0, \frac{-a_1}{a_2^2}, 0, 0, 0 \right).$$

Thus,

$$\hat{\text{var}}[\hat{r}_1] = \frac{1}{\hat{a}_2^2} \text{var}[\hat{a}_1)] + \frac{\hat{a}_1^2}{\hat{a}_2^4} \text{var}[\hat{a}_2].$$

The $(1 - 2\alpha) \times 100\%$ CI is obtained as

$$\left(\frac{\hat{\hat{a}}_1}{\hat{\hat{a}}_2} - z_{1-\alpha}\sqrt{\hat{\text{var}}[\hat{r}_1]}, \ \frac{\hat{\hat{a}}_1}{\hat{\hat{a}}_2} + z_{1-\alpha}\sqrt{\hat{\text{var}}[\hat{r}_1]} \right).$$

Fieller's theorem (1944) can also be used to construct a two-sided $(1 - 2\alpha) \times 100\%$ $(1 - 2\alpha) \times 100\%$ interval for this ratio. Since CIs based on Fieller's theorem are exact, they potentially may have better performance than the approximate intervals described above. The $(1 - 2\alpha) \times 100\%$ CIs for r_2 and r_3 can be similarly constructed, using the following facts (Sondag et al. 2015):

$$g_2'(\theta) = \left(-\frac{1}{d_2 - a_2}, 0, 0, \frac{1}{d_2 - a_2}, \frac{d_1 - a_1}{(d_2 - a_2)^2}, 0, 0, \frac{d_1 - a_1}{(d_2 - a_2)^2} \right)$$

$$g_3'(\theta) = \left(-\frac{b_1}{(d_2 - a_2)b_2}, \frac{d_1 - a_1}{(d_2 - a_2)b_2}, 0, \frac{b_1}{(d_2 - a_2)b_2}, \right.$$

$$= -\frac{(d_1 - a_1)b_1}{(d_2 - a_2)^2 b_2}, -\frac{(d_1 - a_1)b_1}{(d_2 - a_2)^2 b_2}, 0, -\left. \frac{(d_1 - a_1)b_1}{(d_2 - a_2)^2} \right).$$

3.3.2.2.3 A Bayesian Approach

Both the significance and equivalence tests described previously are indirect approaches for testing parallelism, as they establish similarity between two curves through statistical inference on dose–response model parameters. As previously discussed, an apparent drawback of this approach is that the difference in model parameters cannot be directly translated into the difference in the dose–response curve. Therefore, similarity in model parameters does not necessarily provide any assurance of the similarity of the curves of the reference standard and test sample. In addition, the statistical tests discussed so far do not account for the variability in the model parameters. As mentioned in Section 3.1, Novick et al. (2012) suggested an alternative metric of parallelism and proposed a Bayesian approach that directly tests the hypothesis that the dose–response curve of the test sample is a copy of the reference standard dose–response curve after a horizontal shift. This method is conceptually appealing as it is consistent with the similarity concept summarized by Wood (1946). With this approach, the hypotheses of interest become

$$H_0 : \min_{\rho} \max_{x \in [x_L, x_U]} \left| f(\theta_1, x) - f(\theta_2, x + \rho) \right| \geq \delta$$

versus

$$H_1 : \min_{\rho} \max_{x \in [x_L, x_U]} \left| f(\theta_1, x) - f(\theta_2, x + \rho) \right| < \delta. \tag{3.16}$$

As previously discussed, when the dose–response curves are linear, the value of the parameter ρ that minimizes the measure of parallelism is given in Equation 3.4. As a result, the above hypotheses become

$$H_0: |a_1 - a_2| \geq \delta^* \text{ versus } H_1: |a_1 - a_2| < \delta^*, \tag{3.17}$$

with $\delta^* = 2\delta/(x_U - x_L)$. Thus, in essence, the proposed metric results in the same hypotheses as those in Equation 3.10, which centered on demonstration of closeness between the slopes of two lines. However, for a nonlinear dose–response relationship, such a closed-form solution in general does not exist. Instead, a numerical min–max algorithm by Novick et al. (2012) can be used to evaluate the measure of parallelism and test the hypotheses in Equation 3.16. The idea is to determine the min–max value over a fine grid of x and ρ. For this purpose, Novick et al. (2012) developed a two-dimensional optimization routine and made it available in the appendix of their article. The algorithm has a satisfactory speed and provides accurate estimation.

3.3.2.2.4 Test for Parallel Equivalence Using Bayesian Approach
Now, we let

$$p(\delta, x_L, x_U) = \Pr\left[\min_{\rho} \max_{x \in [x_L, x_U]} \left| f(\theta_1, x) - f(\theta_2, x + \rho) \right| < \delta \middle| \text{data} \right]$$

be the posterior probability that the difference between two dose–response curves will be completely confined within the range of $(-\delta, \delta)$. The equivalence limits $(-\delta, \delta)$ are chosen based on practical considerations. Since they are on the raw response scale, selection of the limits is conceivably easier than that for tests of the model parameters. This is doubtlessly another advantage of the new method. The hypotheses in Equation 3.16 are tested based on the following decision rules: reject H_0 if $p(\delta, x_L, x_U) > p_0$, a preselected number such as 0.9; otherwise, accept H_0.

The Bayesian posterior probability is estimated through the following procedure. First of all, the posterior distributions of θ_1 and θ_2 are derived, based on both the prior distributions of θ_1 and θ_2 and the sampling distributions of measurement errors. Depending on the knowledge of the assay, different priors may be chosen (Gelman et al. 2004). Random samples are repeatedly drawn from the posterior distributions. For every random draw from the posterior distributions, the optimization in Equation 3.16 is carried out, and whether the condition $\min_{\rho} \max_{x \in [x_L, x_U]} \left| f(\theta_1, x) - f(\theta_2, x + \rho) \right| < \delta$ is met is recorded. Finally, the posterior probability is estimated by the proportion of draws that satisfy the above condition. The hypotheses in Equation 3.16 are tested by comparing this posterior probability estimate to the prespecified cut point p_0.

3.3.2.2.5 Simulation Studies

Novick et al. (2012) conducted two Monte Carlo simulation studies to compare the performance of this new Bayesian parallelism test with the existing procedures, the first based on the linear model in Equation 3.1 and the second using the 4PL in Equation 3.2. As the results for the linear and 4PL models are very similar, we focus the discussion on the latter. The data were simulated using the format of a real assay, which tests three replicates at the concentrations $0, 10^2, 10^{2.5265}, ..., 10^{6.5}$, resulting in two 10-point dose–response curves. Since both the reference standard and test sample are run on the same plate, it is assumed that the two dose–response curves have the same lower asymptote. The empirical properties evaluated include rates of false claims of parallelism and nonparallelism. Therefore, the simulation was carried out for six cases listed in Table 3.1, with Cases 1 and 2, Cases 3 and 4, Case 5, and Case 6, representing exactly parallel, parallel equivalent, borderline parallel equivalent, and inequivalent, respectively. More specifically, for Case 1, the test sample and reference standard have the exact same dose–response curve, whereas for Case 2, the curve of the test sample is precisely a horizontal shift of that of the reference standard. Thus, in both of those cases, the two curves are exactly equivalent, having a maximum difference of zero. After a proper horizontal shift, the two curves differ in the Hill slope for Case 3 and upper asymptote for Case 4. The parameters were chosen to render a maximum difference of 0.15 in both Cases 3 and 4. Similar to Case 3, for Case 5, the two curves differ in the Hill slope, however, by a greater margin. Last, the two curves in Case 6 are different from each other in both the Hill slope and upper asymptote.

TABLE 3.1

Simulation Conditions for Dose–Response Curves Described through 4PL Models

	Reference Standard				Test Sample				Maximum
Case	a_1	b_1	c_1	d_1	a_2	b_2	c_2	d_2	Difference
1	2	4.5	4	−1	2	4.5	4	−1	0
2					2	4.5	4.7	−1	0
3					2	4.792	4.7	−1	0.15
4					2	4.5	4.7	−1.312	0.15
5					2	4.906	4.7	−1	0.20
6					2	4.792	4.7	−1.305	0.30

Source: Novick, S., Yang, H., and J. Peterson (2012). A Bayesian approach to parallelism testing. *Stat. Biopharm. Res.*, 4(4), 357–374.

Data were generated using a 4PL model, which is parameterized differently from that of Model 3.2 to reflect the 10-fold dilution used by the assay:

$$y_{ij} = a_i + \frac{d_i - a_i}{1 + 10^{b_i(x_j - c_i)}} + \varepsilon_{ij}.$$

The errors in the model are normally distributed with a common variance of σ^2. To assess the effect of assay variability, simulations were done for σ values of 0.02, 0.04, 0.11, and 0.21, which correspond to %CV values of 5%, 10%, 25%, and 50%, respectively, on the log-concentration scale. For the F and χ^2 significance tests, the hypotheses are H_0: $b_1 = b_2$ and $d_1 = d_2$ versus H_1: $b_1 \neq b_2$ or $d_1 \neq d_2$. For the parallel-equivalence test, the range is set to be $x_L = 3.5$ and $x_U = 5$, and the equivalence limit $\delta = 0.2$, which is equal to the maximum difference in the borderline equivalence of Case 5. Because of the equal lower asymptote assumption, the hypotheses in the IUT are

$$H_0: \frac{b_1}{b_2} \leq D_L \text{ or } \frac{b_1}{b_2} \geq D_U \text{ or } \frac{d_1}{d_2} \leq D_L \text{ or } \frac{d_1}{d_2} \geq D_U \text{ versus}$$

$$H_1: D_L < \frac{b_1}{b_2} < D_U \text{ and } D_L < \frac{d_1}{d_2} < D_U. \tag{3.18}$$

We chose the equivalence limits based on the Hill slope values of Case 5, in which the two dose–response curves have a maximum difference of 0.2, representing a practical difference. The limits (D_L, D_U) were calculated to be

$$D_U = \frac{1}{D_L} = \frac{b_1}{b_2} = 0.917.$$

For each simulation run, the two dose–response curves were fit simultaneously. Estimates of the parameters were used to construct the F, χ^2, and IUT tests. Their corresponding hypotheses were tested at the significance level of 0.10. The cut point 0.10 was selected to be consistent with the cut point 0.9 for the Bayesian test (hereafter referred to as the parallel-equivalence test). For the parallel-equivalence test, a vague prior was given to the parameters $(a, b_1, c_1, d_1, b_2, c_2, d_2)$, assuming a normal distribution with mean being the least square estimate and a variance of 100. In addition, a Uniform prior distribution $U(0, 100)$ was placed on the standard deviation σ. The posterior probability $p(\delta, x_L, x_U)$ was estimated based on data from 20,000 random draws from the posterior distribution after a burn-in period of 5000 runs for the model parameters. The null hypothesis (Equation 3.18) is rejected (equivalence is declared) if $p(\delta, x_L, x_U) > 0.90$. For all four tests, the simulation was repeated for 5000 times. The proportion of times for which parallelism was declared was calculated for each test. The results are summarized in Table 3.2.

TABLE 3.2

Summary of Simulation Results of Different Parallelism Tests Using Six Different Cases Based on 4PL Models

			Proportion of Times Parallelism Declared			
Case	Maximum Difference	Percentage of CV	Parallel Equivalence	t Equivalence	F Test	χ^2 Test
1	0	5	1.00	1.00	0.90	0.99
		10	1.00	0.57	0.90	0.99
		25	0.99	0.00	0.90	0.99
		50	0.44	0.00	0.89	0.99
2	0	5	1.00	0.99	0.91	0.99
		10	1.00	0.52	0.90	0.99
		25	0.99	0.00	0.90	0.99
		50	0.37	0.00	0.91	0.99
3	0.15	5	1.00	1.00	0.00	0.00
		10	0.96	0.58	0.00	0.00
		25	0.43	0.00	0.00	0.01
		50	0.10	0.00	0.26	0.58
4	0.15	5	1.00	0.00	0.00	0.00
		10	0.86	0.00	0.00	0.00
		25	0.35	0.00	0.17	0.47
		50	0.08	0.00	0.63	0.89
5	0.20	5	0.09	0.10	0.00	0.00
		10	0.10	0.04	0.00	0.00
		25	0.09	0.00	0.00	0.00
		50	0.02	0.00	0.05	0.21
6	0.30	5	0.00	0.00	0.00	0.00
		10	0.00	0.00	0.00	0.00
		25	0.00	0.00	0.00	0.00
		50	0.00	0.00	0.04	0.17

Source: Novick, S., Yang, H., and J. Peterson (2012). A Bayesian approach to parallelism test-ing. *Stat. Biopharm. Res.*, 4(4), 357–374.

For the exactly parallel Cases 1 and 2, the F test claims parallelism at a rate close to the nominal level of 90%. However, it unduly falsely rejects paral-lelism in the parallel equivalence Cases 3 and 4, particularly when the assay precision has low %CV values ($\leq 10\%$). By comparison, the χ^2 significance test demonstrates higher power than the F test to declare parallelism for the exactly parallel Cases 1 and 2, and similar performance for Cases 3–6. For Cases 1–3, when the %CV is 5%, the two equivalence tests (t test and parallel equivalence) have similar performance; further, while the ability to claim parallelism decreases for both tests as the %CV increases, the effect is more pronounced for the IUT t test. In addition, the IUT t test appears to have less power than the parallel-equivalence method for Case 4. For the borderline equivalence Case 5 and inequivalent Case 6, the equivalence and parallel-equivalence tests have similar performance.

In light of the above results, it appears that the Bayesian test overcomes some of the drawbacks of the frequentist approaches. Since the added computational intensity of the Bayesian test can be effectively addressed through an efficient optimization algorithm, the method presents a viable alternative to the current parallelism testing procedures.

3.4 Method Comparison

As previously discussed, P value–based significance tests for parallelism are flawed because they use lack of statistical significance as an indicator of parallelism. Because of this, they do not protect consumer risk (falsely declaring parallelism). By contrast, equivalence tests are both conceptually appealing and theoretically sound. They are oriented toward the protection of consumer risk by shifting the burden of demonstrating parallelism to the experimenter (producer). However, despite the important conceptual difference between the two types of statistical tests, there are few published works investigating the performance of the methods. Jonkman and Sidik (2009) conducted a simulation study of 4PL curves to compare the empirical properties of the IUT test that they proposed to the traditional F test. In their simulation, the equivalence limits for the ratios of parameters were chosen to be (0.80, 1.25). The study was carried out for five cases: (1) approximately parallel: all three ratios of parameters (lower and upper asymptotes and slope) of the test sample and reference standard dose–response curves are within the limits (0.8, 1.25); (2) exactly parallel: the dose–response curves are exactly the same except for the potency parameter; (3) borderline case where the three parameter ratios are equal to the equivalence limits; (4) unequal lower asymptotes but equal slopes; and (5) unequal upper asymptotes but equal slopes. For each case, the simulation was performed for all combinations of dose levels (8, 10, 12), replicate numbers (3, 4), and levels of assay precision (0.15, 0.2, 0.3). For each combination of model parameter values, numbers of dose levels and replicates, and assay precision, 10,000 sets of paired dose–response curves were generated using Model 3.2. For each data set, the IUT and F test described in Section 3.3 were performed. The probability of declaring parallelism was estimated to be the proportion of times out of 10,000 simulations that parallelism is claimed. The simulation results indicated that the IUT t test provides better performance (i.e., correct test conclusion) for cases either where the assay is precise and the dose–response curves are approximately parallel or where the assay is imprecise and the dose–response curves are not parallel. The results further show that the F test is superior for cases where the dose–response curves are exactly parallel, except for cases where the assay is highly precise and number of dose levels is large.

In general, the performance of any parallelism test is characterized by both the consumer risk (false claim of parallelism) and producer risk (false claim of nonparallelism) of the test. Since these two quantities are dependent on the α level, comparisons between the significance and equivalence tests at a single α level do not make sense. As a result, the simulation study by Jonkman and Sidik (2009) conducted at a single α level of 5% may not be complete. In addition, only one set of equivalence limits (0.8, 1.25) was used in their simulation study. Since both the consumer and producer risks are dependent on the selection of equivalence limits (narrower equivalence range makes it harder to declare parallelism and vice versa), it is unlikely that their results are completely indicative of the overall performance of the two methods. In the following, we describe a method by Yang and Zhang (2012a) that evaluates significance and equivalence tests for parallelism based on ROC curve analysis.

3.4.1 Measures of Performance

3.4.1.1 Consumer and Producer Risks

Yang and Zhang (2012a) introduced two metrics, consumer risk (CR) and producer risk (PR), to measure the performance of a parallelism test. CR and PR are defined as the expected probabilities of false claim of parallelism and false claim of nonparallelism. Mathematically,

$$CR = E_\theta \left(\Pr\left[\text{two curves tested parallel} \middle| \theta \in \Theta_{NP} \right] \right)$$
$$= \int_{\theta \in \Theta_{NP}} \left(\Pr\left[\text{two curves tested parallel} \middle| \theta \right] \right) d\, F^{NP}(\theta)$$

and

$$PR = E_\theta \left(\Pr\left[\text{two curves tested non-parallel} \middle| \theta \in \Theta_{NP} \right] \right)$$
$$= \int_{\theta \in \Theta_P} \left(\Pr\left[\text{two curves tested non-parallel} \middle| \theta \right] \right) d\, F^P(\theta),$$

where Θ_P and Θ_{NP} are parameter spaces of $\theta = (\theta_T, \theta_R)$ corresponding to parallel curves and nonparallel curves, respectively, and $F^P(\theta)$ and $F^{NP}(\theta)$ are the probability functions of (θ_T, θ_R) in the parameter spaces Θ_P and Θ_{NP}. For example, for the linear model in Equation 3.1, these two parameter spaces can be defined as

$$\Theta_P = \{\theta = (\alpha_1, \beta_1, \alpha_2, \beta_2): |\beta_1 - \beta_2| < \delta\} \quad \text{and} \quad \Theta_{NP} = \{\theta: |\beta_1 - \beta_2| \geq \delta\},$$

where δ is a difference in slope between the test sample and reference standard that is of practical significance.

Now, consider the case in which the linear model in Equation 3.1 is used to characterize the dose–response curves. The tests in Equations 3.7 and 3.11 are used to test their corresponding parallelism hypotheses in Equations 3.6 and 3.10. For the significance test in Equation 3.7, the CR and PR can be obtained as

$$CR^{SIG}(\alpha) = E_\theta \left(\Pr \left[|T| < t_{1-\alpha/2,2n-4} \big| \theta \in \Theta_{NP} \right] \right)$$
$$PR^{SIG}(\alpha) = E_\theta \left(\Pr \left[|T| \geq t_{1-\alpha/2,2n-4} \big| \theta \in \Theta_P \right] \right). \tag{3.19}$$

Similarly, CR and PR of the equivalence test can be estimated

$$CR^{EQ}(\alpha) = E_\theta \left(\Pr \left[\hat{\beta}_1 - \hat{\beta}_2 \pm t_{1-\alpha,2n-4} \hat{\sigma} \sqrt{2/S_x} \in (-\Delta, \Delta) \big| \theta \in \Theta_{NP} \right] \right)$$
$$= E_\theta \left(\Pr \left[T_1 < \Delta \big| \theta \in \Theta_{NP} \right] \right)$$
$$PR^{EQ}(\alpha) = E_\theta \left(\Pr \left[\hat{\beta}_1 - \hat{\beta}_2 \pm t_{1-\alpha,2n-4} \hat{\sigma} \sqrt{2/S_x} \notin (-\Delta, \Delta) \big| \theta \in \Theta_P \right] \right)$$
$$= E_\theta \left(\Pr \left[T_1 \geq \Delta \big| \theta \in \Theta_P \right] \right) \tag{3.20}$$

where

$$T_1 = \max \left(\left| \hat{\beta}_1 - \hat{\beta}_2 - t_{1-\alpha,2n-4} \hat{\sigma} \sqrt{2/S_x} \right|, \left| \hat{\beta}_1 - \hat{\beta}_2 + t_{1-\alpha,2n-4} \hat{\sigma} \sqrt{2/S_x} \right| \right).$$

Yang and Zhang (2012a) developed a theoretical result that shows that the equivalence test does not always outperform the significance test in terms of protecting the CR and PR, and vice versa. The result is stated in the following theorem:

Theorem 3.1: Relationship between Significance and Equivalence Tests

Under Model 3.1, there exists α_0, $0 < \alpha_0 < 1$, such that $CR^{SIG}(\alpha) > CR^{EQ}(\alpha)$ for $\alpha < \alpha_0$, $CR^{SIG}(\alpha) = CR^{EQ}(\alpha)$ for $\alpha = \alpha_0$, and $CR^{SIG}(\alpha) < CR^{EQ}(\alpha)$ for $\alpha > \alpha_0$. Similarly, there exists α_1, $0 < \alpha_1 < 1$, such that $PR^{SIG}(\alpha) < PR^{EQ}(\alpha)$ for $\alpha < \alpha_1$, $PR^{SIG}(\alpha) = PR^{EQ}(\alpha)$ for $\alpha = \alpha_1$, and $PR^{SIG}(\alpha) > PR^{EQ}(\alpha)$ for $\alpha > \alpha_1$. ∎

Proof of the theorem is fairly straightforward. We first introduce $F(\alpha) = CR^{SIG}(\alpha) - CR^{EQ}(\alpha)$ and $G(\alpha) = PR^{SIG}(\alpha) - PR^{EQ}(\alpha)$. The two functions are continuous and monotonically decreasing and increasing, respectively, satisfying

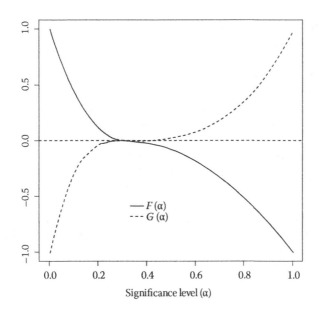

FIGURE 3.3

Plot of difference in consumer and producer risks with respect to significance level α. (From Yang, H. and Zhang, L. (2012a). Evaluations of parallelism testing methods using ROC analysis. *Stat. Biopharm. Res.*, 2(12), 67–74.)

$F(0) = 1$, $F(1) = -1$, $G(0) = -1$, and $G(1) = 1$. By the Intermediate Value Theorem, there exists α_0, $0 < \alpha_0 < 1$, such that $F(\alpha_0) = 0$. Based on the strict monotonicity of $F(\alpha)$, we can conclude that $F(\alpha) > F(\alpha_0) = 0$, for $\alpha < \alpha_0$. Consequently, $CR^{SIG}(\alpha) > CR^{EQ}(\alpha)$. Likewise, the second half of the theorem can be verified.

As an illustration, functions $F(\alpha)$ and $G(\alpha)$ are plotted in Figure 3.3 assuming $\alpha_0 = \alpha_1$. As seen from the plot when $\alpha \leq \alpha_0$, the significance test has a higher CR and a lower PR than the equivalence test. When $\alpha > \alpha_0$, the significance test has a lower CR and a higher PR than the equivalence test.

3.4.1.2 ROC Curve Analysis

The result in Section 3.4.1.1 implies that the performance of significance and equivalence tests is dependent on the selection of α level. Therefore, an objective comparison between the two methods cannot be achieved with α being set at a fixed level. A measure of parallelism free of a particular selection of α level is needed. Because the performance of the equivalence test is also influenced by the selection of the equivalence limits, a comparison between the significance and equivalence tests should also take into account this important fact.

Yang and Zhang (2012a) proposed using ROC curve analysis to compare the performance of the significance and equivalence tests. The ROC curve is a commonly used tool for evaluating diagnostic test accuracy. It plots the sensitivity (true-positive rate) of a diagnostic test against or 1 − specificity (where specificity is the false-positive rate), over a range of response thresholds, such as significance level or equivalence limits. An example ROC plot is shown in Figure 3.4.

In general, the ROC of a test with high discriminatory power tends to bend up toward the upper left-hand corner. A test with an ROC curve corresponding to the 45° diagonal line has zero discriminatory power, as it designates a test sample as either positive or negative with 50% probability. ROC analysis has a wide range of applications in medical research including evaluation of diagnostic tests (Metz 1978), biomarker discovery (Pepe et al. 2010), and comparisons of diagnostic tests (Hanley 1989). The AUC is often used to measure the overall discriminatory power of a diagnostic test. It also has an intuitive interpretation as the probability that the test outcomes of diseased and healthy subjects are in correct order, that is, $P[X_D > X_N]$ (under the assumption that the higher test values represent the more diseased state), where X_D (X_N) represents the test result for the individual randomly selected from the diseased (healthy) population (Swets and Pickett 1982). The fact that the AUC is independent of the decision criterion makes it straightforward to compare different tests with the same intended purpose but different metrics. In a broad sense, a parallelism test method can be viewed as a diagnostic test that has a binary outcome where two dose–response curves are either similar or not similar. The claims of similarity and nonsimilarity are dependent

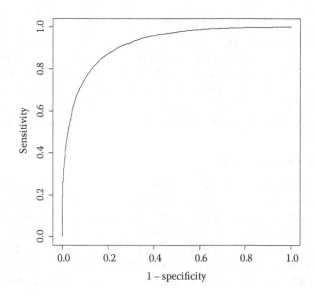

FIGURE 3.4
Plot of ROC curve. (From Yang, H. and Zhang, L. (2012a). Evaluations of parallelism testing methods using ROC analysis. *Stat. Biopharm. Res.*, 2(12), 67–74.)

on the outcomes of the test statistics when compared to the cutoff value. For example, for the significance test described in Section 3.3.2 for comparing two straight lines, the test statistic in Equation 3.7 is compared to the cutoff value $t_{1-\alpha/2,2n-4}$. The parallelism claim is rejected if $|T| \geq t_{1-\alpha/2,2n-4}$; otherwise, it is accepted. It is evident that the performance of the test is dependent on the choice of the significance level α. Therefore, it is sensible to use the AUC obtained over the range of α in $(0,1)$ as an overall measure of performance.

3.4.1.3 Sensitivity versus Specificity

Analogous to the characterization of a diagnostic test, the sensitivity (Se) of a parallelism test can be defined as the expected probability that the test will conclude nonparallelism when the two curves are indeed nonparallel. Similarly, the specificity (Sp) of a parallelism test is defined as the expected probability that the test will claim parallelism when the two curves are parallel. By definition, we have

$$Se = 1 - CR$$
$$Sp = 1 - PR.$$

3.4.1.4 Estimation of Sensitivity, Specificity, and AUC

Estimation of sensitivity and specificity requires one to carry out the integration in Equations 3.19 and 3.20 over the parameter spaces Θ_P and Θ_{NP}. Thanks to the advance in modern statistical computations, the integrals can be estimated through simulation (Robert and Casella 2004). Yang and Zhang (2012a) suggested the following procedure to carry out the estimation. Define

$$Se^{SIG}(\theta; \alpha) = \Pr[|T| \geq t_{1-\alpha/2,2n-4} | \theta \in \Theta_{NP}|]$$

By Equation 3.14,

$$Se^{SIG}(\alpha) = E_\theta[Se^{SIG}(\theta; \alpha)]. \tag{3.21}$$

In other words, the sensitivity $Se^{SIG}(\alpha)$ is viewed as an expectation of the function with θ being a random variable, which is distributed according to $F^{NP}(\theta)$. For random samples θ_i, $i = 1, \ldots m$, which are independently identically distributed according to $F^{NP}(\theta)$, by the Law of Large Numbers, we have

$$\overline{Se}_m^{SIG}(\alpha) = \frac{1}{m} \sum_{i=1}^{m} Se^{SIG}(\theta_i; \alpha) \rightarrow E_\theta[Se^{SIG}(\theta; \alpha)]. \tag{3.22}$$

Therefore, $\overline{Se}_m^{SIG}(\alpha)$ is a consistent estimate of $Se^{SIG}(\alpha)$. Similarly, $Sp^{SIG}(\alpha)$, $Se^{EQ}(\alpha)$, and $Sp^{EQ}(\alpha)$ can be estimated by their corresponding empirical averages:

$$\overline{Sp}_m^{SIG}(\alpha) = \frac{1}{m}\sum_{i=1}^{m} Sp^{SIG}(\theta_i;\alpha) = \frac{1}{m}\sum_{i=1}^{m} Pr\left[|T| < t_{1-\alpha/2,2n-4}\,\middle|\,\theta_i \in \Theta_P\right]$$

$$\overline{Se}_m^{EQ}(\alpha) = \frac{1}{m}\sum_{i=1}^{m} Se^{EQ}(\theta_i;\alpha) = \frac{1}{m}\sum_{i=1}^{m} Pr\left[T_1 \geq \Delta\,\middle|\,\theta_i \in \Theta_{NP}\right] \qquad (3.23)$$

$$\overline{Sp}_m^{EQ}(\alpha) = \frac{1}{m}\sum_{i=1}^{m} Sp^{EQ}(\theta_i;\alpha) = \frac{1}{m}\sum_{i=1}^{m} Pr\left[T_1 < \Delta\,\middle|\,\theta_i \in \Theta_P\right].$$

The ROC curves are created by plotting the paired estimates $\left(\overline{Se}^{SIG}(\alpha),\ 1-\overline{Sp}^{SIG}(\alpha)\right)$ and $\left(\overline{Se}^{EQ}(\alpha),\ 1-\overline{Sp}^{EQ}(\alpha)\right)$ over a fine grid of α values between 0 and 1. Consequently, the AUCs of the significance and equivalence tests are estimated, using the standard trapezoidal method.

3.4.1.5 Simulation

Yang and Zhang (2012a) carried out a simulation study to compare the overall performance of significance and equivalence parallelism tests. Parallel curves and nonparallel curves were simulated using the linear model (Equation 3.1) with $\Theta_P = \{(1, \beta_2):|\beta_2 - 1| < 0.2\}$ and $\Theta_{NP} = \{(1, \beta_2):|\beta_2 - 1| \geq 0.2\}$, respectively. A distribution of θ in each of the spaces of Θ_P and Θ_{NP} was chosen such that $F^P(\theta) = F^P(\beta_2)$ is the probability function of the truncated normal distribution with mean $= 1$, standard deviation $= 0.1$ when $\theta \in \Theta_P$, and $F^{NP}(\theta) = F^{NP}(\beta_2)$ is the probability function of a uniform distribution that assumes a value of 1.25 over the range of $[0.4, 0.8] \cup [1.2, 1.6]$ and a uniform distribution that assumes a value of 0 over the range of $(-\infty, 0.4) \cup (1.6, +\infty)$ when $\theta \in \Theta_{NP}$. To explore the effect of equivalence bound Δ, number of doses J, number of replicates K, and assay variability, the simulation was conducted for $\Delta = 0.01, 0.05, 0.1, 0.2, 0.4, 0.6,$ and 0.8, $J = 4, 5,$ and 6, and $K = 1$ and 2 per dose level, and assay variability $\sigma = 0.1, 0.3, 0.5$. The slope β_1 and equivalence bound Δ were set at 1 and 0.2, respectively.

3.4.1.6 Simulation Results

The results of the simulations are shown in Table 3.3. For each combination of dose level, number of replicates, equivalence limit, and assay variability, the entry in the table is the AUC estimate with associated standard

TABLE 3.3

Summary of AUC Estimates for Various Assay Formats and Variability Based on Equivalence and Significance Parallelism Tests

Assay Format		Equivalence Limit	Assay Variability = 0.1				Assay Variability = 0.3				Assay Variability = 0.5			
			Equivalence Test		Significance Test		Equivalence Test		Significance Test		Equivalence Test		Significance Test	
Dose	Rep.	Δ	AUC	SD	AUC	SD	AUC	SD	AUC	SD	AUC	SD	AUC	SD
4	1	0.01	0.959	0.004	0.949	0.013	0.798	0.009	0.788	0.015	0.667	0.011	0.663	0.011
		0.05	0.969	0.003	0.948	0.013	0.805	0.010	0.788	0.024	0.671	0.011	0.662	0.015
		0.1	0.978	0.003	0.948	0.014	0.813	0.009	0.789	0.013	0.673	0.012	0.660	0.019
		0.2	0.984	0.002	0.943	0.040	0.822	0.009	0.790	0.011	0.678	0.013	0.661	0.013
		0.4	0.955	0.005	0.951	0.009	0.817	0.010	0.791	0.013	0.682	0.010	0.663	0.012
		0.6	0.895	0.007	0.950	0.015	0.784	0.011	0.788	0.021	0.675	0.011	0.662	0.012
		0.8	0.826	0.009	0.949	0.017	0.745	0.012	0.784	0.023	0.660	0.013	0.662	0.013
	2	0.01	0.930	0.007	0.987	0.002	0.900	0.007	0.898	0.007	0.777	0.009	0.775	0.009
		0.05	0.960	0.004	0.987	0.001	0.903	0.007	0.898	0.007	0.775	0.010	0.771	0.010
		0.1	0.978	0.003	0.987	0.002	0.906	0.007	0.898	0.007	0.778	0.011	0.772	0.010
		0.2	0.992	0.002	0.987	0.002	0.908	0.005	0.898	0.005	0.781	0.010	0.772	0.010
		0.4	0.978	0.003	0.987	0.002	0.901	0.008	0.898	0.007	0.779	0.012	0.771	0.012
		0.6	0.900	0.007	0.986	0.002	0.882	0.006	0.898	0.006	0.772	0.009	0.773	0.009
		0.8	0.639	0.015	0.978	0.003	0.849	0.010	0.897	0.006	0.757	0.011	0.772	0.010
5	1	0.01	0.980	0.003	0.978	0.003	0.887	0.007	0.883	0.008	0.764	0.011	0.762	0.011
		0.05	0.986	0.002	0.978	0.003	0.894	0.006	0.884	0.007	0.768	0.011	0.761	0.011
		0.1	0.991	0.001	0.977	0.004	0.900	0.007	0.883	0.008	0.773	0.011	0.761	0.011
		0.2	0.994	0.001	0.978	0.003	0.907	0.006	0.885	0.007	0.778	0.010	0.760	0.011
		0.4	0.974	0.004	0.977	0.003	0.893	0.008	0.883	0.007	0.777	0.010	0.762	0.011
		0.6	0.892	0.006	0.978	0.003	0.859	0.009	0.885	0.007	0.762	0.011	0.762	0.011

(Continued)

TABLE 3.3 (CONTINUED)

Summary of AUC Estimates for Various Assay Formats and Variability Based on Equivalence and Significance Parallelism Tests

| Assay Format | | Equivalence Limit | Assay Variability = 0.1 | | | | Assay Variability = 0.3 | | | | Assay Variability = 0.5 | | | |
| | | | Equivalence Test | | Significance Test | | Equivalence Test | | Significance Test | | Equivalence Test | | Significance Test | |
Dose	Rep.	Δ	AUC	SD	AUC	SD	AUC	SD	AUC	SD	AUC	SD	AUC	SD
2	2	0.8	0.712	0.007	0.978	0.003	0.816	0.009	0.885	0.007	0.735	0.011	0.760	0.010
		0.01	0.434	0.015	0.993	0.001	0.951	0.005	0.951	0.005	0.867	0.007	0.866	0.007
		0.05	0.550	0.016	0.993	0.001	0.955	0.004	0.951	0.005	0.870	0.008	0.866	0.008
		0.1	0.674	0.013	0.993	0.001	0.957	0.004	0.952	0.004	0.873	0.008	0.867	0.008
		0.2	0.887	0.009	0.993	0.001	0.958	0.004	0.951	0.005	0.874	0.008	0.866	0.007
		0.4	0.978	0.003	0.993	0.001	0.951	0.005	0.952	0.004	0.871	0.008	0.867	0.008
		0.6	0.670	0.017	0.992	0.001	0.926	0.007	0.951	0.004	0.858	0.008	0.867	0.008
		0.8	0.180	0.012	0.993	0.001	0.833	0.007	0.951	0.004	0.837	0.009	0.866	0.009
6	1	0.01	0.964	0.005	0.986	0.002	0.937	0.006	0.934	0.006	0.843	0.007	0.840	0.007
		0.05	0.981	0.003	0.987	0.002	0.942	0.005	0.934	0.005	0.846	0.009	0.839	0.009
		0.1	0.991	0.002	0.987	0.002	0.947	0.005	0.935	0.005	0.853	0.009	0.841	0.009
		0.2	0.996	0.001	0.987	0.002	0.949	0.005	0.934	0.006	0.856	0.009	0.841	0.008
		0.4	0.972	0.004	0.986	0.002	0.937	0.006	0.935	0.005	0.850	0.008	0.840	0.009
		0.6	0.857	0.007	0.987	0.002	0.904	0.007	0.935	0.005	0.829	0.009	0.841	0.009
		0.8	0.725	0.013	0.987	0.002	0.853	0.008	0.935	0.005	0.798	0.011	0.841	0.009
	2	0.01	0.122	0.010	0.995	0.001	0.949	0.006	0.974	0.003	0.923	0.006	0.922	0.006
		0.05	0.219	0.013	0.995	0.001	0.963	0.005	0.975	0.003	0.926	0.006	0.923	0.006
		0.1	0.354	0.017	0.995	0.001	0.973	0.004	0.975	0.003	0.928	0.007	0.923	0.007
		0.2	0.607	0.014	0.995	0.001	0.979	0.003	0.974	0.003	0.930	0.005	0.923	0.005
		0.4	0.925	0.009	0.995	0.001	0.973	0.003	0.974	0.003	0.924	0.006	0.923	0.006
		0.6	0.457	0.016	0.995	0.001	0.920	0.005	0.974	0.003	0.910	0.007	0.922	0.006
		0.8	0.019	0.004	0.995	0.001	0.790	0.012	0.974	0.003	0.856	0.007	0.923	0.006

Source: Yang, H. and Zhang, L. (2012a). Evaluations of parallelism testing methods using ROC analysis. *Stat. Biopharm. Res.*, 2(12), 67–74.

deviation. Several observations can be made. First, in general, the AUC value decreases as the assay standard deviation (σ) increases. In other words, the discriminatory ability of both the significance and equivalence test is affected by the assay precision. Second, among the total of 18 combinations of dose levels and replicates per dose level, the AUC of the equivalence test is dependent on the equivalence limit Δ and achieves its maximum at $\Delta = 0.2$, for most of the times except for the cases $(J, K, \sigma) = (4, 1, 0.5)$, $(5, 2, 0.1)$, and $(6, 2, 0.1)$, where the maxim is attained at $\Delta = 0.4$. This is hardly surprising as 0.2 is the difference of practical significance used in the simulation to generate parallel and nonparallel curves. Last, for all 18 combinations of (J, K, σ) except for two cases $[(J, K, \sigma) = (5, 2, 0.1)$ and $(6, 2, 0.1)]$, the equivalence test has a higher AUC at $\Delta = 0.2$ than the significance test. However, this is not true for other choices of Δ. For instance, when $\Delta = 0.8$, the AUC of the equivalence test is smaller than that of the significance test in each of the 18 cases. These results suggest that the equivalence test does not uniformly outperform the significance test.

The results (replicate = 1, assay variability = 0.3 and 0.5) in Table 3.3 are plotted in Figures 3.5 and 3.6. A close examination of the plots verifies the aforesaid observations.

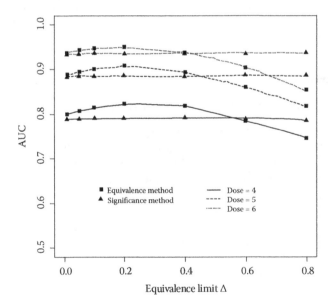

FIGURE 3.5
Estimated AUCs for significance and equivalence tests versus equivalence limit for three assay formats. The assay has one replicate at each dose and SD = 0.3. (From Yang, H. and Zhang, L. (2012a). Evaluations of parallelism testing methods using ROC analysis. *Stat. Biopharm. Res.*, 2(12), 67–74.)

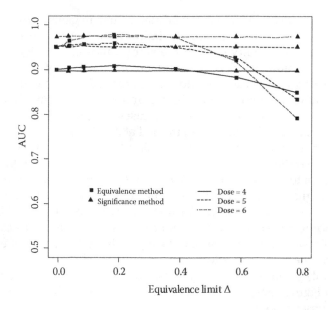

FIGURE 3.6
Estimated AUCs for significance and equivalence tests versus equivalence limit for three assay formats. The assay has two replicates at each dose and SD = 0.3. (From Yang, H. and Zhang, L. (2012a). Evaluations of parallelism testing methods using ROC analysis. *Stat. Biopharm. Res.*, 2(12), 67–74.)

3.5 Determination of Equivalence Limits

As discussed above, selection of the equivalence limits has a significant impact on the performance of the equivalence parallelism test. Ideally, the equivalence limits should be based on the impact of nonparallelism on the quality of product, in terms of product safety and efficacy (Hauck et al. 2005). However, it is not a trivial task to establish a causal relationship between nonparallelism of dose–response curves in a bioassay and product quality. This is, in part, as noted by Hauck et al. (2005), due to the fact that not all important product quality issues may be reflected in a parallelism measure, nor are all deviations from parallelism necessarily indicative of an important quality issue. Nevertheless, several statistical methods for setting the equivalence limits have been described in the literature and are discussed below.

3.5.1 Capability-Based Methods

In the absence of a known causal relationship between nonparallelism and product quality, provisional equivalence limits may be established using capability-based approaches (Hauck et al. 2005). This approach establishes the equivalence limits based on repeated testing of a reference standard against itself. It is foreseeable that such equivalence limits help control false nonsimilarity claims. However, it does not provide any assurance regarding how well the rate of false similarity claims is managed (Liao et al. 2011; Yang and Zhang 2012a). In other words, the capability-based limits protect PR as opposed to CR.

Hauck et al. (2005) proposed two nonparametric methods for setting parallelism test equivalence limits. Of note is the tolerance interval approach based on ranked data. Consider $X_1 \dots X_n$ to be a random sample of ratios of model parameter estimates based on repeated testing of reference standard against itself, and $X^{(1)} \dots X^{(n)}$ their ranked values. Define

$$q = \frac{4n - 2(r + m - 1) - \chi_{2(r+m)}(1 - \alpha)}{4n - 2(r + m - 1) + \chi_{2(r+m)}(1 - \alpha)},$$

where r and m are two integers less than n and $\chi_{2(r+m)}(1 - \alpha)$ is the $(1 - \alpha)$th percentile of a χ^2 distribution with $2(r + m)$ degrees of freedom. It is known that with probability at least $(1 - \alpha)$, the tolerance limits $X^{(r)}$ and $X^{(n+1-m)}$ cover $100q\%$ of the population (Conover 1999). One may use $X^{(r)}$ and $X^{(n+1-m)}$ as the parallelism equivalence limits. The advantage of the method is that it does not require a normality assumption for the ratio estimates. The second method discussed by Hauck et al. (2005) is based on a one-sided tolerance interval bound on the extreme value from the CIs of the ratio.

3.5.2 ROC Curve Method

To determine equivalence limits that protect both CR and PR, Yang and Zhang (2012a) suggested a method based on ROC curve analysis. Suppose that paired parallel and nonparallel samples are available. By varying the equivalence bound Δ, sensitivity and specificity in Equation 3.20 as functions of the equivalence limit can be estimated. Figure 3.7 displays a pair of such curves. In general, sensitivity, which is the average probability of correctly claiming nonparallelism, is an increasing function of the equivalence limit, whereas specificity, which is the average probability of correctly declaring parallelism, increases as Δ gets larger.

These two properties enable one to determine equivalence bound Δ_0 such that it renders the best trade-off between sensitivity and specificity. The following are two procedures suggested by Yang and Zhang (2012a):

1. Choose Δ_0 such that $\hat{Se}^{EQ}(\Delta_0) \geq \lambda_1$ and $\hat{Sp}^{EQ}(\Delta_0) \geq \lambda_2$, where λ_1 and λ_2 are two prespecified numbers, satisfying $0 < \lambda_1, \lambda_2 < 1$.

2. Choose Δ_0 such that

$$\max\left[1 - \hat{Se}^{EQ}(\Delta_0),\ 1 - \hat{Sp}^{EQ}(\Delta_0)\right] = \min_{\{\Delta \geq 0\}}\left\{\max\left[1 - \hat{Se}^{EQ}(\Delta),\ 1 - \hat{Sp}^{EQ}(\Delta)\right] \leq \lambda\right\}$$

where $0 < \lambda < 1$.

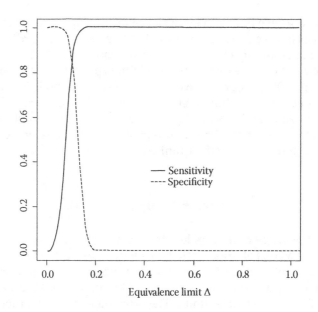

FIGURE 3.7

Plot of sensitivity and specificity of an equivalence parallelism test as functions of equivalence limit. (From Yang, H. and Zhang, L. (2012a). Evaluations of parallelism testing methods using ROC analysis. *Stat. Biopharm. Res.*, 2(12), 67–74.)

The first method chooses Δ_0 in the way that allows sensitivity and specificity to meet predetermined thresholds, thus achieving direct control over false claims on nonparallelism and parallelism. As an illustration, suppose that λ_1 and λ_2 are set at 0.80. From Figure 3.7, it can be seen that by choosing $\Delta_0 = 0.12$, both sensitivity and specificity are greater than 80%. This also implies that the rates of false claim of nonparallelism and parallelism are both kept under 20%. More assurance of the sensitivity and specificity can be obtained by selecting Δ_0, based on the lower confidence limits of the curves in Figure 3.7. The second procedure is intended to choose Δ_0, such that the larger of the CR and PR is minimized. For the above example, the solution is also $\Delta_0 = 0.12$. It can be shown that the two procedures give rise to the same solution of Δ_0 if $\lambda_1 = \lambda_2$. When λ_1 and λ_2 differ from each other, the solution of the second procedure is not unique.

Note that the above two procedures give equal consideration to CR and PR. However, under certain circumstances, being out of compliance by failing to reject nonparallelism may be of more concern than falsely rejecting assays for which parallelism holds. In those cases, a higher cost can be assigned to a false parallelism claim than to a false nonparallelism declaration. As pointed out by Yang and Zhang (2012a), this can be achieved through a decision theory framework. Specifically, Table 3.4 can be constructed to allow for different costs (weights) to be assigned to each decision.

TABLE 3.4

Decision Costs

| | True State | |
Parallelism Test	Parallel	Nonparallel
Parallel	L_1	L_3
Nonparallel	L_2	L_4

It can be shown that the overall expected cost is given by

$$C(\Delta) = p_0\{L_1 Se(\Delta) + L_2[1 - Se(\Delta)]\} + (1 - p_0)\{L_3[1 - Sp(\Delta)] + L_4 Sp(\Delta)\},$$

where p_0 is the probability of the assay passing parallelism. $C(\Delta)$ usually can be estimated using historical data. Thus, the optimum Δ_0 can be chosen such that it minimizes the above overall cost.

3.5.3 Limits Based on AUC

Another alternative is to determine the equivalence bound Δ, based on the AUC (Yang and Zhang 2012a). As previously discussed, the AUC of an equivalence test varies according to the selection of the equivalence bound Δ and Type I error α. When parallel and nonparallel samples are available, the ROC curve and AUC can be estimated over a range of Δ values. Plotting AUC against Δ creates a plot in Figure 3.8. Using the plot, one may determine a value Δ_0 such that AUC achieves its maximum at Δ_0.

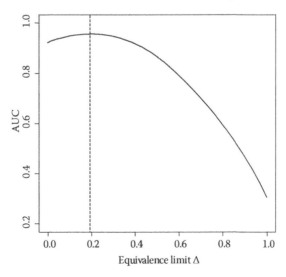

FIGURE 3.8
AUC is plotted against equivalence limit for an equivalence parallelism test. The maximum AUC is achieved at $\Delta = 0.19$. (From Yang, H. and Zhang, L. (2012a). Evaluations of parallelism testing methods using ROC analysis. *Stat. Biopharm. Res.*, 2(12), 67–74.)

3.6 Concluding Remarks

Since parallelism is a necessary condition for the relative potency of a bioassay to be meaningful, verification of parallelism before data interpretation is critical in ensuring the validity of the assay reportable value. In the literature, both significance tests and equivalence tests are described for parallelism testing. However, recent research results revealed that the significance test may reject parallelism even for marginal insignificant differences when the sample size is large or the assay is precise and that it may accept parallelism of nonparallel curves when the sample size is small or the assay is imprecise. Therefore, the method rewards nonparallel assays with small sample sizes and large variability and does not offer adequate protection to CR. These findings spurred interest in developing alternative parallelism tests. Equivalence tests in general address the issues encountered by the significance tests and are adopted in USP Chapters <1032> and <1034> to provide better control over CR. The current equivalence tests only indirectly tackle the parallelism problem, as the hypotheses of parallelism concern similarity of model parameters. A direct method was suggested by Novick et al. (2012) using the Bayesian framework. By incorporating the uncertainty in the model parameters in the posterior probability calculations, the approach provides a better level of assurance of parallelism claim than the other approaches. Its computational expenditure is offset by a fast optimization algorithm, which is readily available to practitioners of bioassay.

4

Validation of Method Linearity

4.1 Introduction

Quantitative analytical methods such as high-performance liquid chromatography use a calibration relationship between the measured response and analyte concentration to quantify the amount of analyte in a test sample. The relationship is normally established during method development through fitting a regression model to test results of reference standards of known amounts of analyte. Depending on the true nature of the calibration relationship, fewer or more reference standard concentrations may need to be tested in each run along with the test sample, in routine use. For example, if the relationship is linear, potentially two reference standards at different concentrations would suffice. However, if the true relationship is nonlinear, more reference standards are needed to capture the curvature of the dose–response curve. Therefore, a linear calibration relationship is operationally desirable. When the calibration relationship is nonlinear, approximating it with a linear model will cause bias in the measured analyte concentration, thus affecting the performance of the analytical method. Suffice it to say, it is important to evaluate assay linearity. In fact, validation of analytical method linearity is a regulatory requirement (CLSI 2003; ICH Q2(R1) 2005; USP <1225> 1989). ICH Q2(R1) clearly states, "A linear relationship should be evaluated across the range of the analytical procedure."

As noted by LeBlond et al. (2013), there are at least two different types of "linearity" concepts that are not well differentiated in scientific and regulatory publications. The first type concerns the calibration relationship between the instrument signal and true analyte concentration, which is used to estimate the analyte concentration in a test sample through reverse projection. In this case, linearity refers to whether the calibration relationship is linear. The second type of linearity refers to whether the relationship between the true and measured analyte concentrations is linear. This type of linearity is closely related to method accuracy. LeBlond et al. (2013) refer the former as "calibration linearity" and the latter as "relative accuracy." Although different statistical methods may be needed for testing these two types of linearity, the distinction is not always well defined in regulatory documents

(USP <1210>). For example, on one hand, the guidance states that "Linearity should be evaluated by visual inspection of a plot of signals as a function of analyte concentration or content," which appears that the guidance refers to the second type of linearity. On the other hand, ICH Q2(R1) (ICH 2005) defines linearity of an analytical procedure as "its ability (within a given range) to obtain test results which are directly proportional to the concentration (amount) of analyte in the sample." It implies the first type of linearity. By contrast, CLSI EP06-A clearly specifies that "(a) Linearity typically refers to overall system response (i.e., the final analytical answer rather than the raw instrument output. (b) The linearity of a system is measured by testing levels of an analyte which are known by formulation or known *relative to each other* (not necessarily known absolutely). (c) When the system results are plotted against these values, the degree to which the plotted curve conforms to a straight line is a measure of system linearity." Despite the difference in definitions, statistical methods applicable to one type may also be applied to the other.

This chapter is primarily focused on statistical methods for testing conformance of a response curve (whether system response or measured concentration) to a straight line. These methods are applicable to the evaluation of either calibration linearity or relative potency. In the literature, various methods of varying degrees of statistical rigor have been suggested for the evaluation of linearity. They range from graphical inspection and descriptive summaries to inferential analyses. It is our intent to provide a comprehensive review of the existing methods and suggest other statistical techniques, such as orthogonal regression for validation of linearity.

4.2 Study Design

As mentioned above, linearity needs to be evaluated across the range of the analytical procedure (ICH 2005). Both ICH Q2(R1) and CLSI guideline EP6-A (2003) state that a minimum of five concentrations is recommended for establishing linearity. In addition, CLSI guideline EP6-A (2003) also recommends that at least two samples per concentration be tested. Mathematically, let Y_{ij} represent the jth replicate measurement at concentration level i and x_i be the true value of the ith concentration, with $i = 1,..., l; j = 1,..., n$, where l is the number of concentration levels and n is the number of replicates for each concentration level. It is assumed that the numbers l and n are chosen in accordance with both product-use and regulatory requirements and that the experiment is carried out to ensure that the measurements Y_{ij} are independent of each other.

4.3 Calibration Model

In theory, the calibration relationship between the measured response and analyte concentration can take any monotonic functional form. Rarely is the calibration relationship perfectly linear. Intuitively by confining the concentration levels within a narrow range, the calibration relationship can be well approximated by a linear function. However, to make the calibration model useful, the range needs to be sufficiently wide to cover the practical range of the analyte in test samples. Such a range is usually chosen through experimentation during prevalidation method development. Validation of method linearity is intended to demonstrate that approximating the true calibration relationship with a linear model does not result in any unacceptable bias within the specified range. Mathematically, evaluation of linearity can be formulated as a hypothesis-testing problem with the hypotheses being defined as

H_0: The calibration model is linear: $g_1(x) = a + bx$ versus

H_1: The calibration model is a nonlinear function: $g(x)$. (4.1)

As most nonlinear functions can be well approximated by a high-order polynomial using a Taylor expansion, we assume that the calibration relationship is a polynomial function. Thus, the two models of interest are the linear and higher-order polynomial models given below:

$$Y_{ij} = \alpha_0 + \alpha_1 x_i + \varepsilon_{ij} = g_1(x_i) + \varepsilon_{ij} \tag{4.2}$$

and

$$Y_{ij} = \beta_0 + \beta_1 x_i + \ldots + \beta_k x_i^k + \varepsilon_{ij} = g_k(x_i) + \varepsilon_{ij}, \tag{4.3}$$

where ε_{ij}, $i = 1,\ldots, l; j = 1,\ldots, n$, are measurement errors, assumed to be independently and identically normally distributed with a mean of 0 and a variance of σ^2.

4.4 Current Statistical Methods

A variety of statistical methods have been proposed in literature for testing linearity, ranging from visual inspection (ICH Q2(R1) 2005) and descriptive summaries, such as Pearson's correlation coefficient (r) (Massart et al. 1997), to various inferential statistical tests (Brüggemann et al. 2006; Hsieh and Liu 2008; Hsieh et al. 2009; Kroll et al. 2000; Krouwer and Schlain 1993; Novick and Yang 2013; van Loco et al. 2002; Yang et al. 2015a).

4.4.1 Descriptive Summary

4.4.1.1 Visual Inspection

Often, the system response values are plotted against the analyte concentrations. If the values fluctuate around a straight line, it is indicative of linearity. Visual inspection can be an effective means for detecting obvious deviation from linearity. It is advisable to use this method to assess linearity before any more formal test with respect to some acceptance criterion is used.

4.4.1.2 Pearson's Correlation Coefficient

Pearson's correlation coefficient is defined as

$$r = \frac{\sum_{i,j}(x_i - \bar{x})(Y_{ij} - \bar{Y})}{\sqrt{\sum_{i,j}(x_i - \bar{x})^2 \sum_{i,j}(Y_{ij} - \bar{Y})^2}},$$

where $\bar{x} = \dfrac{\sum_{i=1}^{l} X_i}{l}$ and $\bar{Y} = \dfrac{\sum_{i=1}^{l}\sum_{j=1}^{n} Y_{ij}}{nl}$. The quantity r, having a value between -1 and 1, is commonly used as a metric for linearity, with $r = 1$ or -1 corresponding to a perfectly linear relationship between two variables. However, as noted by several researchers (Anscombe 1973; van Loco et al. 2002), data sets with very different patterns may have the same correlation coefficient. A correlation coefficient close to 1 may be obtained from data sets that demonstrate apparent nonlinear relationships. Therefore, it is challenging, if not impossible, to establish a meaningful cut point for the correlation coefficient above which linearity is claimed (LeBlond et al. 2013). In addition, because r is merely a point estimate, it does not provide statistical assurance that the relationship is either linear or nonlinear even if its value is close to 1 or 0.

4.4.2 Significance Tests

4.4.2.1 Lack-of-Fit Test

Another commonly used method is the lack-of-fit (LOF) test (Brüggemann et al. 2006; van Loco et al. 2002). To perform the test, the data are fit to Model

4.2. The total variation, estimated as the total sum of squares, is apportioned to the sum of squares due to deviation of the model predicted mean value to the mean value at each concentration and the sum of squares due to measurement variability.

$$\sum_{i=1}^{l}\sum_{j=1}^{n}(Y_{ij}-\hat{Y}_{ij})^2 = \sum_{i=1}^{l}n(\bar{Y}_i-\hat{Y}_i)^2 + \sum_{i=1}^{l}\sum_{j=1}^{n}(Y_{ij}-\bar{Y}_i)^2$$

The first term on the right-hand side of the above equation is also referred to as the sum of squares due to LOF. Under the null hypothesis in Equation 4.1, the test statistic

$$F = \frac{\sum_{i=1}^{l}n(\bar{Y}_i-\hat{Y}_i)^2/(l-2)}{\sum_{i=1}^{l}\sum_{j=1}^{n}(Y_{ij}-\bar{Y}_i)^2/l(n-1)}$$

follows the F distribution with degrees of freedom of $l-2$ and $l(n-1)$. The null hypothesis in Equation 4.1 is rejected if $F > F_{\alpha,l-1,l(n-1)}$, where $F_{\alpha,l-1,l(n-1)}$ is the $100 \times (1-\alpha)$th percentile of the above F distribution.

4.4.2.2 Mendel's Method

Mendel's test is used to examine whether or not there is a statistically significant difference between linear and quadratic fits. The test statistic, constructed as

$$F_M = \frac{\sum_{i=1}^{l}\sum_{j=1}^{n}\left(Y_{ij}-\hat{Y}_{ij}^L\right)^2 - \sum_{i=1}^{l}\sum_{j=1}^{n}\left(Y_{ij}-\hat{Y}_{ij}^Q\right)^2}{\sum_{i=1}^{l}\sum_{j=1}^{n}(Y_{ij}-\bar{Y}_i)^2/l(nl-3)}$$

has an F distribution with degrees of freedom of 1 and $nl-3$, where $\hat{Y}_{ij}^L$ and $\hat{Y}_{ij}^Q$ are the fitted values of the linear and quadratic models, respectively. The null hypothesis in Equation 4.1 is rejected at a significance level of α if $F_M > F_{\alpha,l-1,l(n-1)}$.

4.4.2.3 Kroll's Method

More recently, a method for linearity testing was described in EP6-A (CLSI 2003). The method is centered on evaluation of the magnitude of nonlinearity, which is defined as the maximum difference in predicted means between the linear and best-fit polynomial models at the concentration levels of a linearity experiment. Linearity is claimed if either the best-fit model, measured by a P value greater than 0.05 from a LOF test, is linear, or if the best-fit model is not linear but the difference in predicted means between the linear and best-fit models is within prespecified limits across all concentration levels. As noted by several authors (Hsieh and Liu 2008; Hsieh et al. 2009), the EP6-A–recommended method is likely to inflate Type I error, the probability of false claim of linearity. This is because the point estimate of the difference between the linear and best-fit polynomial model means is compared to the acceptable limits, which does not account for sampling error; that is, a point estimate is more likely to be contained within the acceptable limits than a metric that takes into account the variability in the difference estimate. Therefore, it is more likely to claim linearity when the linear relationship does not exist than if a metric is used that takes into account the estimation uncertainty. Kroll et al. (2000) proposed an alternative procedure, based on the average deviation from linearity (ADL) defined as

$$\theta = ADL = \frac{\sqrt{\sum_{i=1}^{l} (\mu_{Pi} - \mu_{Li})^2}}{\mu}, \tag{4.4}$$

where μ_{Li} and μ_{Pi} are the mean values of the linear and polynomial models, respectively, and μ is the mean concentration for all solutions of the assay. Linearity is ascertained through testing the hypotheses:

$$H_0: \theta \le \theta_0 \text{ versus } H_1: \theta > \theta_0, \tag{4.5}$$

where θ_0 is the maximum acceptable limit of ADL. Kroll et al. suggested using

$\hat{\theta} = \dfrac{\sqrt{\sum_{i=1}^{l} (\hat{Y}_{Pi} - \hat{Y}_{Li})^2 / l}}{\mu}$ as the test statistic for testing (Equation 4.5), noting

that $\sum_{i=1}^{l} (\hat{Y}_{Pi} - \hat{Y}_{Li})^2$ follows a noncentral χ^2 distribution with degrees of freedom of $nl - k - 1$ and a noncentrality parameter of $nl\theta_0^2 \left(\dfrac{\mu}{\sigma}\right)^2$ under H_0. H_0 is rejected at the 5% significance level if $\hat{\theta} < \dfrac{\sigma}{\mu} \sqrt{\dfrac{q_{0.95}}{nl}}$, with $q_{0.95}$ being the 95th percentile of the noncentral χ^2 distribution with degrees of freedom $nl - k - 1$.

4.4.3 Equivalence Tests

The statistical procedures for assessing linearity described so far use test statistics that follow either an F or a t distribution under the null hypothesis that the calibration model is linear. A small P value is indicative of a significant deviation from linearity and rejection of the null hypothesis. However, there is a major drawback concerning these significance-based tests, as the *P* value is susceptible to the influence of assay precision and sample sizes; specifically, these statistical tests penalize assays with smaller variability or studies with larger sample sizes and reward those with large variability or small sample sizes. In addition, even if a deviation from linearity is detected by these methods, it is not assessed for practical significance. Thus, it can be reasonably argued that application of significance tests to ascertain linearity might be fundamentally flawed. Several alternative statistical approaches have been considered in the literature and are described in the following sections.

4.4.3.1 Krouwer and Schlain's Method

Krouwer and Schlain (1993) proposed a method to determine the magnitude of deviation from assay linearity. The premise of their method is that the dose–response curve without the last concentration level is linear. Therefore, deviation from linearity is primarily caused by the last point added to the analysis. To estimate the amount of deviation, the design matrix of the linear regression based on the first $n - 1$ concentration levels is augmented by a column, which is orthogonal to the design matrix. The column is constructed through a regression analysis. It decomposes an indicator function, which assumes values of 0 or 1 when the last concentration is not included and included in the model, respectively, into its projection in the space spanned by the columns of the design matrix and a residual vector. The residual vector is orthogonal to the design matrix and is used as the last column in the expanded design matrix. In doing so, the deviation from a linear curve estimated from the first $n - 1$ concentrations is quantified, along with a 95% confidence interval (CI).

As an illustration, Krouwer and Schlain (1993) considered the data set in EP6-P (NCCLS 1986), which are results of a manual ammonia assay. The data are listed in Table 4.1 and plotted in Figure 4.1.

TABLE 4.1

Data from EP6 Manual Ammonia Example

Concentration of Standard	Observed Values			
	Replicate 1	Replicate 2	Replicate 3	Replicate 4
1	0.7	0.9	1.2	1.1
4	4.6	4.1	3.2	4.8
7	6.5	6.9	7.2	7.7
12	11.0	12.2	11.7	12.6
20	18.2	17.5	16.8	16.0

Source: Krouwer, J. and Schlain, B. (1993). A method to quantify deviations from assay linearity. *Clin. Chem.*, 39(8), 1689–1693.

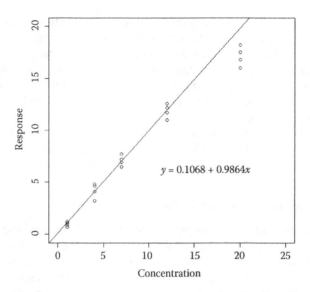

FIGURE 4.1
Plot of ammonia data. The straight line is the regression fit based on data from the first four concentrations. Values from the last concentration appear to deviate from the regression line. (From Krouwer, J. and Schlain, B. (1993). A method to quantify deviations from assay linearity. *Clin. Chem.*, 39(8), 1689–1693.)

From Figure 4.1, the dose–response curve appears to be linear in the range of the first four concentration levels. However, there is apparent nonlinearity when the results from the last concentration are added to the data set. Define

$$D_5 = \begin{cases} 1 & \text{if } x = 20 \\ 0 & \text{if } x \neq 20 \end{cases}.$$

The deviation from linearity can be quantified through estimating the coefficient of D_5 in the following regression model:

$$Y_{ij} = \alpha_0 + \alpha_1 x_i + \delta D_5 + \varepsilon_{ij}.$$

Expanding a method by Daniel (1985), Krouwer and Schlain (1993) suggested to re-parameterize the above model as

$$Y_{ij} = (\alpha_0 + \hat{\gamma}_0) + (\alpha_1 + \hat{\gamma}_1)x_i + \delta(D_5 - \hat{\gamma}_0 - \hat{\gamma}_1 x_i) + \varepsilon_{ij}.$$

$$Y_{ij} = \alpha_0^* + \alpha_0^* x_i + \delta LPO_5 + \varepsilon_{ij}, \tag{4.6}$$

where $LPO_5 = D_5 - \hat{\gamma}_0 - \hat{\gamma}_1 x_i (i = 1,...,5)$ is the residual of the regression model $D_5 = \gamma_0 + \gamma_1 x_i$. It is a well-known fact that the column consisting of LPO_5 values is orthogonal to the design matrix of the regression model

$$Y_{ij} = \alpha_0^* + \alpha_0^* x_i + \varepsilon_{ij}, \tag{4.7}$$

with $i = 1,...,4$. As a result, the least square estimates (LSEs) from fitting the full data set to Model 4.6 are the same as the LSEs from fitting data from the first four concentrations to Model 4.7. Therefore, the deviation from linearity due to the addition of the last concentration level is fully characterized by the estimate of the coefficient δ in Equation 4.6. Using the data in Table 4.1, it is estimated that $\hat{\delta} = -2.71\,\mu mol/L$ with two-sided 95% CI $(-4.07, -1.35)$. On the basis of these estimates and scientific knowledge of the assay, one may judge if the deviation is practically significant or not.

By using weighted regression, Krouwer and Schlain (1993) showed that their statistical method can be extended to the cases where variances are not constant across the concentration range. Further, the authors demonstrated that the above procedure can be applied iteratively to deviations from linearity at the last two or more concentrations. The method definitely represents an improvement over the significance tests described in Section 4.3. However, it relies heavily on the assumption that the dose–response curve without the last point(s) is linear, which usually is unknown. Although the authors suggested that either a LOF test or testing for the significance of a quadratic term be used to confirm the assumption, it is somewhat paradoxical as the original intent of their effort is to provide an alternative approach to the significance tests. A method that obviates this assumption was suggested by Novick and Yang (2013), which is discussed in Section 4.5.

4.4.3.2 Corrected Kroll Method

As discussed in Section 4.4.2.3, Kroll et al. (2000) assessed linearity through a composite test statistic based on the ADL. The null hypothesis of linearity is formulated as ADL being no greater than a maximum allowable deviation from linearity and is tested at a significance level of 5%. Like the LOF test, the method has a major drawback of conducting hypothesis testing with the linearity claim as the null hypothesis. Hsieh and Liu (2008) proposed a corrected ADL statistic by simply reformulating linearity as the alternative hypothesis:

$$H_0: \theta \geq \theta_0 \text{ versus } H_1: \theta < \theta_0. \tag{4.8}$$

The null hypothesis H_0 is rejected at the 5% significance level if $\hat{\theta} < \dfrac{\sigma}{\mu}\sqrt{\dfrac{q_{0.95}}{nl}}$ with $q_{0.95}$ being the 95th percentile of the noncentral χ^2 distribution with degrees of freedom. They referred to this procedure as the corrected Kroll method.

4.4.3.3 Liu and Hsieh's Methods

Several other methods were proposed by Hsieh and Liu (2008), Hsieh et al. (2009), and Liu and Hsieh (2010), which are based on various metrics of deviation from linearity. The first method is based on two one-sided tests (TOST) to evaluate deviation from linearity at each concentration. The second, called the sum of squares of deviation from linearity (SSDL), is the sum of the squared differences between the mean test results predicted by the linear model and by the best-fit polynomial model, at each of the concentration levels in the linearity experiment. This is an unscaled aggregate criterion. The third method uses the scaled metric, the coefficient of variation of the deviation from linearity (CVDL), which was also suggested by Kroll et al. (2000). Unlike the ADL, which is scaled by the mean concentration, CVDL is scaled by the variability of the best-fit polynomial model.

4.4.3.3.1 Two One-Sided Tests

Hsieh and Liu (2008) suggested performing a point-wise TOST procedure to examine the deviation between linearity and the best model fit at each concentration used in the linearity experiment. The point-wise TOST procedure is a reasonable approach in which linearity is declared if the null hypothesis is rejected:

$$H_0: |g_k(Xx_i) - g_1(x_i)| < \lambda \text{ for all } i = 1, 2, \ldots, l, \text{ versus}$$
$$H_1: |g_k(x_i) - g_1(x_i)| \geq \lambda \text{ for at least one } i, i = 1, 2, \ldots, l, \quad (4.9)$$

where $g_1()$ and $g_k()$ denote the linear and best-fit polynomial models, respectively, and λ is the maximum acceptable deviation from linearity. The test procedure consists of l two-sided $(1 - 2\alpha) \times 100\%$ CIs on the mean differences, $g_k(x_i) - g_1(x_i)$:

$$\hat{Y}_{Pi} - \hat{Y}_{Li} \pm t_{\alpha, nl-k-1} \hat{\sigma}_{di}, i = 1, \ldots, l,$$

where $\hat{Y}_{Li}$ and $\hat{Y}_{Pi}$ are predicted mean values from the linear and best-fit polynomial models, respectively, $\hat{\sigma}_{di}$ is the standard deviation of the difference between $\hat{Y}_{Li}$ and $\hat{Y}_{Pi}$, and $t_{\alpha, nl-k-1}$ is the upper 100αth percentile of the t distribution with a degree of freedom of $nl - k - 1$. The null hypothesis is rejected on the basis that all the above intervals are contained within the acceptable limits $(-\lambda, \lambda)$. As this is an intersection–union test, it has a size of α (Berger and Hsu 1996). The method was motivated by the desire to improve a test suggested in CLSI EP6-A (2003) and described in Section 4.4.2.3, which does not take into account sampling error at all and thereby conceivably inflates the Type I error. The TOST definitely represents an improvement, as shown through a simulation study by Liu and Hsieh (2010).

One point worth making is that although the TOST consists of l two-sided tests, the P value is typically driven by the concentration level with the largest deviation from linearity. The point-wise TOST can, however, suffer from design issues, should no element in the set of X_i lie close enough to the location of the largest deviation between $g_1()$ and $g_k()$, resulting in a false claim of linearity.

4.4.3.3.2 Sum of Squares of Deviation from Linearity

In a later paper, Hsieh et al. (2009) proposed a linearity test based on the SSDL, $\tau = SSDL = l^{-1} \sum_{i=1}^{1} \{g_k(x_i) - g_1(x_i)\}^2$. The null and alternative hypotheses of nonlinearity are

$$H_0: \tau \geq \lambda^2 \text{ versus } H_1: \tau < \lambda^2. \tag{4.10}$$

A test statistic of τ is given by $\sum_{i=1}^{L} (\hat{Y}_{Pi} - \hat{Y}_{Li})^2 / L$. Since the distribution of this test statistic is rather complex, Hsieh et al. (2009) suggested a generalized pivotal quantity (GPQ) approach.

Let $\mathbf{Y} = (Y_{11}, \dots Y_{1r}, \dots Y_{L1}, \dots, Y_{Lr})^T$ be the vector of measured assay responses and

$$\mathbf{X}_k = \begin{pmatrix} 1 & x_1 & \cdots & x_1^k \\ \vdots & \vdots & \cdots & \vdots \\ 1 & x_L & & x_L^k \end{pmatrix}, k \geq 1 \text{ be the design matrix of the Regression Models 4.2}$$

and 4.3. Let $\mathbf{W}_L = \mathbf{X}_1 (\mathbf{X}_1' \mathbf{X}_1)^{-1} \mathbf{X}_1$ and $\mathbf{W}_P = \mathbf{X}_k (\mathbf{X}_k' \mathbf{X}_k)^{-1} \mathbf{X}_k$ be the projection matrices of the linear model and the best-fit polynomial model, respectively. Let $\mathbf{W} = \mathbf{W}_P - \mathbf{W}_L$, and let $\hat{\mathbf{Y}}_L = \mathbf{W}_L \mathbf{Y}$ and $\hat{\mathbf{Y}}_P = \mathbf{W}_P \mathbf{Y}$ be the predicted mean values of Models 4.2 and 4.3, respectively. Thus, $\hat{\mathbf{Y}}_P - \hat{\mathbf{Y}}_L = \mathbf{WY}$ follows a multivariate normal distribution $\text{MVN}(\mu_P - \mu_L, \sigma^2 \mathbf{WW'})$. Define

$$R(\mathbf{Y}, \mathbf{y}, \mu_L, \mu_P) = \mathbf{Wy} - \frac{\mathbf{WY} - \mu_P - \mu_L}{\sigma} / \sqrt{SSE(\mathbf{Y})/\sigma^2} \sqrt{SSE(y)},$$

where $SSE(\mathbf{Y}) = Y^T(\mathbf{I}_N - \mathbf{W}_P)Y$. Note that

$$Z = \frac{\mathbf{WY} - \mu_P - \mu_L}{\sigma} \sim N(0, \mathbf{WW'}) \text{ and } U = \frac{SSE(\mathbf{Y})}{\sigma^2} \sim \chi^2(nl - (k+1)).$$

The distribution of $R(\mathbf{Y}, \mathbf{y}, \mu_L, \mu_P)$ is free of unknown parameters. Furthermore,

$$R(y, y, \mu_L, \mu_P) = \mu_P - \mu_L.$$

$R(Y, y, \mu_L, \mu_P)$ is a GPQ for $\mu_P - \mu_L$ (Weerahandi 1993). Therefore, a GPQ for SSDL is given by

$$R_{SSDL} = \frac{R(Y, y, \mu_L, \mu_P)' R(Y, y, \mu_L, \mu_P)}{l}.$$

Consequently, a generalized $100(1 - \alpha)\%$ confidence interval (GCI) of $\mu_P - \mu_L$ can be obtained from the following procedure:

Step 1. For $i = 1, \ldots, m$, simulate (Z^i, U^i) as distributed in Equation 4.6.

Step 2. Calculate R^i using Equation 4.7.

Step 3. Let $R^{(1-\alpha)}$ be the $100(1 - \alpha)$th percentile of $\{R^i, i = 1, \ldots m\}$. $R^{(1-\alpha)}$ is an estimate of the upper limit of the $(1 - \alpha) \times 100\%$ GCI of $\mu_P - \mu_L$.

The null hypothesis in Equation 4.10 is rejected if $R^{(1-\alpha)} < \lambda^2$, for some pre-specified limit λ^2. Hsieh et al. (2008) showed that the GPQ approach controls the test size and provides sufficient power for linearity assessment. Using GPQ methods, the authors also show a similar testing profile using the corrected ADL statistic.

4.4.3.3.3 Coefficient of Variation of Deviation from Linearity

Another metric for assessing linearity was suggested by Liu and Hsieh (2010). Similar to ADL, it is the square root of the sum of squared differences between the linear and best-fit polynomial model at the concentration levels used in the linearity study, scaled by the standard deviation of the best-fit model:

$$\eta = CVDL = \frac{\sqrt{\sum_{i=1}^{l} \{g_k(x_i) - g_1(x_i)\}^2 / l}}{\sigma}. \tag{4.11}$$

The associated hypotheses are as follows:

$$H_0: \eta \geq \eta_0 \text{ versus } H_1: \eta < \eta_0, \tag{4.12}$$

where η_0 is the acceptable limit of CVDL. Since $\hat{\sigma} = \sqrt{\dfrac{U}{u}}$ is a GPQ for σ, where $u = SSE(y)$, a GPQ for η is given by

$$R_{CVDL} = \sqrt{R_{SSDL} / \hat{\sigma}}.$$

Using the simulation procedure discussed above, the hypotheses in Equation 4.12 can be tested at a prespecified significance level α.

Define

$$\hat{\mu} = \bar{y} - \frac{1}{\sqrt{nl}} \sqrt{\frac{U}{u}} \frac{(\bar{Y} - u)}{\sqrt{\sigma^2/nl}}.$$

Liu and Hsieh (2010) showed that $\hat{\mu}$ is a GPQ for μ. Therefore, a GPQ for ADL is obtained as

$$R_{ADL} = \sqrt{R_{SSDL}/\hat{\mu}}.$$

4.4.3.3.4 Simulation Studies

Two simulation studies were carried out by Liu and Hsieh (2010) to compare the TOST method (Section 4.4.3.3) with the EP6-A (Kroll's) method (Section 4.4.2.3) and to evaluate the performance of the PQ-based SSDL, ADL, and CVDL methods. Empirical size and power are two characteristics frequently used to measure the performance of a statistical test. For the comparison between the TOST and EP6-A methods, the empirical size is used as the performance characteristic. However, both empirical size and power were used to compare the three GPQ-based methods. In principle, the closer the empirical size of a test to its nominal level, and the higher the power, the better the method is. Twelve combinations of numbers of concentrations (5 or 7), replicates at each concentration (2, 3, or 4), and assay variability (SD = 0.1 or 0.2) were used for the simulations.

For the comparison between the TOST and EP6-A methods, for each of the 12 combinations, 5000 random samples were generated, each representing a run of a linearity experiment. For each run, the hypotheses in Equation 4.9 were tested based on the TOST and EP6-A methods. The nominal significance level of the TOST was set at 0.05. The empirical size was estimated to be the proportion of runs in which the null hypothesis in Equation 4.9 is rejected. Let R be the number of times that the null hypothesis is rejected; R follows a binomial distribution $B(5000, 0.05)$, which with $n = 5000$ can be approximated by a normal distribution with mean 0.05 and standard deviation $\sqrt{0.05 \times 0.95/5000} = 0.031$. It is expected that among all the estimates of the empirical size of a test, approximately 95% (mean ±1.95 × SD) should fall within 0.04396 and 0.05604. Table 4.2 presents the estimates of empirical sizes of the TOST and EP6-A methods.

It is apparent that the empirical sizes of the EP6-A are close to 50% for all 12 simulation scenarios, regardless of the number of concentrations or replicates, or the assay variability. Therefore, the method does not provide control over the rate of false claims of linearity. The TOST method produces empirical test size estimates close to the nominal level of 0.05. In fact, only in 1 out of 12 scenarios (8.33%) is the empirical size estimate for the TOST procedure outside of the predicted range (0.04396, 0.05604).

TABLE 4.2

Estimates of Empirical Sizes of EP6-A and TOST Methods from a Simulation Study

Number of Concentrations	Number of Replicates	Assay Variability	EP6-A	TOST
5	2	0.1	0.4985	0.0522
		0.2	0.5050	0.0506
	3	0.1	0.4930	0.0440
		0.2	0.5050	0.0486
	4	0.1	0.5048	0.0490
		0.2	0.5066	0.0560
7	2	0.1	0.4972	0.0512
		0.2	0.5024	0.0484
	3	0.1	0.4978	0.0478
		0.2	0.4946	0.0504
	4	0.1	0.5044	0.0504
		0.2	0.5066	0.0494

Source: Liu, J. and Hsieh, E. (2010). Evaluation of linearity in assay validation. In *Encyclopedia of Biopharmaceutical Statistics*. 2nd ed., Informa Healthcare, 467–474.

Another simulation study was performed to compare the SSDL, ADL, and CVDL methods. This time, 10,000 random experimental data sets were generated for each of the 12 scenarios, and both empirical size and power were estimated for each statistical test. The range that is expected to cover 95% of the empirical size estimates was estimated to be (0.04930, 0.5066). The estimated empirical sizes are summarized in Table 4.3.

TABLE 4.3

Estimates of Empirical Sizes of SSDL, ADL, and CVDL Methods from a Simulation Study

Number of Concentrations	Number of Replicates	Assay Variability	SSDL	ADL	CVDL
5	2	0.1	0.0462	0.0467	0.0540
		0.2	0.0523	0.0517	0.0467
	3	0.1	0.0499	0.0502	0.0513
		0.2	0.0522	0.0517	0.0511
	4	0.1	0.0498	0.0505	0.0489
		0.2	0.0504	0.0508	0.0509
7	2	0.1	0.0504	0.0501	0.0409
		0.2	0.0495	0.0494	0.0504
	3	0.1	0.0505	0.0509	0.0473
		0.2	0.0495	0.0498	0.0504
	4	0.1	0.0498	0.0498	0.0529
		0.2	0.0498	0.0510	0.0452

Source: Liu, J. and Hsieh, E. (2010). Evaluation of linearity in assay validation. In *Encyclopedia of Biopharmaceutical Statistics*. 2nd ed., Informa Healthcare, 467–474.

The above results show that the empirical size estimates of all three methods are very close to the nominal level 0.05 and within the expected range of (0.04930, 0.5066). None of the effects due to number of concentrations of replicates or assay variability is prominent. The three methods provide comparable protection for the rate of false claims of linearity.

Liu and Hsieh (2010) also compared the empirical power of the three methods through a simulation study. The results showed that the ADL method is uniformly more powerful than the CVDL and SSDL and that CVDL is more powerful than SSDL.

4.4.3.4 Novick and Yang's Method

As pointed out by Novick and Yang (2013), while testing linearity over an analytical range is of interest, most statistical approaches proposed so far in the literature are dependent on and affected by the specific concentration levels at which the linearity experiment is conducted. It is conceivable that there may be a meaningful difference between the linear and best-fit models at particular concentration levels, whereas an overall measure of deviation remains statistically insignificant. Therefore, a test may conclude that there is no statistically significant deviation from linearity, yet provide little assurance regarding the closeness between the linear and best-fit models at all concentration levels. They reformulated the goal of linearity testing as demonstrating that the maximum difference between a straight line and a polynomial curve fit is bounded by an equivalence limit, over the entire test range of the analytical method, with a certain probability. A method based on GPQ analysis was suggested to estimate the probability of equivalence. To ease computational intensity, they re-parameterized Models 4.2 and 4.3, using orthogonal polynomial regression, which is described below.

4.4.3.4.1 Orthogonal Polynomial Regression Model

Consider $f_k(x_i)$ to be orthogonal polynomials of degree $k(k \geq 0)$. Thus,

$$\sum_{i=1}^{I} f_j(x_i) f_{j'}(x_i) = \begin{cases} 0 & \text{if } j \neq j' \\ 1 & \text{if } j = j' \end{cases}$$

Let $\theta = (\theta_0, \theta_1, ..., \theta_k)^T$ be unknown parameters. The models in Equations 4.2 and 4.3 can be rewritten as

$$Y_{ij} = \theta_0 f_0(x_i) + \theta_1 f_1(x_i) + ... + \theta_k f_k(x_i) + \varepsilon_{ij}, \tag{4.13}$$

where ε_{ij} are independently identically distributed according to a normal distribution with a mean of 0 and variance of σ^2. There are several ways in which the orthonormal polynomials $f_k(x_i)$ can be constructed. A method developed by Robson (1959) and Narula (1979) creates the $f_k(x_i)$ recursively from the relationship between the orthonormal polynomial function $f_k(x_i)$ and lower-order orthonormal polynomials:

$$f_k(x_i) = \frac{1}{c_k}\left[x_i^k - \sum_{v=0}^{k-1} f_v(x_i)\sum_{j=1}^{l} x_j^k f_v(x_j) \right],$$

where $c_k = \left\{\sum_{i=1}^{l}\left[x_i^k - \sum_{v=0}^{k-1} f_v(x_i)\sum_{j=1}^{l} x_j^k f_v(x_j) \right]\right\}^{1/2}$ is a normalizing

constant.

As an example, we have

$$f_0(x_i) = \frac{1}{\sqrt{l}}$$

$$f_1(x_i) = \frac{x_i - \bar{x}}{\sqrt{\sum_{j=1}^{l}(x_j - \bar{x})^2}}$$

$$f_2(x_i) = \frac{1}{c_2}\left[x_i^2 - \frac{1}{l}\sum_{j=1}^{l} x_j^2 - (x_i - \bar{x})\frac{\sum_{j=1}^{l} x_j^2 (x_j - \bar{x})}{\sum_{j=1}^{l}(x_j - \bar{x})^2} \right],$$

with $\bar{x} = \frac{1}{l}\sum_{i=1}^{l} x_i$. We define $\mathbf{Y} = (Y_{11},...Y_{1r}...Y_{l1},...,Y_{l,r})^T$ and

$$\mathbf{F} = \begin{pmatrix} f_0(X_1) & f_1(X_1) & \cdots & f_k(X_1) \\ \vdots & \vdots & \cdots & \vdots \\ f_0(X_{l \times n}) & f_1(X_{l \times n}) & & f_k(X_{l \times n}) \end{pmatrix}$$

as the measured responses and design matrix, respectively. The LSEs of the regression coefficients θ can be obtained as

$$\hat{\boldsymbol{\theta}} = (\mathbf{F}^T\mathbf{F})^{-1}\mathbf{F}^T\mathbf{Y} = \mathbf{F}^T\mathbf{Y}.$$

Because of the orthogonality of the design matrix F, $E[\hat{\theta}] = (F^T F)\theta = \theta$ and $Var[\hat{\theta}] = F^T Var[Y]F = \sigma^2 I_{k+1}$, where I_{k+1} is a $(k+1) \times (k+1)$ identify matrix. An unbiased LSE of σ^2 is given by

$$\hat{\sigma}^2 = \frac{Y^T(I_N - F^T F)Y}{N-(k+1)} = \frac{\displaystyle\sum_{i=1}^{l}\sum_{j=1}^{n}(Y_{ij} - \hat{Y}_{ij})^2}{N-(k+1)},$$

where $N = l \times n$ is the total number of response values. Consequently, an unbiased estimator of $Var[\hat{\theta}]$ is obtained as $Var[\hat{\theta}] = \hat{\sigma}^2 I'_{k+1}$.

4.4.3.4.2 Testing the Linearity Hypothesis

Novick and Yang (2013) suggested that the deviation from linearity be assessed through testing the hypotheses of

$$H_0 : |g_k(x) - g_1(x)| \geq \delta \text{ for at least one } x \in [X_L, X_U] \text{ versus}$$
$$H_1 : |g_k(x) - g_1(x)| < \delta \text{ for all } x \in [X_L, X_U], \tag{4.14}$$

where $[X_L, X_U]$ is a prespecified concentration range and δ is the maximum allowable bias in assay response. Using the model in Equation 4.13,

$$g_k(x) - g_1(x) = \sum_{r=2}^{k} \theta_r f_r(x)$$

As a consequence, the above hypotheses are equivalent to

$$H_0 : \max_{x \in [X_L, X_U]} \left| \sum_{r=2}^{k} \theta_r f_r(x) \right| \geq \delta$$

versus

$$H_1 : \max_{x \in [X_L, X_U]} \left| \sum_{r=2}^{k} \theta_r f_r(x) \right| < \delta. \tag{4.15}$$

The above hypotheses can be graphically illustrated. Figure 4.2 exhibits a linear and a quadratic function. The maximum difference between the two curves is indicated by a vertical line, which represents the maximum bias as a result of approximating the quadratic calibration relationship using a linear model. The null hypothesis in Equation 4.14 is rejected if the maximum bias is shown to be bounded by δ within the prespecified range $[X_L, X_U]$.

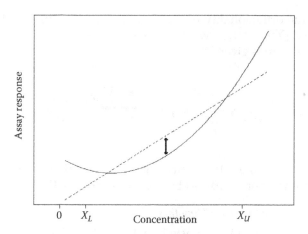

FIGURE 4.2
Maximum bias between two curves is indicated by the vertical line segment.

Thus, it may be concluded that the linear model is suitable for describing the calibration model.

4.4.3.4.3 A GPQ Test

A statistical test for the hypotheses in Equation 4.14 was developed by Novick and Yang (2013). It is based on a GPQ analysis. Define R(Y, y, θ) as

$$R(\mathbf{Y}, \mathbf{y}, \boldsymbol{\theta}) = F^T \mathbf{y} - \frac{F^T \mathbf{Y} - \boldsymbol{\theta}}{\sigma} \Big/ \sqrt{SSE(\mathbf{Y})/\sigma^2} \sqrt{SSE(\mathbf{y})}, \tag{4.16}$$

where $SSE(\mathbf{Y}) = \mathbf{Y}^T(I_N - FF^T)\mathbf{Y}$.

The distribution of R(Y, y, θ) is free of unknown parameters because $\frac{F^T \mathbf{Y} - \boldsymbol{\theta}}{\sigma} \sim N(0, I_{k+1})$ and $\frac{SSE(\mathbf{Y})}{\sigma^2} \sim \chi^2(N - (k+1))$. Note that R(y, y, θ) = θ. Thus, R is a GPQ for θ (Weerahandi 1993).

By considering the distribution of $\boldsymbol{\theta}_{\mathbf{GPQ}} = (\theta_{GPQ,0}, \theta_{GPQ,1}, \ldots, \theta_{GPQ,k})$ given the data, the proposed metric to measure linearity is the conditional probability

$$p(\delta, x_L, x_U) = Pr\left\{ \max_{x \in [x_L, x_U]} \sum_{r=2}^{k} \theta_{GPQ,r} f_r(x) < \delta \,\middle|\, data \right\}. \tag{4.17}$$

The test is constructed such that it rejects the null hypothesis in Equation 4.14 if $p(\delta, x_L, x_U) > p_0$, a predefined cut point. Novick and Yang (2013) suggested a computational method to estimate the above probability, based on a large random sample of $\boldsymbol{\theta}_{GPQ}$ and search algorithm that estimates the maximum inside the probability (Equation 4.17) over a grid of concentration values $\{x_L, x_1,...,x_U\}$. The probability $p(\delta, x_L, x_U)$ is estimated as the percentage of times that $\displaystyle\max_{x\in\{x_L,x_1,x_2,...,x_U\}} \sum_{r=2}^{k} \theta_{GPQ,r} f_r(x) < \delta.$

Similarly, a conditional probability metric based on the SSDL method was suggested by Novick and Yang (2013) such that

$$SSDL(\psi) = Pr\left\{\left[\sum_{i=2}^{l}\sum_{r=2}^{k}\theta_{GPQ,r}f_r(x_i)\right]^2 < \psi | data\right\}. \tag{4.18}$$

4.4.3.4.4 Comparison of Statistical Test Methods

The performance of these statistical test methods can be either assessed theoretically or empirically. For the special case where $k = 2$, Novick and Yang (2013) found that with proper selection of the equivalence limits, δ and ψ, the proposed method and the SSDL method are identical and, thus, have the same performance, whereas the TOST method discussed in Section 4.4.3.3 can have either the same performance as Novick and Yang's method or a worse performance than Novick and Yang's method. The results are summarized in Theorem 4.1.

Theorem 4.1

For $k = 2$, $SSDL(\psi) = p(\delta^*, x_L, x_U)$ with $\delta^* = m(x)\sqrt{\psi/S(X)}$, $m(x) = \displaystyle\max_{x\in[x_L,x_U]}|f_2(x)|$, and $S(X) = \displaystyle\sum_{i=1}^{l} f_2^2(X_i)$. The TOST is too liberal in claiming linearity when $\lambda > T(X)\delta/m(x)$; too strict when $\lambda < T(X)\delta/m(x)$; and equally sized as Novick and Yang's method when $\lambda = T(X)\delta/m(x)$ where $T(X) = \displaystyle\max_{x\in\{x_1,x_2,...,x_l\}}|f_2(x)|.$ ∎

Detailed steps that lead to the proof of Theorem 4.1 can be found in Novick and Yang (2013). When the maximum difference between the linear and quadratic models is achieved at one of the study design concentrations, $T(X) = m(x)$. By Theorem 4.1, when the equivalence limit λ is chosen to be the same as δ, the TOST and Novick and Yang's methods are also equivalent. For the general $k > 2$ case, there are no theoretical results concerning the relative performance of the above three methods.

4.4.3.4.5 Simulation Results

Novick and Yang (2013) carried out two Monte Carlo simulation studies to investigate the performance of the $p(\delta, x_L, x_U)$, $SSDL(\psi)$, and TOST methods. The first study compared the methods when the true dose–response curve is quadratic, and the second investigated the performance of the methods when the true dose–response curve was cubic. As the results of simulation for $k = 2$ are consistent with those in Theorem 4.1, we only describe here the second simulation for $k > 2$ and discuss the associated results in detail.

Two data sets were generated, the first to represent the situation in which the maximum difference occurs at one of the experiment concentrations, and the second to represent situations in which the maximum difference occurs at a point between two experimental concentrations. Duplicate response values were simulated from a normal distribution with mean $g_3(x) = 10 + (1 + 800\beta)x - 60\beta x^2 + \beta x^3$, with $\beta = 0$, 0.0005, 0.0010, 0.0015, or 0.0020, corresponding to varying degrees of nonlinearity, and a standard deviation $\sigma = 1$ or 1.5.

For the first data set, the experimental concentrations were {1, 9.9, 20.5, 30, 35, 40}, and the maximum difference between the linear and cubic fits occurred at $x = 9.9$. To ensure a fair comparison, the equivalence limits λ, ψ, and δ were carefully chosen to be 3.2, 5.5, and 3.2, respectively, so that the parameters hypothesized in Equations 4.9, 4.17, and 4.18 are on the border of H_0/H_1 when $\beta = 0.0015$. Concentrations {1, 7.5, 14, 20.5, 35, 40} were used to generate the second data set. The maximum difference between the linear and cubic fits occurred at $x = 30.2$, which is not a point of the experimental concentrations. Likewise, the δ, ψ, and λ were tuned with $\delta = 3.9$, $\psi = 4.2$, and $\lambda = \delta = 3.9$ to ensure that the hypothesized parameters are on the border of H_0/H_1 when $\beta = 0.0015$.

For each data set, and each combination of β and σ values, 20,000 GPQ statistics were simulated using the distribution of θ_{GPQ}. Linearity was respectively declared when, for the p-TOST test, the P value < 0.05, $p(\delta, x_L, x_U) > 0.95$, SSDL$(\psi) > 0.95$. The simulation was repeated 10,000 times with the estimated probability to declare linearity recorded. The results are summarized in Table 4.4.

TABLE 4.4

Power Results of Monte Carlo Simulation to Compare Method Performance

β	σ	Concentration Set 1			Concentration Set 2		
		TOST	SSDL	P Equiv.	TOST	SSDL	P Equiv.
0	1.0	1.00	1.00	1.00	1.00	1.00	1.00
	1.5	0.97	0.98	0.92	1.00	0.90	0.93
0.0005	1.0	0.99	1.00	0.98	1.00	0.99	0.98
	1.5	0.80	0.88	0.70	0.99	0.73	0.75
0.0010	1.0	0.59	0.74	0.50	1.00	0.60	0.58
	1.5	0.27	0.38	0.20	0.89	0.28	0.30
0.0015	1.0	0.02	0.04	0.01	0.86	0.03	0.05
	1.5	0.02	0.03	0.01	0.51	0.03	0.04
0.0020	1.0	0.00	0.00	0.00	0.18	0.00	0.00
	1.5	0.00	0.00	0.00	0.10	0.00	0.00

Source: Novick, S. and Yang, H. (2013). Directly testing the linearity assumption for assay validation. *J. Chemom.*, 27(5), 117–123.

For the first concentration set, the SSDL(ψ) method is slightly more power-ful than the TOST method, which, in turn, is more powerful than the new equivalence test. All three methods have conservative test size, less than the nominal level of 0.05. It is also evident that the power of the three tests decreases as the model departs from the linear model, which is character-ized by larger β values. Last, as expected, the standard deviation has a nega-tive effect on the power of the test. It is unclear why the test size of $p(\delta, x_L, x_U)$ was so conservative over this set of conditions, but there is some solace in knowing that the other two test methods were also conservative.

For the second concentration set, because the maximum difference between the cubic and linear models occurs between two concentrations, the TOST method is most powerful. However, it also has a much inflated test size of 0.86 for the H_0/H_1 borderline case $\beta = 0.0015$ and $\sigma = 1.0$. The $p(\delta, x_L, x_U)$ test retains the test size at the nominal level of 0.05 in this borderline case with $\beta = 0.0015$ and $\sigma = 1.0$, whereas SSDL(ψ) has a conservative test size of 0.03. The degree of deviation from linearity and standard deviation has the same effect on the power of the three tests as in the first concentration set.

4.5 Test Linearity on Concentration Scale

There exist situations in which the instrument signal cannot be directly con-verted to the final analytical measurement. Under such circumstances, as signal scale units are technology dependent, it is impossible to set uniform or fit-for-purpose acceptable limits for linearity metrics, based on the metrics of linearity that are constructed, using the signal scale rather than the con-centration scale.

4.5.1 Extension of Novick and Yang's Method

Novick and Yang (2013) suggested a method to examine the closeness between the straight line and a higher-order polynomial in the X (concentra-tion) space. The method follows a similar thought process to that described in Section 4.4.3.4. For each $x \in [X_L, X_U]$, it calculates the difference between the true concentration x and the concentration value predicted by the higher-order polynomial g_k in Equation 4.3. An equivalence test is used to test the hypotheses

$$H_0 : |z_k(x) - x| \geq \delta \text{ for at least one } x \in [X_L, X_U] \text{ versus}$$
$$H_1 : |z_k(x) - x| < \delta \text{ for all } x \in [X_L, X_U],$$

where $z_k(x) = [g_k(x) - \alpha_0]/\alpha_1$ and $z_k(x) - x = [g_k(x) - \alpha_0 - \alpha_1 x]/\alpha_1$ is the bias in concentration due to approximation of the higher-order polynomial g_k

using the linear model. Alternatively, if examination of the *relative* closeness between $z_k(x)$ and x $\left(\text{i.e.,} \dfrac{z_k(x)}{x} \right)$ is of more interest, these values may be log-transformed and the hypotheses of interest are

$$H_0 : |\log[z_k(x)] - \log(x)| \geq \delta \text{ for at least one } x \in [X_L, X_U] \text{ versus}$$
$$H_1 : |\log[z_k(x)] - \log(x)| < \delta \text{ for all } x \in [X_L, X_U].$$

As in Section 4.4.3.4, a test procedure for the above hypotheses was suggested (Novick and Yang 2013). It concludes linearity if $\Pr\{\max_{x \in [X_L, X_U]} |\log[z_k(x)] - \log(x)| \langle \delta | \text{data}\} > p_0$, where p_0 is a prespecified number, say, 0.95. The conditional probability can be estimated using the simulation method described in Section 4.4.3.4 (for details, see Novick and Yang 2013). The statistical properties of the test procedure were evaluated and may be controlled in much the same way as for the test described in Section 4.4.3.4.

4.5.1.1 Alternative Test

Conceptually, the direct testing method suggested by Novick and Yang (2013) is more rigorous than other linearity tests proposed in the literature and thus represents an improvement. However, one thing that may make its application difficult is that the method is computationally intensive. For statistically unsophisticated users, it is challenging to implement. As a remedy, LeBlond et al. (2013) developed a method that assesses deviation from linearity based on TOST for the bias on the concentration scale. However, a notable drawback of this approach is that it does not control the *overall* Type I error, though the test has a size of 5% at each concentration level. More recently, Yang et al. (2015a) proposed a simple alternative approach based on the construction of a CI for the maximum bias on the concentration scale. Linearity is claimed if this interval is contained within acceptable limits. The CI is an exact test when the true calibration relationship is quadratic. However, for higher-order polynomials, such an exact test is unattainable. Instead, a CI for an upper confidence limit of the maximum bias is constructed using GPQ analysis. The test is conservative, as its size does not reach the nominal significance level. As Yang et al. (2015a) pointed out, the method can be computationally easily implemented owing to the closed-form solution for the CI.

4.5.1.2 Bias on Concentration Scale

In order to formulate the linearity problem in terms of testing hypotheses related to the maximum bias on the concentration scale, it is important to establish the relationship between the bias on the concentration scale $bias_x(x)$ and that on the instrument signal scale $bias_y(x) = g_k(x) - g_1(x)$. This can be accomplished through the aid of a graph such as that in Figure 4.3 (LeBlond

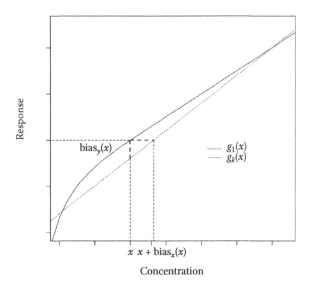

FIGURE 4.3
Relationship between bias in response and bias in concentration. (From LeBlond, D., Tan, C., and Yang, H. (2013). Confirmation of analytical method calibration linearity. *Pharmacopeial Forum*, May–June Issue, 39(3).)

et al. 2013). As seen from the plot, $bias_x(x)$ and $bias_y(x)$ have the following relationship:

$$bias_x(x) = \frac{bias_y(x)}{\beta_1},$$ (4.19)

where β_1 is the slope of the straight line.

It can be verified that the slope of the linear model (Equation 4.2) and coefficient θ_1 in Equation 4.13 satisfy

$$\beta_1 = \frac{\theta_1}{m},$$ (4.20)

with $m = \sqrt{\sum_{i=1}^{n}(x_i - \bar{x})^2}$. By Equations 4.19 and 4.20, we have

$$bias_x(x) = m\frac{\left|\sum_{r=2}^{k}\theta_r f_r(x)\right|}{\theta_1}$$

Therefore, the linearity can also be assessed through testing the following hypotheses:

$$H_0 : \frac{m}{|\theta_1|} \left(\max_{x \in [X_L, X_U]} \left| \sum_{r=2}^{k} \theta_r f_r(x) \right| \right) \geq \delta_1 \text{ versus}$$

$$H_0 : m \left| \frac{\theta_2}{\theta_1} \right| \left(\max_{x \in [X_L, X_U]} |f_2(x)| \right) \geq \delta_1$$

(4.21)

where δ_1 is the maximum allowable concentration bias.

4.5.2 Statistical Test Methods

Yang et al. (2015a) proposed two test methods for testing the hypotheses in Equation 4.21, one for $k = 2$ and the other for $k > 2$. An exact test was obtained for $k = 2$ and a more conservative test was suggested for $k > 2$.

4.5.2.1 Linear versus Quadratic Models

When $k = 2$, the hypotheses in Equation 4.21 become

$$H_0 : m \left| \frac{\theta_2}{\theta_1} \right| \left(\max_{x \in [X_L, X_U]} |f_2(x)| \right) \geq \delta_1 \text{ versus}$$

$$H_1 : m \left| \frac{\theta_2}{\theta_1} \right| \left(\max_{x \in [X_L, X_U]} |f_2(x)| \right) < \delta_1.$$

(4.22)

Because the expression $m \left| \frac{\theta_2}{\theta_1} \right| \left(\max_{x \in [X_L, X_U]} |f_2(x)| \right)$ is a function of the ratio of two parameters (θ_1, θ_2) and their LSEs $(\hat{\theta}_1, \hat{\theta}_2)$ are normally distributed with mean (θ_1, θ_2) and variance matrix $\sigma^2 I_2$, using Fieller's theorem, a 90% CI $(bias_{xL}, bias_{xU})$ of $bias_x(x)$ is given as

$$bias_{xL} = m_0 \left[\frac{\hat{\theta}_2}{\hat{\theta}_1} - \frac{t_{N-3,0.95} \hat{\sigma}}{\hat{\theta}_1} \sqrt{(1-g) + \left(\frac{\hat{\theta}_2}{\hat{\theta}_1} \right)^2} \right] \Big/ (1-g)$$

$$bias_{xU} = m_0 \left[\frac{\hat{\theta}_2}{\hat{\theta}_1} + \frac{t_{N-3,0.95} \hat{\sigma}}{\hat{\theta}_1} \sqrt{(1-g) + \left(\frac{\hat{\theta}_2}{\hat{\theta}_1} \right)^2} \right] \Big/ (1-g),$$

(4.23)

where $g = \dfrac{t^2_{N-3,0.95}\hat{\sigma}^2}{\hat{\theta}^2_1}$, with $t_{N-3,0.95}$ being the 95th percentile of the Student t distribution with $N - 3$ degrees of freedom. A test procedure was constructed to reject H_0 in Equation 4.21 if the interval (Equation 4.23) is entirely contained within $(-\delta_1, \delta_1)$. This is an exact test, having a size of 5% (Chow and Liu 2008).

4.5.2.2 Linear versus Higher-Order Polynomials

Now consider $k > 2$. Since the expression $\sum_{r=2}^{k} \theta_r f_r(x)$ in the hypotheses in Equation 4.21 involves unknown parameters θ, there is no closed-form solution for the maximization problem. An alternative solution was suggested by Yang et al. (2015a). Instead of testing the hypotheses in Equation 4.21, linearity is assessed based on testing the null hypothesis that an upper bound of the maximum bias in Equation 4.21 is below acceptable limit. As shown below, the upper bound can be expressed as a product of a function of θ, which does not involve concentration x, and a constant. The result is stated in the following theorem:

Theorem 4.2

The maximum bias $\dfrac{m}{|\theta_1|}\left(\max_{x\in[X_L,X_U]}\left|\sum_{r=2}^{k} \theta_r f_r(x)\right|\right)$ *on the centration is bounded by* $m_1 h(\theta)$ *such that* $h(\theta)$ *and* m_1 *are given as follows:*

$$h(\theta) = \left[\frac{\sqrt{\sum_{r=2}^{k}\theta_r^2}}{|\theta_1|}\right]$$

$$m_1 = m\left(\max_{x\in[X_L,X_U]}\sum_{r=2}^{k}f_r^2(x)\right).$$

∎

The theorem can be verified by applying the Cauchy and Schwarz inequality (Strang 2005). It is evident for each $x \in[X_L, X_U]$

$$\left[m\frac{\left|\sum_{r=2}^{k}\theta_r f_r(x)\right|}{|\theta_1|}\right] \leq \left[m\frac{\sqrt{\sum_{r=2}^{k}\theta_r^2}\sum_{r=2}^{k}f_r^2(x)}{|\theta_1|}\right] \leq m_1 h(\theta).$$

Consequently,

$$\frac{m}{|\theta_1|}\left(\max_{x\in[X_L,X_U]}\left|\sum_{r=2}^{k}\theta_r f_r(x)\right|\right)\leq m_1 h(\theta).$$

The linearity hypotheses are re-formulated as

$$H_0 : m_1 h(\theta) \geq \delta_1 \text{ versus } H_1 : m_1 h(\theta) < \delta_1. \tag{4.24}$$

The theoretical result in Theorem 4.2 makes it possible to construct a test procedure for the hypotheses in Equation 4.24. Define $\mathbf{A} = \begin{bmatrix} 0_2 & 0 \\ 0 & I_{k-2} \end{bmatrix}$ and $\mathbf{B} = (0, 1, 0, ..., 0)$, a $(k + 1)$ dimension vector and let

$$H(\mathbf{Y},\mathbf{y},\theta) = \frac{\sqrt{(R(\mathbf{Y},\mathbf{y},\theta)\mathbf{A})^T (R(\mathbf{Y},\mathbf{y},\theta)\mathbf{A})}}{BR(\mathbf{Y},\mathbf{y},\theta)}, \tag{4.25}$$

where, as previously discussed, $R(\mathbf{Y}, \mathbf{y}, \theta)$ is a GPQ for θ. Using algebraic manipulations, it can be shown that $H(\mathbf{Y}, \mathbf{y}, \theta)$ is the GPQ for $h(\theta)$. Following the standard procedure by Weerahandi (1995a,b, 2004), a test procedure using $H(\mathbf{Y}, \mathbf{y}, \theta)$ was constructed by Yang et al. (2015a). It first estimates an upper 95% confidence limit of $h(\theta)$, based on random draws from the distribution of the GPQ $H(\mathbf{Y}, \mathbf{y}, \theta)$. An approximate 95% upper confidence limit of $h(\theta)$ is then obtained, using the following algorithm:

Step 1. Draw random samples $\mathbf{Z}_i$ from $N(0, I_{k+1})$ and $\mathbf{U}_i$ from $\chi^2(N - (k + 1))$, $i = 1, ..., n$, respectively.

Step 2. Calculate $R(\mathbf{Y}_i, \mathbf{y}, \theta) = \mathbf{F}^T \mathbf{y} - \mathbf{Z}_i \sqrt{\dfrac{SSE(y)}{U_i}}$ and $H(\mathbf{Y}_i, \mathbf{y}, \theta)$ using Equation 4.25.

Step 3. Rank the $H(\mathbf{Y}_i, \mathbf{y}, \theta)$ and let $H(\mathbf{Y}, \mathbf{y}, \hat{\theta})$ be the 95th percentile of $\{H(\mathbf{Y}_i, \mathbf{y}, \theta)\}$. $H(\mathbf{Y}, \mathbf{y}, \hat{\theta})$ is the upper 95% confidence limit on $H(\mathbf{Y}, \mathbf{y}, \theta)$.

The maximum bias on the concentration scale is bounded by $H(\mathbf{Y}, \mathbf{y}, \hat{\theta})m_1$ with at least 95% confidence. A test for hypotheses (Equation 4.24) can be constructed such that it rejects H_0 in Equation 4.24 if

$$H(\mathbf{Y}, \mathbf{y}, \hat{\theta})m_1 < \delta_1. \tag{4.26}$$

This test has a size no greater than 5%. Thus, it is a conservative test that protects the consumer risk.

Yang et al. (2015a) also discussed a possible alternative method to construct the one-sided 95% CI for $h(\theta)$. When $k > 2$, a maximum likelihood estimator of $h(\theta)$ in Theorem 4.1 is obtained as

$$h(\hat{\theta}) = \left[\frac{\sqrt{\sum_{r=2}^{k} \hat{\theta}_r^2}}{|\hat{\theta}_1|} \right] = \sqrt{\frac{\sum_{r=2}^{k} \hat{\theta}_r^2}{\hat{\theta}_1^2}}.$$

Because $\hat{\theta} \sim N(\theta, \sigma^2 I_{k+1})$, $h(\hat{\theta})$ is the square root of the ratio of two independent noncentral χ^2 variables with degrees of freedom of $k + 1$ and 1, respectively. Therefore, the exact distribution of $h(\hat{\theta})$ can be derived. However, the distributions and moments of $h(\hat{\theta})$ are very complex (Finney 1938). The method might be computationally more demanding than the GPQ method.

4.5.2.3 Examples

Yang et al. (2015a) used a real-world example to illustrate the use of the statistical tests described in Section 4.5.2 for linearity of an assay. The assay was performed at five concentration levels (0, 20, 50, 70, and 100), with three replicates per level. The data are presented in Table 4.4 and also plotted in Figure 4.4. It is evident that the data show some nonlinear patterns. It is of interest to test whether or not a linear model can be used to adequately describe the data, in lieu of a higher-order polynomial model.

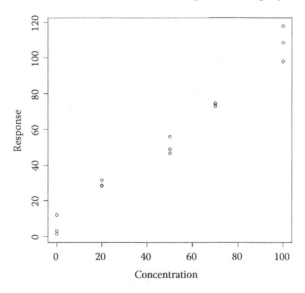

FIGURE 4.4
Plot of response values against concentration.

Using the technique in Section 4.4.3.4, four orthonormal polynomial functions $f_k(x)$, $k = 0, 1, 2, 3$, each of order 3, were constructed. The design matrix

$$F = \begin{pmatrix} f_0(x_1) & f_1(x_1) & f_2(x_1) & f_4(x_1) \\ \vdots & \vdots & \cdots & \vdots \\ f_0(x_{15}) & f_1(x_{15}) & f_2(x_{15}) & f_4(x_{15}) \end{pmatrix} \text{ is listed in Table 4.5.}$$

4.5.2.3.1 Case 1: Linear versus Quadratic (k = 2)

The linear model was first tested against a quadratic alternative. On the basis of practical knowledge, a bias of 10 on the concentration scale is deemed to be significant. Therefore, the equivalence margin δ_1 in Equation 4.22 was chosen to be 10. Using results in Table 4.5, the LSEs of the parameters of Model 4.13 were obtained:

$$\hat{\theta} = F^T Y = (207.29, 136.59, 7.05)$$

$$var[\hat{\theta}] = (5.92)^2 I_3.$$

Thus,

$$\frac{\hat{\theta}^2}{\hat{\theta}_1^2} = \frac{(7.05)^2}{(136.59)^2} = 0.002664038.$$

TABLE 4.5

Raw Data and Design Matrix Based on Orthonormal Polynomials

Sample	Concentration (X)	Response (Y)	Orthonormal Design Matrix F			
			f_0	f_1	f_2	f_3
1	0	12.08	0.2582	−0.3497	0.2925	−0.2258
2	0	1.47	0.2582	−0.3497	0.2925	−0.2258
3	0	3.23	0.2582	−0.3497	0.2925	−0.2258
4	20	28.43	0.2582	−0.2040	−0.0954	0.3868
5	20	31.75	0.2582	−0.2040	−0.0954	0.3868
6	20	28.57	0.2582	−0.2040	−0.0954	0.3868
7	50	56.00	0.2582	0.0146	−0.3090	0.0336
8	50	46.74	0.2582	0.0146	−0.3090	0.0336
9	50	48.89	0.2582	0.0146	−0.3090	0.0336
10	70	73.8	0.2582	0.1603	−0.2057	−0.3347
11	70	74.69	0.2582	0.1603	−0.2057	−0.3347
12	70	72.86	0.2582	0.1603	−0.2057	−0.3347
13	100	97.95	0.2582	0.3788	0.3176	0.1401
14	100	117.79	0.2582	0.3788	0.3176	0.1401
15	100	108.59	0.2582	0.3788	0.3176	0.1401

Other quantities that are necessary for constructing the 90% CI for maximum bias were also estimated:

$$g = \frac{t^2_{N-3,0.95}\hat{\sigma}^2}{\hat{\theta}_1^2} = 0.005964339 \text{ and}$$

$$m|f_2(x)| = 43.59044 \text{ when } x = 100,$$

where we used the fact that

$$f_2(x) = 0.000246x^2 - 0.02431x + 0.29255.$$

As a result, the two-sided 90% CI for the $\text{bias}_x(x)$ is estimated to be

$$(\text{bias}_{xL}, \text{bias}_{xU}) = (-1.12, 5.64).$$

As the interval is contained entirely within $(-10, 10)$, the null hypothesis in Equation 4.14 was rejected and linearity of the assay is claimed.

4.5.2.3.2 Case 2: Linear versus Cubic (k = 3)

The linear model was further tested against a cubic model. To begin, the LSEs of the parameter of the model in Equation 4.13 were obtained along with their variance estimates:

$$\hat{\theta} = (207.29, 136.59, 7.05, 7.00)$$

$$\text{var}[\hat{\theta}] = (5.81)^2 I_3.$$

Using the algorithm described in the previous section, 5000 random samples were drawn from the distribution of $H(\mathbf{Y}, \mathbf{y}, \theta)$. The upper 95th percentile of these samples and the constant m_1 were determined to be 0.163 and 60.1, respectively. Consequently, the upper bound of the one-sided 95% CI for the maximum bias was estimated to be 9.8. Since it is smaller than the equivalence bound 10, the null hypothesis (Equation 4.21) was again rejected and linearity of the assay is claimed.

4.5.3 Single-Point Calibration

Assuming that the true calibration relationship is linear, approximating Linear Model 4.1 with Model 4.27 below is sometimes advantageous as it makes it possible to use a single-point calibration for each run, thus resulting in tremendous savings in resources.

$$Y_{ij} = \beta_1 x_i + \varepsilon_{ij}. \tag{4.27}$$

To ensure that such an approximation does not cause unacceptable bias, the following hypotheses need to be tested:

$$H_0: \max_{x\in[X_L,X_U]} \left|bias_x(x)\right| \geq \delta \text{ versus } H_1: \max_{x\in[X_L,X_U]} \left|bias_x(x)\right| < \delta, \tag{4.28}$$

where $bias_x(x) = |\beta_{0str} + \beta_{1str} \, x - \beta_1 x|$ is the bias at concentration x associated with approximating the linear model with the proportional model, with β_{0str} and β_{1str} being the intercept and slope of the linear model in Equation 4.1, respectively. Using a graphical method, LeBlond et al. (2013) expressed the $bias_x(x)$ as a function of the ratio $\beta_{0str}/\beta_{1str}$. It is illustrated as follows. Let x_{std} denote the concentration of the reference standard, and y_{std} be the theoretical mean response value of the reference standard. It is expected that the two lines in Equations 4.1 and 4.27 intersect each other at x_{std}. Figure 4.5 shows a plot of the two lines. Because the triangle $\triangle ABC$ is congruent to the

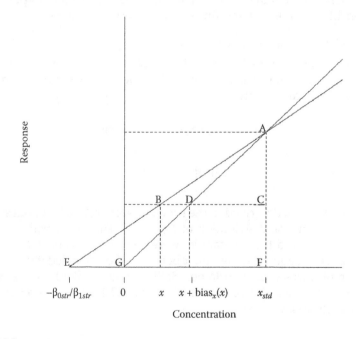

FIGURE 4.5
Bias associated with approximating a linear model with a proportional model. (From Yang, H., Novick, S., and LeBlond, D. (2015a). Testing analytical method linearity within a pre-specified range. *J. Biopharm. Stat.*, 25(2), 334–350.)

triangle $\triangle AEF$, and the triangle $\triangle ABD$ is congruent to the triangle $\triangle AEG$, we have the following relationships:

$$\frac{BC}{EF} = \frac{AB}{AE} = \frac{BD}{EG}.$$

As the straight line $\beta_{0str} + \beta_{1str}x$ crosses the x axis at $-\beta_{0str}/\beta_{1str}$, it is evident that

$$\frac{x_{std} - x}{x_{std} - \left(-\dfrac{\beta_{0str}}{\beta_{1str}}\right)} = \frac{x_0 + bias_x}{0 - \left(-\dfrac{\beta_{0str}}{\beta_{1str}}\right)}. \tag{4.29}$$

Solving Equation 4.29 for $bias_x(x)$, we obtain the bias at a given concentration x_0:

$$bias_x = \frac{\dfrac{\beta_{0str}}{\beta_{1str}}(x_{std} - x_0)}{x_{std} + \dfrac{\beta_{0str}}{\beta_{1str}}}.$$

Since both β_{0str} and β_{1str} are positive, the maximum bias $M(x) = \max_{x \in [X_L, X_U]} |bias_x(x)|$ is given by

$$M(x) = \frac{\dfrac{\beta_{0str}}{\beta_{1str}} \max\{|x_{std} - x_L|, |x_U - x_{std}|\}}{x_{std} + \dfrac{\beta_{0str}}{\beta_{1str}}}.$$

Let $(\hat{\beta}_{0str}, \hat{\beta}_{1str})$ be the LSEs of $(\beta_{0str}, \beta_{1str})$ and $s^2 \begin{pmatrix} v_{11} & v_{12} \\ v_{12} & v_{22} \end{pmatrix}$ be the corresponding variance–covariance matrix of $(\hat{\beta}_{0str}, \hat{\beta}_{1str})$ with s^2 being the mean squared error of Model 4.1 with $N - 2$ degrees of freedom. Applying Fieller's theorem, a two-sided 90% CI for $\beta_{0str}/\beta_{1str}$ can be obtained as

$$\left(\frac{\beta_{0str}}{\beta_{1str}}\right)_L, \left(\frac{\beta_{0str}}{\beta_{1str}}\right)_U = \frac{\hat{\beta}_{0str}}{\hat{\beta}_{1str}} \pm \frac{t_{N-2,0.95}}{\hat{\beta}_{1str}} \sqrt{s^2 v_{11} - 2m_{lin}s^2 v_{12} + m_{lin}^2 s^2 v_{22}}. \tag{4.30}$$

Because $M(x) = \dfrac{\dfrac{\beta_{0str}}{\beta_{1str}}\max\{|x_{std} - x_L|,|x_U - x_{std}|\}}{x_{std} + \dfrac{\beta_{0str}}{\beta_{1str}}}$ is a monotonically increas-

ing function in $\beta_{0str}/\beta_{1str}$, a two-sided 90% CI for $M(x)$ is given by

$$\left[\frac{\left(\dfrac{\beta_{0str}}{\beta_{1str}}\right)_L \max\{|x_{std} - x_L|,|x_U - x_{std}|\}}{x_{std} + \left(\dfrac{\beta_{0str}}{\beta_{1str}}\right)_L}, \frac{\left(\dfrac{\beta_{0str}}{\beta_{1str}}\right)_U \max\{|x_{std} - x_L|,|x_U - x_{std}|\}}{x_{std} + \left(\dfrac{\beta_{0str}}{\beta_{1str}}\right)_U}\right].$$

A test procedure can be devised by rejecting the null hypothesis in Equation 4.28 if the above CI is within the acceptance limit $(-\delta,\delta)$.

4.6 Concluding Remarks

Linearity is an important characteristic of any analytical method. Deviation from linearity may cause both bias and imprecision of the assay. Therefore, it is critical to evaluate the magnitude and impact of deviations from the linearity assumption. Most statistical tests to assess linearity proposed in the literature are aimed at demonstrating linearity based on a bias evaluation in the response space. They run into the challenge in defining meaningful fit-for-purpose acceptance limits in the instrument response space, which is technology dependent. Furthermore, those test methods make inference about linearity only at the concentrations used in the experiment. Therefore, they are influenced by the validation study design. The test suggested by Novick and Yang (2013) addresses these issues. However, it is computationally intensive and cannot be easily implemented by statistically unsophisticated users. The method suggested by Yang et al. (2015a) is both methodologically rigorous and can be implemented easily. Therefore, it is a viable alternative to all the current methods.

Section III

Process Development

5

Residual Host Cell DNA Risk Assessment

5.1 Introduction

As shown in Figure 5.1, product purification is a key step in downstream process development. One objective of the purification process is to remove residual host cell DNA so as to mitigate its potential risk to the patient. The assessment of the effectiveness of DNA removal relies on experimental design and statistical analysis. For this purpose, several statistical methods have been developed. We begin with some background of the issue before introducing these statistical techniques.

Cell cultures are conventionally used for production of biologicals. In recent years, responses to emerging diseases such as pandemic influenza catalyzed cell-based biological product development. Cell culture production has several advantages over other media. First of all, it has the potential to deliver a large number of doses in a short period. Second, it allows for better control of product consistency and quality. In the past decade, there has been increasing utilization of continuous cell lines (CCLs) for biologic product manufacturing (Petricciani and Loewer 2001). In addition, a number of new CCLs are being employed for the development of new biologicals (World Health Organization [WHO] 2007). However, despite various purification steps used in biological product manufacturing, residual cell DNA may still be present in the final product. As some cell lines are known to contain oncogenes and viral agents (Petricciani and Loewer 2001), it is theoretically possible, however remotely so, that the residual DNA may transmit an activated oncogene or infectious viral DNA to product recipients (Lewis et al. 2001). Therefore, it is necessary to consider the safety issues related to the residual DNA in biologic development.

Various studies have been conducted to assess the risk of residual DNA. As early as the 1960s, it was found that viral nucleic acids could be infective (Petricciani and Loewer 2001). Subsequent in vitro studies further revealed that DNA from various viruses turned the infected organism's cells into tumorigenic. Perhaps of more significance were the findings that viral DNA could cause infections in animals and that the purified oncogene v-src was tumor causing. More recently, Sheng et al. (2008) demonstrated that two

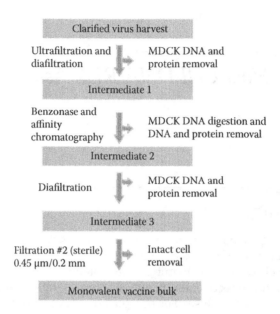

FIGURE 5.1

Overview of downstream manufacturing process for a viral vaccine.

cellular oncogenes (activated human H-ras and c-myc), when inoculated together, could induce sarcomas in two different mouse strains (NIH Swiss and C57BL/6). Peden et al. (2006) also observed that infectivity could be reduced after endonuclease digestion of a mixture of cloned HIV (plasmid) and hcDNA. If residual DNA were digested to a mean size of 650 bp, then complete loss of infectivity of 0.15 μg of cloned viral DNA was achieved. Taken together, these studies confirm the oncogenicity and infectivity of residual DNA.

Because of the oncogenic and infective potential of residual DNA, several regulatory guidelines related to residual DNA risk assessment and the development of risk mitigation strategies were issued (Food and Drug Administration [FDA] 2010; WHO 2007). The FDA guidance (2010) states, "The risks of oncogenicity and infectivity of your cell-substrate DNA can be lessened by decreasing its biological activity. This can be accomplished by decreasing the amount of residual DNA and reducing the size of the DNA (e.g., by DNAse treatment or other methods) to below the size of a functional gene (based on current evidence, approximately 200 base pairs)...." A meeting report issued by a WHO Study Group on Cell Substrates for Production of Biologicals concurred that decreasing the size of residual DNA to below 200 bp mitigates the oncogenic and infective risks of residual DNA. The study group also agreed that 10 ng of host cell DNA per dose is an appropriate upper limit for biologicals produced in

CCLs. Although neither WHO nor FDA guidelines mandate manufacturers to conform to the limits for DNA content and size (10 ng per dose or less and 200 bp or less, respectively), these limits are generally viewed as regulatory specifications.

In this chapter, a probabilistic model to estimate the risk due to residual DNA is discussed. The model takes into account enzyme inactivation and allows for more accurate risk assessment when compared to methods currently in use. An application of this model to determine the safety factor for host cell DNA in a vaccine product is provided. The model is further applied to establish acceptable limits of residual DNA that may differ from the current regulatory specifications. An extension of the model based on Bayesian inference is also discussed.

5.2 DNA Inactivation and Removal

To control the risk of residual DNA in biological products and ensure product quality, a cell culture–based manufacturing process utilizes modern manufacturing technologies to remove intact host cells and reduce the amount and size of residual DNA. Figure 5.1 shows an overview of a typical downstream manufacturing process for a viral vaccine.

5.2.1 Filtration

Various filtration steps are used to remove host cells during the downstream process. Residual DNA is fractionated through application of enzymatic treatment and fragments and reduced using affinity chromatography.

5.2.2 DNA Inactivation

Enzymatic degradation of DNA to a size below that of a functional gene is known to reduce DNA activity (Peden et al. 2006). Figure 5.2 depicts an enzymatic inactivation process. As an illustration, it is assumed that the host cell genome contains one oncogene. Fractionation of the DNA is a chance event, in which each phosphate ester bond between two nucleotides is disrupted by an enzyme with a certain probability. The more effective the enzyme is in degrading the DNA, the fewer intact oncogenes or infective agents will remain in the final dose. The fractionation results in a reduced likelihood of having an oncogenic or infective event. However, how to take into account residual DNA in product and process risk assessment can be very challenging.

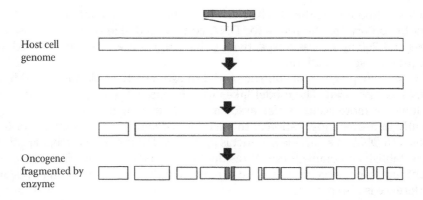

Host cell
genome

Oncogene
fragmented by
enzyme

FIGURE 5.2
Diagram of DNA inactivation using enzyme. An oncogene sequence is either intact or fractionated at the end of enzymatic reaction.

5.3 Risk Assessment

Oncogenic and infective risks of the residual DNA are usually quantified through a metric called the safety factor, which is defined as the total number of doses needed to induce an oncogenic (infective) event in a product recipient. The measure has been broadly used in research for DNA risk assessment (Krause and Lewis 1998; Peden et al. 2006; Sheng et al. 2008). When estimating the safety factor, consideration needs to be given to the amount and size of residual DNA and to the characteristics of the host genome, oncogenes, and infective agents that reside in the host cell. It is also important to take into account the number of oncogenes or infective agents needed to induce an oncogenic or infective event. In the literature, several estimation methods have been proposed and are described in detail in this section.

5.3.1 Peden, Sheng, and Lewis' Method

Assuming that each host cell genome contains I different oncogenes (infective agents), each of size m_i (number of base pairs [bp]), with I_i copies of oncogene (infective agent) i, $i = 1\ldots I$. Then, the total number of oncogenes (infective agents) I_0 and the average oncogene size m, respectively, are

$$I_0 = \sum_{i=1}^{I} I_i \quad \text{and} \quad m = \sum_{i=1}^{I} I_i m_i / I_0.$$ (5.1)

Peden et al. (2006) suggested using the following formula to estimate the safety factor (SF):

$$SF_{PSL} = \frac{O_m}{(m/M)I_0E[U]} , \tag{5.2}$$

where O_m is the amount of oncogenes (infective agents) required for inducing an oncogenic (infective) event, M is the genome size (total bp) in one copy of the host cell, and $E[U]$ is the average amount of residual DNA per dose of the product. These parameters involved in SF estimation can be either experimentally determined or extracted from the literature. It is worth noting that the expression

$$(m/M)I_0E[U] = \left(\sum_{i=1}^{I} I_i m_i/M \right) E[U] \tag{5.3}$$

in Equation 5.2 represents the genomic mass equivalent of oncogenes (infective agents) in a dose. However, there is a serious deficiency with this estimation method; that is, it does account for the effect of DNA inactivation as evidenced by the fact that the denominator in Equation 5.2 includes genomic mass of both fractionated and unfractionated oncogenes. As a result, the risk estimate based on this method is likely to be inflated.

5.3.2 Krause and Lewis' Method

Krause and Lewis (1998) published an alternative approach aimed at evaluating the safety of viral DNA in biological product. Their method attempts to incorporate only unfractionated DNA in the risk calculations, by reducing the denominator in Equation 5.2 by the percentage of DNA shown to be smaller than the infective viral genome in the host cell. Specifically,

$$SF_{KL} = \frac{O_m}{P(m/M)I_0E[U]} , \tag{5.4}$$

where P is the percentage of DNA with size greater than or equal to that of the viral genome. It is evident that the method is applicable to oncogenic risk assessment of residual DNA.

5.3.3 Yang, Zhang, and Galinski's Method

As pointed out by Yang et al. (2010), SF_{PSL} does not account for disruption of the oncogene sequences, nor does it take into account the possibly unequal sizes of individual oncogenes. It was also noted that SF_{KL} does not consider the sizes of individual oncogenes or infective agents (Yang 2013b). As a result, neither of the two methods can provide an accurate estimate of the safety factor when DNA inactivation is employed with multiple oncogenes or infective agents of varying sizes. On the basis of mechanistic modeling of the relationship between the risk and process parameters and host cell characteristics, Yang et al. (2010) suggested a new method, which provides an effective remedy to the deficiencies of the above two methods.

5.3.3.1 Modeling of DNA Inactivation

In the following, we discuss the method by Yang et al. (2010) in the context of the assessment of residual DNA oncogenicity. The method is directly applicable for infectivity evaluation. Central to the method is to model the enzymatic DNA inactivation process. It is conceivable that the size of residual DNA in the final product is dependent on the cutting efficacy of enzyme. The more efficient an enzyme is, the shorter is the residual DNA. Enzymatic disruption of DNA is a chance event, as the enzyme cleaves the ester phosphate bond between any two adjacent nucleotides with a certain probability. It is crucial to establish a direct relationship between enzyme cutting efficiency and the residual DNA size.

To that end, Yang et al. (2010) introduced a method based on a probabilistic model of the enzyme digestion process. Let Φ, Ω, and c denote the host cell genome, the oncogene DNA sequence residing in the host genome, and the phosphate ester bond between two nucleotides, respectively. Φ and Ω can be expressed as

$$\Phi = B_1 c B_2 c ... c B_M, \quad \Omega = B_l c B_{l+2} c ... c B_{l+m-1}, \tag{5.5}$$

where M and m represent haploid size of host genome and oncogene size, respectively, and $l \geq 1$, $m > 1$, and $l + m - 1 < M$. The $m - 1$ bond c's within Ω are denoted as $c_1, c_2 ... c_{m-1}$. Define X_i as binary random variables with outcomes of either 0 or 1 such that

$$P[X_i = 1] = P[c_i \text{ is disrupted by the enzyme}] = p,$$

where p represents the cutting efficiency of the enzyme. An intact oncogene would imply that none of the ester phosphate bonds within the oncogene is cut. Mathematically, it is equivalent to

$$X_1 = X_2 ... = X_{m-1} = 0.$$

Assuming that the X_i are independently identically distributed, the probability for Ω not to be disrupted is

$$P[X_1 = X_2 ... = X_{m-1} = 0] = (1 - p)^{m-1}. \tag{5.6}$$

5.3.3.2 Residual DNA from Oncogenes

The above modeling approach provides a way to separate fractionated residual DNA from unfractionated DNA, for each oncogene in the host cell genome, in the risk assessment. Consider a general case in which the host cell genome Φ contains a total of I_0 oncogenes (each oncogene is denoted Ω_i) of size m_i:

$$\Omega_i = B_{l_i} c B_{l_i+1} c ... c B_{l_i+m_i-1}, \ 1 \le i \le I_0.$$

Some Ω_i may be identical copies of the same oncogene. By Equation 5.6, the probability for Ω_i to remain unfractionated is given by

$$p_i = (1-p)^{m_i-1}. \tag{5.7}$$

Yang et al. (2010) developed a method to estimate the amount of unfractionated oncogene in the final dose through a series of probabilistic derivations. The method models the numbers of fractionated and unfractionated oncogenes as random Poisson variables and derives the total amount of unfractionated oncogene through a conditional probability calculation. Specifically, let U denote the total amount of residual host cell DNA per dose; let V_i, W_i, and Z_i be the total number of copies of oncogene Ω_i (either fractionated or unfractionated), the total number of copies of unfractionated oncogene Ω_i, and the total number of copies of fractionated oncogene Ω_i in a dose, respectively. Clearly, $V_i = W_i + Z_i$. Finally, let Y be the total amount (weight) of unfractionated oncogene in a dose. Thus,

$$Y = \sum_{i=1}^{I_0} d_i W_i ,$$

where d_i is the weight of a single (unfractionated) oncogene Ω_i. It is assumed that, conditional on U, V_i has a Poisson distribution:

$$V_i \sim P\left(\frac{m_i}{M}(U/d_i) \right),$$

where U/d_i represents the maximum number of oncogene Ω_i, in a dose. It is also reasonable to assume that conditional on V_i, W_i is distributed according to a binomial distribution $B(p_i, W_i)$ with p_i being given in Equation 5.7. It can be shown that

$$E\left[V_i|U\right] = \frac{m_i}{M}(U/d_i)$$

$$E\left[W_i|V_i\right] = p_iV_i$$

$$E[W_i] = E_{V_i}\left(E_W\left[W_i|V_i\right]\right) = E_{V_i}[p_iV_i] = E_U\left(E_{V_i}\left[p_iV_i|U\right]\right) = \left(p_i\frac{m_i}{M}\right)/d_iE[U].$$

As a consequence, the expected value of total amount of unfractionated oncogene Y in a dose can be obtained by

$$E[Y] = \sum_{i=1}^{I_0} d_iE[W_i] = \sum_{i=1}^{I_0} p_i\frac{m_i}{M}E[U]. \tag{5.8}$$

Equation 5.8 indicates that the total amount of unfractionated oncogene in the final dose is related to the size of the host cell genome, the number of oncogenes, their sizes, the total amount of residual DNA per final dose, and enzyme cutting efficiency.

5.3.3.3 Safety Factor Estimation

Since the safety factor (SF) is defined as the number of doses required to produce an oncogenic amount O_m of unfractionated oncogene, the safety factor satisfies

$$\sum_{j=1}^{SF} Y_j = O_m,$$

where Y_j is the amount of unfractionated oncogene in dose j, $j = 1, ..., SF$.

As SF is usually large, by the Strong Law of Large Numbers (Billingsley 1986), we obtain

$$\frac{\sum_{j=1}^{SF} Y_j}{SF} \approx E[Y],$$

which is equivalent to

$$SF = \frac{\sum_{j=1}^{SF} Y_j}{E[Y]} \; .$$

Taken together, the safety factor, SF, can be estimated by

$$SF = \frac{O_m}{\sum_{i=1}^{I_0} (1-p)^{m_i-1} \frac{m_i}{M} E[U]} \; . \tag{5.9}$$

The above formula establishes a mathematical relationship between the safety factor and all other parameters of interest. Of particular note is that the safety factor is directly affected by the enzyme cutting efficiency and total amount of residual DNA. As the latter can be controlled through process, the estimation can be used to guide process improvement. Assume that the host cell genome harbors I different oncogenes of varying sizes m_i and that there are I_i copies of oncogene i, $i = 1, ..., I$. Thus, the total number of oncogenes I_0 can be re-expressed as $I_0 = \sum_{i=1}^{I} I_i$. After some algebraic manipulations, the safety factor in Equation 5.9 can be rewritten as

$$SF = \frac{O_m}{\sum_{i=1}^{I} I_i(1-p)^{m_i-1} \frac{m_i}{M} E[U]} \; . \tag{5.10}$$

It is also worthy pointing out that when $p = 0$,

$$SF = \frac{O_m}{\sum_{i=1}^{I} I_i \frac{m_i}{M} E[U]} = \frac{O_m}{(m/M)I_0 E[U]} = SF_{PSL} \; ,$$

where we use the fact that

$$m = \sum_{i=1}^{I} I_i m_i / I_0 .$$

The above result implies that the method suggested by Peden et al. (2006) is a special case where no DNA inactivation steps are taken. This indirectly verifies the method by Yang et al. (2010).

Another point to make is that calculation of SF involves p, which, in general is unknown, and furthermore p cannot be directly estimated through experimentation. This issue was resolved through a modeling approach to estimate enzyme cutting efficiency, suggested by Yang et al. (2010).

5.3.3.4 Determination of Enzyme Efficiency

After enzyme digestion, a DNA segment can be expressed as

$$B_{r+1}cB_{r+2}c...cB_{r+X},$$

where r $(1 \le r \le M)$ is an integer representing the start of the segment and X $(1 \le X \le M - 1)$ is an integer representing the length of the segment (bp); M is an integer representing the size of the genome. The segment can be viewed as a random outcome of a stochastic process, in which it takes an enzyme X number of tries before succeeding in cutting through an ester phosphate bond to obtain a DNA segment expressed as above. In essence, then, X is a random variable that can be described by a negative binomial distribution:

$$\Pr[X = k] = (1 - p)^{k-1}p, k = 1, 2,..., M - 1.$$

As a direct consequence, the theoretical median of X is given by

$$\text{Median} = -\frac{\log 2}{\log(1-p)}. \tag{5.11}$$

Various analytical methods such as agarose, polyacrylamide, and capillary electrophoresis are readily available for estimation of the size distribution of residual DNA. Since the size distribution of the residual DNA can be experimentally estimated, Equation 5.11 renders a way to indirectly estimate the enzyme cutting efficiency. Figure 5.3 displays the relationship between the median size of residual DNA and enzyme cutting efficiency. For instance, a median residual DNA size of 200 bp corresponds to an estimated enzyme cutting efficiency (the probability for each ester phosphate bond to be cut) of 0.0035. The strictly monotonic decreasing trend reflects the assumption that the more efficient the enzyme is, the smaller the size of the residual DNA.

Let Med_0 denote the median size of residual DNA in the final dose. Solving Equation 5.11 for p gives rise to

$$p = 1 - 2^{-1/\text{Med}_0}.$$

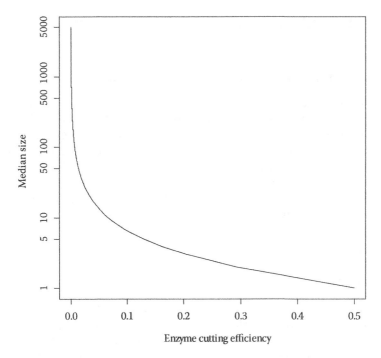

FIGURE 5.3
Relationship between median DNA size and enzyme cutting efficiency. (From Yang, H., Zhang, L., and Galinski, M. (2010). A probabilistic model for risk assessment of residual host cell DNA in biological products. *Vaccine*, 28(19), 3308–3311.)

Substituting it for p in Equation 5.10, we obtain

$$\text{SF}_{\text{YZG}} = \frac{O_m}{\sum_{i=1}^{I} I_i 2^{-\frac{m_i-1}{\text{Med}_0}} \frac{m_i}{M} E[U]} \cdot \qquad (5.12)$$

Similarly, a formula for safety factor concerning infectivity can be obtained:

$$\text{SF}_{\text{YZG}}^{I} = \frac{Q_m}{\sum_{i=1}^{J} J_i 2^{-\frac{n_i-1}{\text{Med}_0}} \frac{n_i}{N} E[U]}, \qquad (5.13)$$

where Q_m is the viral genome amount required to induce an infection, J represents the total number of proviruses contained in Madin–Darby canine kidney (MDCK) cell genome with sizes n_i, with J_i copies of provirus i, $i = 1,..., J$, and N is the diploid size of the viral genome.

5.3.4 Safety Factor Estimation Method Comparisons

As previously discussed, the SF estimation methods by Peden et al. (2006) and Krause and Lewis (1998) are inaccurate as they do not take into account all factors that have an impact on the patient risk due to residual DNA or infectious agents. Yang (2013b) compared the three methods (Krause and Lewis 1998; Peden et al. 2006; Yang et al. 2010) through both theoretical argument and empirical evaluations. The main results are discussed below. To ease the discussion, we hereafter refer to these three methods as SF_{PSL}, SF_{KL}, and SF_{YZG}, respectively.

5.3.4.1 Theoretical Results

Theorem 5.1

The three methods SF_{PSL}, SF_{KL}, and SF_{YZG} have the following properties: (1) When there is no DNA inactivation step, $SF_{PSL} = SF_{YZG}$. However, when there is DNA inactivation, $SF_{PSL} < SF_{YZG}$; (2) When there is one and only one oncogene on the host genome, $SF_{KL} = SF_{YZG}$; when the host genome contains more than one oncogene, $SF_{KL} > SF_{YZG}$ if $m > (2/\ln 2)Med_0$; otherwise, $SF_{KL} \leq SF_{YZG}$. ∎

The results in Theorem 5.1 indicate that both SF_{PSL} and SF_{KL} are special cases of SF_{YZG}. In general, SF_{PSL} underestimates the safety factor compared to SF_{YZG}, and SF_{KL} can either underestimate or overestimate the safety factor compared to SF_{YZG}. The proof of the theorem is briefly outlined below.

Proof of the first part: When there is no DNA inactivation, $p = 0$. By Equation 5.10, $SF_{PSL} = SF_{YZG}$. When $p > 0$, it is obvious that

$$SF_{YZG} = \frac{O_m}{\sum_{i=1}^{I} I_i (1-p)^{m_i - 1} (m_i/M) E[U]}$$

$$> \frac{O_m}{\sum_{i=1}^{I} I_i (m_i/M) E[U]} = SF_{PSL}.$$

Proof of the second part: Recall that m in Equation 5.1 is the average size of oncogenes on the host genome.

Define

$$f(x) = 2^{-\frac{x-1}{Med_0}} (x/M)E[U].$$

From Equations 5.4 and 5.6,

$$SF_{KL} = O_m/f(m). \tag{5.14}$$

When $I = 1$, it can be easily verified that

$$SF_{KL} = \frac{O_m}{(m/M)E[U]} = SF_{YZG}.$$

For $I > 1$, the second-order derivative of $f(x)$

$$f''(x) = \frac{2^{-\frac{x-1}{Med_0}} (\ln 2)^2 E[U]}{Med_0 M} [x - (2/\ln 2)Med_0]$$

satisfies

$$f''(x) \begin{cases} > 0 & \text{if } x > (2/\ln 2)Med_0, \\ \leq 0 & \text{if } x \leq (2/\ln 2)Med_0. \end{cases}$$

Note that $f(x)$ is concave and convex over the intervals $[0, (2/\ln 2) Med_0]$ and $((2/\ln 2) Med_0, \infty)$, respectively (Boyd and Vandenberghe 2004). Let

$$\bar{f} = \sum_{i=1}^{I_0} f(m_i)/I_0.$$

By Jensen's inequality,

$$f(m) \begin{cases} < \bar{f} & \text{if } m > (2/\ln 2)Med_0, \\ \geq \bar{f} & \text{if } m \leq (2/\ln 2)Med_0. \end{cases} \tag{5.15}$$

Combining Equations 5.14 and 5.15 and noting the fact that $SF_{YNG} = O_m / \bar{f}$, we obtain

$$SF_{KL} \begin{cases} > SF_{YZG} & \text{if } m > (2/\ln 2)\text{Med}_0, \\ \leq SF_{YZG} & \text{if } m \leq (2/\ln 2)\text{Med}_0. \end{cases}$$

5.3.4.2 Empirical Comparisons

To gain a sense about how the three methods compare to one another, Yang (2013b) applied them to a realistic problem concerning oncogenic risk assessment for a cell-based live attenuated influenza vaccine. The manufacturing process utilizes various purification steps, such as tangential flow filtration and chromatography assay, to remove residual DNA. Remaining DNA, which is not removed by the purification steps, is degraded through treatment with benzonase. The amount of residual DNA in the final product was quantified through a PCR assay and determined to be less than 1 ng per dose.

Since an MDCK cell was used as the substrate, the host genome size is $M = 5 \times 10^9$ bp. Although whether the MDCK cell contains any oncogenes is unknown, for illustration, two sets of calculations were carried out: one based on the assumption that there are three copies of a single oncogene with a size of 2000 bp on the host cell genome, and the other assuming that the genome contains three oncogenes of different sizes (1000, 2000, and 3000 bp), which have an average size of 2000 bp. The average size of 2000 bp was chosen to be close to the average size of human oncogenes of 1925 bp (Yang et al. 2010).

Calculation of SF_{PSL}, SF_{KL}, and SF_{YZG} requires an estimate of the amount of oncogene O_m that is cancer causing. A study conducted by Sheng et al. (2008) showed that a combined amount of 25 μg of two 12.5 μg of plasmids, each containing an activated oncogene (activated human H-ras and c-myc), caused tumors in mice. Assuming that both H-ras and c-myc in the study conducted by Sheng et al. (2008) have a size of 1925 bp, that implies that 37.7% of the plasmids (3186 bp) harbored oncogenes. Hence, the total oncogene contribution is 9.4 μg (25 μg × 37.7% = O_m). It was further assumed that the median size of residual DNA is 2000 bp. On the basis of the above assumptions, the safety factor was estimated using the three methods. The results are shown in Table 5.1.

As expected, for the first scenario, the SF_{PSL} method underestimates the safety factor by more than 1000-fold, while SF_{KL} and SF_{YZG} produce the same estimate. For the second scenario, SF_{PSL} underestimates the safety factor by 60-fold compared to SF_{YZG}, and by contrast, SF_{KL} overestimates it compared to SF_{YZG} by 17-fold.

TABLE 5.1

Estimates of Oncogenicity Safety Factor by Three Methods

No. of Different Oncogenes	Copies of Oncogene	Size(s) of Oncogene(s)	Estimation Method		
			SF_{PSL}	SF_{KL}	SF_{YZG}
1	3	2000	2.35×10^9	2.40×10^{12}	2.40×10^{12}
3	1	1000, 2000, 3000	2.35×10^9	2.40×10^{12}	1.41×10^{11}

Source: Yang, H. (2013b). Establishing acceptable limits of residual DNA (2013). *PDA J. Pharm. Sci. Technol.*, March–April Issue, 67, 155–163.

5.4 Risk Control

The risk and acceptable limits of residual DNA have long been subjects of debate (Petricciani and Loewer 2001). From both a historical and a scientific perspective, Petricciani and Loewer (2001) provided an excellent overview of issues concerning residual DNA. Initially 10 pg/dose was considered an acceptable limit by a group of scientists, based on available data at the time, including the knowledge that a marketed polio vaccine produced in VERO cells used 10 pg/dose as the limit of residual DNA. In 1986, this limit was modified to 100 pg/dose by a group of experts commissioned by the WHO. Upon further evaluations of emerging data, the limit was revised to 10 ng/dose in 1998. Ever since, this limit has been widely viewed as a regulatory requirement. Subsequent publications by both the WHO (2007) and FDA (2010) reiterated that oncogenic and infective risk due to residual DNA can be mitigated by reducing both the amount of DNA (to ≤10 ng/dose) and the size (to approximately 200 bp) in the final dose. However, neither WHO nor FDA guidelines require manufacturers to conform to these limits. Instead a risk-based approach was recommended for setting these limits. For example, the WHO (2007) guideline states, "a risk assessment should be done in order to define the DNA upper limit for a particular vaccine or biological product, based on the following parameters: nature of the cell substrate, inactivation process, the method used to assess DNA content, and the size distribution of DNA fragments." Likewise, the FDA also encourages manufacturers to discuss risk assessment and acceptable limits of residual DNA with the agency, should an alternative approach or limits be used (FDA 2010).

While the risk-based approach makes perfect scientific sense and may provide potential regulatory flexibility, determining such limits can be challenging. In this section, we discuss various strategies through which alternate limits for DNA content and size can be established.

5.4.1 Specifications Based on Current Standards

5.4.1.1 Method

A method suggested by Yang (2013b) determines the acceptable limits by comparing the safety factor of any combination of DNA content (ng/dose) and median size (bp) to that obtained when the DNA content and size are 10 ng/dose and 200 bp, respectively, which are regulatory specifications. A combination ($E[U]$, Med$_0$) is deemed acceptable if the safety factor evaluated at this combination is greater than or equal to the safety factor achieved at (10 ng/dose, 200 bp), using the method by Yang et al. (2010). In other words, ($E[U]$, Med$_0$) meets the following conditions:

$$\frac{O_m}{\sum_{i=1}^{I_0} 2^{-\frac{m_i-1}{Med_0}}(m_i/M)E[U]} \geq \frac{O_m}{\sum_{i=1}^{I_0} 2^{-\frac{m_i-1}{200}}(m_i/M)10} \tag{5.16}$$

$$\frac{Q_m}{\sum_{i=1}^{J_0} 2^{-\frac{n_i-1}{Med_0}}(n_i/N)E[U]} \geq \frac{Q_m}{\sum_{i=1}^{J_0} 2^{-\frac{n_i-1}{200}}(n_i/N)10} . \tag{5.17}$$

After some algebraic manipulations, the two inequalities can be rewritten as

$$E[U] \leq \frac{10\sum_{i=1}^{I_0} 2^{-\frac{m_i-1}{200}}}{\sum_{i=1}^{I_0}\left(2^{-\frac{m_i-1}{Med_0}}\right)} \quad \text{and} \quad E[U] \leq \frac{10\sum_{j=1}^{J_0} 2^{-\frac{n_j-1}{200}}}{\sum_{J=1}^{J_0}\left(2^{-\frac{n_j-1}{Med_0}}\right)} . \tag{5.18}$$

As an illustration, Yang (2013b) provided the following example. Consider a host cell containing one oncogene of size 2000 bp and one viral gene of size 3569 bp, the size of the smallest viral genome MS2. Substituting these numbers into Equation 5.18 results in

$$E[U] \leq 10 \cdot 2^{-1999\left(\frac{1}{200}-\frac{1}{Med_0}\right)} \quad \text{and} \quad E[U] \leq 10 \cdot 2^{-3568\left(\frac{1}{200}-\frac{1}{Med_0}\right)} . \tag{5.19}$$

A plot of the two curves that delineate the boundaries of the two regions defined through the above two inequalities is shown in Figure 5.4. The solid and dashed lines correspond to the curves $E[U] = 10 \cdot 2^{-1999\left(\frac{1}{200}-\frac{1}{Med_0}\right)}$ and

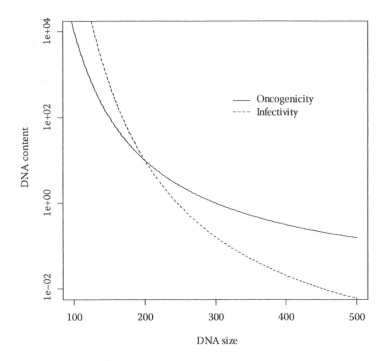

FIGURE 5.4

Combinations of DNA content and size under the solid and dotted curves give rise to safety factors greater than those at regulatory limits (content ≤ 10 ng/dose and median size = 200 bp). (From Yang, H. (2013b). Establishing acceptable limits of residual DNA (2013). *PDA J. Pharm. Sci. Technol.*, March–April Issue, 67, 155–163.)

$E[U] = 10 \cdot 2^{-3568\left(\frac{1}{200} - \frac{1}{Med_0}\right)}$, respectively. DNA content and size that are below both curves would have safety factors of oncogenicity and infectivity greater than their respective counterpart when the content is 10 ng/dose and the median size of DNA is equal to 200 bp.

5.4.1.2 Example

Yang (2013b) illustrated the use of the above method through an example. The safety factor (SF_{YZG}) was calculated for various combinations of DNA content and size (see Table 5.2). The ranges of DNA content and size cover the regulatory limits of (≤10 ng/dose, 200 bp). Also note that the limit 0.1 ng/dose or 100 pg/dose is the original WHO specification for DNA content. For each combination of DNA content and size, the calculated safety factor of oncogenicity or infectivity was expressed as the ratio between the estimated safety factor and that evaluated at (10 ng/dose, 200 bp). If the ratio is greater than or equal to 1, the safety factor is considered to be acceptable. For the combination of DNA content and size as a whole to be acceptable, both the

TABLE 5.2

Ratio of Residual DNA Content and Size Calculated Based on SF_{YZG} Compared to Regulatory Limits

DNA Content (ng/dose)	Median Size (bp)	Relative Safety Factor[a]	
		Oncogenicity	Infectivity
10	200	1.00	1.00
10	250	0.25	0.08
1000	120	1.01	38.5
100	150	1.01	6.17
30	250	0.08	0.03
20	145	6.94	55.5
20	200	0.50	0.50
1	245	2.80	1.03
0.1	318	7.63	1.02
0.01	450	21.3	1.04

Source: Yang, H. (2013b). Establishing acceptable limits of residual DNA (2013). *PDA J. Pharm. Sci. Technol.*, March–April Issue, 67, 155–163.

[a] Relative safety factor is defined as the ratio of safety factor with the DNA content (ng/dose) and median size (bp) to that obtained when the DNA content and size are 10 ng/dose and 200 bp, respectively.

ratio of oncogenicity safety factor and that of infectivity safety factor have to be at least 1. The results are summarized in Table 5.2.

From Table 5.2, a couple of conclusions can be drawn. First, DNA content may exceed its regulatory limit 10 ng/dose, but the risk may be mitigated by reducing the size of DNA below the regulatory limit 200 bp so as to warrant the same level of safety assurance as the combination (10 ng/dose, 200 bp). Likewise, the median DNA size may be greater than the regulatory limit 200 bp without compromising overall safety assurance if DNA content is controlled below the regulatory limit of 10 ng/dose. For example, for a median DNA size of 120 bp, the limit of DNA content can be as low as 1000 ng/dose, and for a DNA content of 0.01 ng/dose, the DNA size can be as large as 450 bp without incurring unacceptable patient risk. Second, when at least one of DNA content and size is above its regulatory limit, and the other is also either at or above its regulatory limit, the overall level of risk is unacceptable. The combinations of DNA content and size are displayed in Figure 5.4. The three combinations (10, 250), (30, 250), and (20, 200) are outside of the boundaries of acceptable safety factor regions. The rest of the combinations are all within Figure 5.5.

An alternative strategy is to define acceptable $(E[U], Med_0)$ based on absolute limits for the safety factors. Let SF_O and SF_I be the safety factors of oncogenicity and infectivity, respectively. The content and DNA size $(E[U], Med_0)$ are deemed acceptable if the following is true:

$$SF_O \geq a \quad \text{and} \quad SF_I \geq b, \tag{5.20}$$

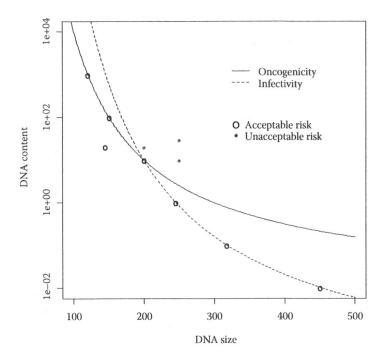

FIGURE 5.5
Combinations of DNA content and size marked by "o" have acceptable safety factors; combinations marked by "*" have unacceptable safety factors. (From Yang, H. (2013b). Establishing acceptable limits of residual DNA (2013). *PDA J. Pharm. Sci. Technol.*, March–April Issue, 67, 155–163.)

where the limits *a* and *b* are chosen based on understanding of the product, scientific justifications, and regulatory requirements. It is conceivable that these limits may change from product to product. For example, if the product is a vaccine intended to be used by a very large healthy population that is less risk tolerant, *a* and *b* should be large; these limits may be very different for a vaccine than for an oncology product. Regulatory precedent and published literature may also be of use in selecting these limits. For instance, in 2005, the FDA Vaccines and Related Biological Products Advisory Committee considered an oncogenic SF greater than or equal to 10^7 as acceptable.

5.4.2 Specifications Based on Acceptable Patient Risk

A more direct method for setting acceptable limits for DNA content and size was suggested by Yang et al. (2015b), which approaches the issue from a patient risk control point of view. Here, risk is defined as the probability of getting an unwanted serious adverse event such as cancer or infection due to residual DNA. The acceptable range of DNA size and content is determined such that this probability is bounded below an acceptable level.

While the method was developed in consideration of oncogenic, infective, and immunogenic risk, to simplify the discussion of the method, we will focus on establishing the range to minimize oncogenicity and infectivity potentials.

5.4.2.1 Acceptable Ranges

Let X_i and Y_i, $i = 1, ..., N$ be the amounts of intact oncogenes and infective agent in the final dose, respectively, where N is the maximum number of doses produced annually of the product. Let θ_S and θ_U be the size (bp) and content (ng/dose) of residual DNA in a dose, respectively. Furthermore, we define

$$\tilde{X} = \sum_{i=1}^{N} X_i \quad \text{and} \quad \tilde{Y} = \sum_{i=1}^{N} Y_i. \tag{5.21}$$

Hence, $\tilde{X}$ and $\tilde{Y}$ are the total numbers of intact oncogenes and infective agent in all N doses. It is clear that $\tilde{X}$ and $\tilde{Y}$ are dependent on both the size θ_S and content θ_U of residual DNA in a single dose. Suppose that x_0 and y_0 are the numbers of intact oncogenes and infective agents needed to induce an oncogenic or infective event, respectively. The acceptable limits for size θ_S and content θ_U were defined as (Yang et al. 2015b)

$$A = \left\{ \theta \equiv (\theta_S, \theta_U) : \Pr\left[(\tilde{X} \geq x_0) \cup (\tilde{Y} \geq y_0) \middle| \theta \right] < r_0 \right\}, \tag{5.22}$$

where r_0 is a prespecified maximum acceptable risk of either an oncogenic or infective event. The numbers x_0 and y_0 can often be determined through properly designed studies, while the selection of r_0 is driven more by regulatory requirements.

As discussed in Section 5.3.3.2, X_i and Y_i follow Poisson models. Therefore, $\tilde{X}$ and $\tilde{Y}$ also follow Poisson distributions (Haight 1967). It can be shown that the means of $\tilde{X}$ and $\tilde{Y}$ are given by (Yang et al. 2015b)

$$\lambda_{\tilde{X}}(\theta) = \frac{2^{-1/\text{Med}_0} m \theta_U}{d_O M} \quad \text{and} \quad \lambda_{\tilde{Y}}(\theta) = \frac{2^{-1/\text{Med}_0} n \theta_U}{d_I M}, \tag{5.23}$$

where Med_0 is the median size of residual DNA in a final dose, d_O and d_I are the molecular weights, and m and n are the sizes of the oncogene and infective agent, respectively. Combining Equations 5.22 and 5.23, the acceptable range is

$$A = \left\{ \theta : 1 - \sum_{i=0}^{x_0-1} \frac{[N\lambda_{\tilde{X}}(\theta)]^i e^{-N\lambda_{\tilde{X}}(\theta)}}{i!} \sum_{j=0}^{y_0-1} \frac{[N\lambda_{\tilde{Y}}(\theta)]^j e^{-N\lambda_{\tilde{Y}}(\theta)}}{j!} < r_0 \right\}. \tag{5.24}$$

5.4.2.2 Applications

Yang et al. (2015b) applied the above method to establish acceptable ranges for the content and size of residual DNA for two products: a cell-based live, attenuated influenza vaccine and a monoclonal antibody. A detailed description of the application in the cell-based live, attenuated influenza vaccine is provided in Section 5.4.2.2.1.

5.4.2.2.1 Cell-Based Influenza Vaccine

The product is a cell-based live attenuated influenza vaccine with MDCK cell as the substrate for production. It was previously discussed in Section 5.3.4.2. The values of the parameters necessary for determining the acceptance range based on Equation 5.24 are listed in Table 5.3. The amounts of oncogenes and infective agent capable of inducing an oncogenic event and an infective event are assumed to be 9.4 and 2.5 µg, based on the research results by Sheng et al. (2008) and Peden et al. (2006), respectively. Suppose that there is one oncogene of size 1925 bp and one infective agent of size 7000 bp on the host genome. On the basis of these assumptions, estimates of x_0 and y_0 are 4.8×10^{12} molecules and 3.21×10^{12} molecules, respectively.

A plot of the probability function $\Pr\left[(\tilde{X} \geq x_0) \cup (\tilde{Y} \geq y_0) \middle| \theta\right]$ is shown in Figure 5.6. It is an increasing function in both DNA size and content. Assuming that the maximum risk is $r_0 = 10^{-9}$, which corresponds to a chance of 1 out of 100 million of having an event, the acceptable range is determined using Equation 5.24 and is depicted in Figure 5.7. It is interesting to note that the regulatory limit $\theta = (200 \text{ bp}, 10 \text{ ng})$ only has a probability less than 10^{-15} to have a serious adverse event.

The plot showing the acceptable range (Figure 5.7) is created as follows. Let $f(\theta) = \Pr\left[(\tilde{X} \geq x_0) \cup (\tilde{Y} \geq y_0) \middle| \theta\right]$. We define an indicator function $I(\theta)$ such that

TABLE 5.3

Quantities Used in Determining DNA Acceptable Ranges for Cell-Based, Live Attenuated Influenza Vaccine Example

Parameter	Value
Total number of annual doses (N)	50×10^6
Size of oncogene (m)	1925 bp
Size of infective agent (n)	7000 bp
Haploid size of MDCK genome (M)	2.41×10^9 bp
Number of intact oncogenes to induce an oncogenic event	4.8×10^{12} molecules
Number of intact infective agents to induce an infection	3.21×10^{12} molecules

Source: Yang, H., Wei, Z., and Schenerman, M. (2015b). A statistical approach to determining criticality of residual host cell DNA. *J. Biopharm. Stat.*, 25(2), 234–246.

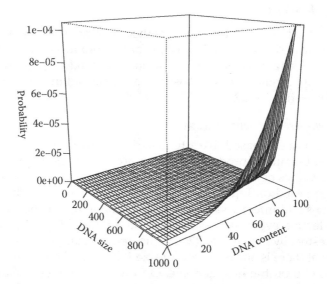

FIGURE 5.6
Plot of the probability for a cell-based influenza vaccine to cause either an oncogenic or an infective event out of a maximum of 50 million doses produced and used annually. That is, $N = 50 \times 10^6$ in Equation 5.21. (From Yang, H., Wei, Z., and Schenerman, M. (2015b). A statistical approach to determining criticality of residual host cell DNA. *J. Biopharm. Stat.*, 25(2), 234–246.)

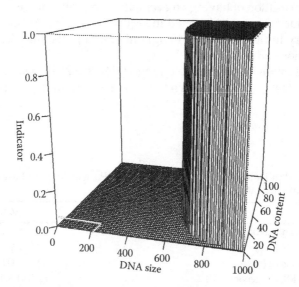

FIGURE 5.7
Acceptable range (dark area at the bottom of the plot) that corresponds to DNA size and content such that the indicator function $I(\theta) = 0$. It is much wider than the range shown as a rectangle defined by the regulatory limits. (From Yang, H., Wei, Z., and Schenerman, M. (2015b). A statistical approach to determining criticality of residual host cell DNA. *J. Biopharm. Stat.*, 25(2), 234–246.)

$$I(\theta) = \begin{cases} 0 & \text{if} & f(\theta) < 10^{-9}, \\ 1 & \text{if} & f(\theta) \geq 10^{-9}. \end{cases}$$

The acceptable range corresponds to $\theta = (\theta_S, \theta_U)$ satisfying $I(\theta) = 0$ and is shown in Figure 5.7. The range is considerably wider than the range defined by the regulatory limits, $\{(\theta_S, \theta_U): (\theta_S, \theta_U) \in [0, 200] \times [0, 10]\}$.

5.5 Bayesian Approach

The above methods are all based on the point estimate of a safety factor, which does not take into account variability in the estimates of the parameters involved in the calculations. Several remedies, such as bootstrapping, were suggested by Yang et al. (2010) to the estimate errors associated with the parameter estimates. The Taylor expansion can then be used to construct a confidence interval for the safety factor. Alternatively, a Bayesian analysis was used by Yang and Zhang (2016) to estimate the posterior probability that the safety factor will exceed a preselected limit. This method has the advantage of incorporating prior information regarding the parameters in the safety factor estimation. In addition, it also lends a probabilistic interpretation to the SF estimate.

5.5.1 Posterior Distribution

Let X, Y, and N be the amount of oncogene needed to induce an oncogenic event, the amount of oncogene in a final dose, and number of DNA segments in the final dose, respectively. It is further assumed that there are k genomes that go through the DNA inactivation process. Yang and Zhang (2016) modeled the total number of DNA segments in a final dose (N) using a binomial distribution with parameters $(k(M - 1), p)$, where p is the enzyme cutting efficiency and M is the total number of ester phosphate bonds in the host cell genome. Under the assumption that X_i, Y_i, and N_i are independently identically distributed, $i = 1, ..., n$, the joint distribution of X_i, Y_i, and N_i is the product of the distributions of the three component distributions:

$$X_i | O_m \sim N(O_m, 1/\tau),$$

$$Y_j | U \sim N(U, \delta),$$

$$f\left(N = t \mid p\right) = \Pr\left[N = t \mid p\right] = \binom{k(M-1)}{t-k} p^{t-k}(1-p)^{kM-t}, \ t = k, \ k+1, ..., kM,$$

where τ, expressed as the reciprocal of variance, is referred to as precision in the literature. Now, consider the parameters $\theta = (O_m, \tau, U, \tau_1, p)$ to follow the conjugate prior distributions

$$O_m \mid \tau \sim N(O_0, n_0\tau),$$

$$\tau \sim \text{Gamma } (\alpha, \beta),$$

$$U \mid \tau_1 \sim N(U_0, n_1\tau_1),$$

$$\tau_1 \sim \text{Gamma } (\alpha_1, \beta_1), \text{ and}$$

$$p \sim \text{Beta } (a, b),$$

where n_0 and n_1 are hyper-parameters. It can be easily verified that

$$O_m \mid X, \ \tau \propto N\left(\frac{n}{n+n_0}\bar{X} + \frac{n_0}{n+n_0}O_0, \ n\tau + n_0\tau\right),$$

$$\tau \mid X \propto \text{Gamma}\left(\alpha + \frac{n}{2}, \ +\beta + \frac{1}{2}\sum_{i=1}^{n}(X_i - \bar{X})^2 + \frac{nn_0}{2(n+n_0)}(\bar{X} - O_0)^2\right),$$

$$U \mid Y, \ \tau_1 \propto N\left(\frac{n}{n+n_1}\bar{Y} + \frac{n_1}{n+n1}U_0, \ n\tau_1 + n_1\tau_1\right),$$

$$\tau_1 \mid Y \propto \text{Gamma}\left(\alpha_1 + \frac{n}{2}, \ +\beta_1 + \frac{1}{2}\sum_{i=1}^{n}(Y_i - \bar{Y})^2 + \frac{nn_1}{2(n+n_1)}(\bar{Y} - U_0)^2\right), \text{ and}$$

$$p \mid N \propto \text{Beta}(a + N - k, \ b + kM - N) \tag{5.25}$$

are posterior distributions of the parameters $\theta = (O_m, \tau, U, \tau_1, p)$. As pointed out by Yang and Zhang (2016), a positive restriction can be placed on the normal prior distributions of O_m and U, as the two parameters must be positive. The posterior distribution of θ, $f(\theta \mid \tilde{X})$, can be calculated as the product of the density functions in Equation 5.25. This allows for estimating the posterior probability

$$\Pr\left[\text{SF} \geq \text{SF}_0 \middle| \tilde{X}\right] \geq P_0, \tag{5.26}$$

where P_0 is a preselected number between 0 and 1. The above probability can be estimated through simulation, in which random draws from the posterior distribution of θ are obtained, and the percentage of times that the inequality $\text{SF} \geq \text{SF}_0$ holds is calculated and compared to P_0. This percentage is an estimate of the probability in Equation 5.26. Because of the Law of Large Numbers Theorem, the estimate is consistent.

5.5.2 Example

Use of the method is illustrated through an example, with the following assumptions: the amount of oncogene (µg) needed to induce an oncogenic event follows the distribution $N(9.4, 2)$ and the amount of oncogene (ng/dose) in a final dose follows the distribution $N(1, 100)$, each quantity being measured for 20 times. In addition, the median size of residual DNA in a final dose is assumed to be 650 bp, while the haploid genome size of the MDCK genome is $M = 2.41 \times 10^9$ bp. Furthermore, we suppose that only one oncogene of size 1925 bp resides in the host cell genome. The prior distributions are chosen to be

$$O_m | \tau \sim N(0, 0.5\tau),$$

$$\tau \sim \text{Gamma}\,(0.001, 0.001),$$

$$U | \tau_1 \sim N(0, 0.5\tau_1),$$

$$\tau_1 \sim \text{Gamma}\,(0.001, 0.001),$$

$$p \sim \text{Beta}\,(0.5, 0.5). \tag{5.27}$$

On the basis of Equations 5.26 and 5.27, the posterior distributions in Equation 5.25 are obtained, as well as their joint distribution. Ten thousand random draws are made, and the safety factor SF is estimated. Assume that the acceptance limit SF_0 is 10^{11} and the cutoff value is $P_0 = 0.999$. The estimated posterior probability on the left-hand side of Equation 5.26 is 1. Therefore, the oncogenic risk is deemed to be acceptable.

To ascertain robustness of this approach with respect to prior specification, Yang and Zhang (2016) conducted a sensitivity analysis, in which various

TABLE 5.4

Results of Sensitivity Analysis Evaluating the Effects of Hyper-Parameter Prior Specification on the Posterior Probability Estimation $\Pr\left[\,SF \geq SF_0 \big| \tilde{X}\,\right]$

Prior Distribution Specification	Scenario									
	1	2	3	4	5	6	7	8	9	10
O_0	0	0	0	0	0	0	10	0	0	0
n_0	0.5	0.5	0.5	0.5	0.5	0.01	0.5	0.5	0.5	5
U_0	0	0	0	0	0	0	0	5	3	0
n_1	0.5	0.5	0.5	0.5	0.5	0.5	0.5	0.5	5	0.5
α	0.001	0	1	0.001	0.001	0.001	0.001	0.001	0.001	0.001
β	0.001	0	0.1	0.001	0.001	0.001	0.001	0.001	0.001	0.001
α_1	0.001	0	0.001	1	0.1	0.001	0.001	0.001	0.001	0.001
β_1	0.001	0	0.001	0.1	1	0.001	0.001	0.001	0.001	0.001
a	0.5	5	0.5	0.5	0.5	0.5	0.5	0.5	0.5	0.5
b	0.5	1	0.5	0.5	0.5	0.5	0.5	0.5	0.5	0.5
SF(Mean) ($\times 10^{10}$)	22.57	22.57	22.57	22.58	22.70	23.12	23.17	20.42	16.05	18.51
SF(SD) ($\times 10^{10}$)	1.32	1.32	1.29	1.38	2.19	1.04	1.04	3.06	10.17	2.34
Prob ($SF \geq SF_0$)	1.00	1.00	1.00	1.00	1.00	1.00	1.00	1.00	0.9998	0.9996

Source: Yang, H. and Zhang, J. (2016). A Bayesian approach to residual host cell DNA safety assessment. *PDA J. Pharm. Sci. Technol.*, 70, 157–162.

specifications of the hyper-parameter distributions were evaluated (see Table 5.4). The results show the following: (1) the hyper-parameters a and b have the least effect on the results; (2) the safety factor was also insensitive to the hyper-parameters ($\alpha\beta\alpha_1$, and β_1); (3) the greatest impact was found when the pair (O_0, n_0) or (U_0, n_1) was set such that the prior for O_m or U was informative as in scenarios 7–9; and finally (4) even when the posterior distribution of the safety factor changed quite a bit as a result of changing the priors, the probability $\Pr\left[\,SF \geq SF_0 \big| \tilde{X}\,\right]$ was above the acceptance limit of 0.999 in all cases.

5.6 Concluding Remarks

Because it is theoretically possible that cell substrates contain oncogenes and viral genes, the residual DNA in a biological product has the potential to transmit genetic information for cancer-causing and infective agents to the product recipient. To mitigate such risks, various purification steps are taken during manufacturing to remove residual DNA. It is also a regulatory requirement to assess oncogenic and infective risk associated with residual

DNA in the final product. Although the regulatory guidelines recommend limits of 10 ng/dose for content and 200 bp for size of residual DNA in the final product, scientific justification of these limits remains unclear. In recent years, there has been an increasing regulatory trend toward using risk-based methods to assess oncogenic and infective potentials of residual DNA in biological products. This makes it possible to potentially have different acceptance limits for different products, in light of enhanced technology, deeper understanding, and scientifically relevant data. However, the burden lies with the manufacturer to provide adequate justification for limits that differ from those conventionally used.

Several strategies for risk assessment of oncogenicity and infectivity including estimation of safety factors and establishment of acceptable limits for the size and content of residual DNA are described in this chapter, based on statistical modeling. In practice, application of these models requires careful consideration of the validity of the model based on both experimental data and mechanistic understanding of the manufacturing processes.

6

Evaluations of Viral Clearance

6.1 Introduction

Another objective of the downstream purification process is viral clearance. Most biological products are produced from cell substrates and raw materials known to harbor adventitious agents. In addition, viral contamination may arise from other sources. For example, adventitious viruses can be introduced into the final product during production, and viral contamination imposes a serious manufacturing risk and needs to be strictly controlled. Therefore, there is a potential for viral contamination of biological products, and it is necessary to assess the capability of the purification process.

Various regulatory guidelines that stress the importance of viral safety evaluation in biological products when derived from cell lines of either human or animal origin exist (European Medicines Agency [EMA] 1996, 1997, 2001; Food and Drug Administration [FDA] 1993, 1997, 2010). Although originally only a small number of known viruses in production cell lines were of regulatory concern, today viral testing is required to be performed to detect a broad range of viruses in cell banks, unprocessed bulk products, and fortified bulk products (Darling 2000). In ICH Q5A (R1) (EMA 1997), three principal approaches are specifically recommended to mitigate the risk of viral contamination. They include (1) testing cell lines and other raw materials, (2) assessing the effectiveness of the production process to remove or inactivate viral contaminants, and (3) testing the product at various steps of production to detect viral presence. Similar recommendations are made by the FDA (1997). There are also two EMA guidelines on virus safety: (1) Virus Safety Evaluation of Biotechnological Investigational Medicinal Products (EMA 2006), requiring that before Phase I studies, it must be demonstrated that any virus or viral particle known to be present in the bulk harvest has been effectively inactivated or removed during downstream processing, and (2) Guideline on Quality of Biotechnological Products: Viral Safety Evaluation of Biotechnology Products Derived from Cells or Animal Origin (EMA 1997), which recommends that a specific level of viral reduction be achieved.

Viral clearance studies are intended to assess the capability of a manufacturing process to inactivate or remove potential viral contaminants. These studies are carried out using materials artificially spiked with infectious viruses. Viral clearance evaluation plays a central role in the overall viral risk control, as detection of viruses at low viral concentrations is challenging in cell line characterization, in raw material qualification, and at various steps of production. To enable accurate assessment of production capability, the spiked samples used in viral clearance studies are typically at concentrations much higher than what would be encountered in ordinary circumstances. Analytical methods are used to quantify infectious viruses before and after each step of the purification process. The process capability is characterized either by the viral reduction factor (RF), which is the ratio of the amounts of viruses before and after each step, or log reduction (LR), defined as the difference in log10 virus titers before and after each step. These estimates are often variable owing to inherently large variability in the viral detection methods. To render a conservative estimate of process capability, it is required that the lower bound of the two-sided 95% confidence interval (CI) on RF or LR be used as the estimate of process effectiveness per ICH Q5A (R1) (EMA 1997). In this chapter, we primarily concern ourselves with statistical methods for assessing the capability of the production process in viral removal. Statistical methods robust to both missing data and zero viral counts postprocess are presented along with results of simulation studies conducted to compare the performance of current and new statistical methods. These results provide practical guidance on the selection of statistical methods for assessing process capability for viral clearance.

6.2 Viral Clearance Studies

The purpose of a viral clearance study is to provide documented evidence that a purification process is capable of inactivating or removing infectious viruses. These studies are conducted at selected steps in the process, using spiked samples with large amounts of infectious viruses. The studies are, in general, composed of several steps, including (1) selection of appropriate viruses, (2) selection of process steps at which virus spike takes place, (3) scale-down of the process steps, (4) evaluation of cytotoxicity and viral interference, (5) spiking experiments and collection of process samples, and (6) calculation of overall reduction factor or log reduction, expressed as the sum of the logarithm of the reductions at each step. Careful implementation of the above steps amounts to a cost-effective and high-quality viral clearance study.

The spiked virus is usually less than 10% of the volume of the starting material (Darling et al. 1998). Central to the determination of the optimum spiked virus volume is the balance between maximization of the amount of virus and retention of characteristics of the starting materials, in terms of pH, ionic strength, and protein concentration, as noted by Darling et al. (1998). Viral loads before and after each step of the purification process are estimated, and the effectiveness of the process is characterized, using the log difference in viral load, which is referred to as the viral reduction factor (RF). Per regulatory requirements, the lower bound of the two-sided 95% CI of RF should be used as an estimate of the process capability, which represents a more conservative estimate of the process effectiveness than the point estimate.

6.2.1 Choices of Viruses for Viral Clearance Evaluation

The selection of viruses for the viral clearance study requires several considerations, including the nature and origin of starting and raw materials, reagents used in the purification process, and stage of clinical development (Darling 2000; Zhou 2011). Where possible, viruses closely resembling those that were found to contaminate the cell substrate or any other reagents or materials used in the product process should be used. When such viruses are either not available or unsuited (e.g., because of low titers), model viruses should be used. In addition, it is also advisable that viruses representing a wide range of physicochemical properties are used to test the ability of the process to inactivate or remove viral material. The number of viruses used for the viral clearance study correlates with the stage of the clinical development. In general, the later the phase of the clinical studies, the broader the range of virus types that are required.

6.2.2 Selection of Process Steps

Usually, multiple viral clearance steps are used in a biological product manufacturing process. Considerations for selecting the process steps for a virus-spiking experiment include the mechanism(s) of clearance, expected effectiveness of the step, its reproducibility, and ease of scale-down. As noted by Darling (2000), pH inactivation, heat treatment, solvent detergent treatment, and physical removal by sterilizing grade filters are robust purification steps for which validation and scale-down are relatively simple to accomplish. A robust step not only has the ability to remove a wide range of viruses but also is less influenced by process parameters such as pH, protein concentration, and buffer types (Zhou 2011) than a less robust step. To ensure adequate assessment of each step, a sufficient concentration of viruses should be added to the material of the step to be tested.

6.2.3 Scale-Down of Process Steps

Since current good manufacturing processes prohibit viral clearance evaluation using the actual production scale, it is necessary to scale down the process steps so that effectiveness of the steps can be assessed in a laboratory setting. The ability to extrapolate results from the scale-down model to the actual production scale is influenced by how closely the scale-down steps mimic the full-scale manufacturing process. Therefore, it is critical to demonstrate the validity of the scale-down steps. For example, to scale down a chromatographic test, column bed size, flow rate, flow rate–to–bed size ratio, buffer and gel types, pH, temperature, and concentration of protein, salt, and product should be shown to be representative of full-scale production (ICH Q5A (R1) 1997). The impact of scale on viral clearance must be discussed, should there be any deviations.

6.2.4 Evaluation of Cytotoxicity and Viral Interference

The product and buffer(s) may be cytotoxic to the cells used in the assay detection system, thus resulting in overestimation of the efficiency of the process step. In addition, viruses that are present in the product may interfere with the assay system to cause an unduly optimistic estimate of the process step's viral clearance efficiency. Therefore, it is necessary to evaluate the effect of the test samples on the assay system. This in general is done through serial dilutions of the test samples. The diluted samples are incubated with the host cells in the assay system to determine cytotoxicity and interference. Dilution levels at which either cytotoxic or viral interfering effects are observed are excluded while those with no observed negative effect will be used for spiking experiments.

6.2.5 Spiking Experiments and Collection of Process Samples

Viral spiking experiments are performed using the scale-down process steps. For each step, samples spiked with a high volume of virus are processed. Both the original spiked samples and the processed samples are diluted to reduce cytotoxic and viral interfering effect, as noted in Section 6.2.4, before being assayed. Depending on the type of process step being evaluated, different sample collection schemes may be required. For example, for virus inactivation studies, it is of interest to study the kinetics of the inactivation step. Therefore, samples are collected both before the treatment and at various times posttreatment. By contrast, for virus removal experiments, it is important to examine the distribution of virus through testing for virus in the spiked samples and in product fractions. It is important to note that the process samples should be titrated immediately after collection to ensure accurate assessment of virus titers. If this is not possible, samples should be frozen before titration, with proper controls.

6.2.6 Calculation of Process Capability

Statistical methods should be used to evaluate results from viral clearance studies (ICH Q5A (R1)). Virus titers both before and after each process step studied should be estimated. To account for variability in both the sample and assay system, it is required that the results are reported using a 95% CI.

6.3 Assays for Viral Quantification

Various assays have been used for detection and quantification of viral loads. Most common are the plaque-forming assay and the cytopathic effect (CPE) assay. Since the validity of the statistical evaluations of viral clearance data is dependent on the assay used for quantifying viral titer, the assay must be validated for various performance characteristics including accuracy, precision, linearity, limit of quantification, and limit of detection. For this purpose, statistical methods described in Chapters 2 through 4 can be used. To minimize the variability of the assay results, replication strategies can be used (Darling 2000).

6.3.1 Plaque-Forming Assay

As mentioned above, plaque-forming assay is one of the most commonly used methods for determining the quantity of infectious virus in a sample. To perform the assay, a series of 10-fold dilutions of the original sample are made. Aliquots of the preparations, often in duplicate or triplicate, are inoculated onto susceptible cell monolayers. Consequently, plaques are formed as a result of viral infections. The number of plaques are counted, each representing one plaque-forming unit (PFU), to determine the viral titer as the number of PFUs per sample volume (PFU/mL). Figure 6.1 depicts the steps

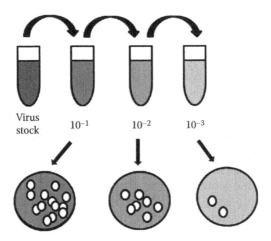

FIGURE 6.1
Plaque assay.

TABLE 6.1

Results of a Plaque Assay (Sample Aliquot Volume = 0.2 mL)

Dilution	Number of PFU/Plate		
10^{-3}	40	39	36
10^{-4}	6	2	2
10^{-5}	1	0	0
10^{-6}	0	0	0

involved in a plaque assay. At lower dilutions, the plaques can be too numerous to count and it may take two to five 10-fold dilutions to yield countable plaques (including 0). The virus titer in the original sample is calculated as PFU/mL, using the observations at the higher dilutions, where counting is possible.

A titer estimation method using a plaque-forming assay was described by Darling through an example (1998). In general, we assume that the assay consists of J dilutions and K aliquots at the jth dilution, each having a volume of v_j of the original sample. The method is illustrated using the data in Table 6.1. Since each aliquot has a volume of 0.2 mL at each dilution level, assuming that the jth dilution is obtained through j 10-fold dilutions of the original sample, a 0.2-mL sample at this dilution level is equivalent to $v_j = 0.2 \times 10^{-j}$ mL of the original stock.

The titer T_0 is determined as the ratio of the total number of plaques to the total volume of the original sample. That is,

$$T_0 = \frac{\sum_{j=1}^{J} \sum_{k=1}^{K} X_{ij}}{K \sum_{j=1}^{J} v_j}. \tag{6.1}$$

6.3.2 CPE Assay

The CPE assay, also referred to as the 50% tissue culture infectivity dose ($TCID_{50}$) assay, is a useful alternative to the plaque-forming assay when the virus does not cause plaques. It is an indirect assay as its titer does not directly relate to the amount of the virus in the original sample. Instead, it determines a dose level as the reciprocal of the dilution that infects 50% of inoculated cell monolayers, where infection is reflected by a positive CPE result. The $TCID_{50}$ is usually reported on the log scale ($\log_{10} TCID_{50}$) and is estimated using the Karber method, which will be described in Section 6.3.2.1.

6.3.2.1 Karber Method

Let X_i be the ith 1:10 dilution of the original undiluted test sample X_0. Define p_i to be the percentage of wells with positive CPE at the ith dilution and X_f and X_l denote the first and last dilutions such that $p_f = 0$ at X_f, $p_l = 1$ X_l. Using the Karber method, the $\log_{10}$ TCID$_{50}$ titer of the original test sample X_0 is given by (Finney 1978)

$$\log_{10} \text{TCID}_{50} = k - \left(0.5 - \sum_{i=f}^{l} p_i \right).$$

Since for the TCID$_{50}$ assay, at each dilution level, there are 8 wells tested for CPE, an estimate of p_i can be obtained as

$$\hat{p}_i = \text{total number of CPE positive wells/8}.$$

Hence, the $\log_{10}$ TCID$_{50}$ titer estimate for X_0 can be estimated by

$$\log_{10} \text{TCID}_{50} = k - \left(0.5 - \sum_{i=f}^{l} \hat{p}_i \right).$$

An example is given in Figure 6.2.

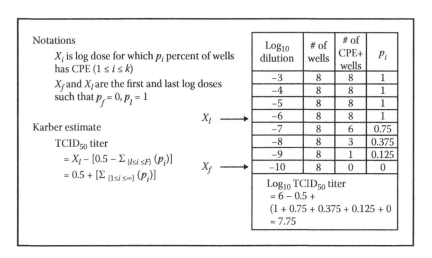

FIGURE 6.2
Calculation of viral titer based on the Karber method.

6.4 Virus Titer Estimation for Plaque-Forming Assays

The validity of the virus titer estimation depends on the appropriate use of statistical methods. In this section, several statistical methods are described. To provide practical guidance for selection of statistical methods, we also describe a simulation study by Li and Yang (2012) to compare the performance of various methods. It is also assumed that a plaque-forming assay is used for virus safety assessment although the statistical methods can be generalized to other assay systems.

6.4.1 Estimation Method Based on Normal Distribution

Assuming that the viral counts X_{jk} in Equation 6.1 are normally distributed, Darling et al. (1998) proposed that the viral titer be estimated using the formula in Equation 6.1. To assess the accuracy of the viral detection method, it is necessary to construct a CI for the viral titer. Let T be the viral titer of the original stock. Define $S_x = \sum_{J=1}^{J} \sum_{K=1}^{K} X_{jk}$ and $S_v = K \sum_{j=1}^{J} v_j$ as the total PFU count and total volume of the original sample used in the assay, respectively. Without loss of generality, we assume $K = 3$. Under the assumption that the PFU counts X_{jk} ($k = 1, 2, 3$) are independently and identically normally distributed as

$$X_{jk} \sim N\left(v_j, \sigma_j^2\right),$$

we have

$$S_x \sim N\left(3T \sum_{j=1}^{J} v_j, \ 3 \sum_{j=1}^{J} \sigma_j^2\right),$$

where T is the virus titer of the original stock.

Thus, the estimator T_0 for T in Equation 6.1 is also normally distributed:

$$T_0 \sim N\left(T, \ 3 \sum_{j=1}^{J} \sigma_j^2 / S_v^2\right).$$

Darling et al. (1998) suggested using the following as an approximate two-sided 95% CI estimate of the titer T_0:

$$T_0 \pm t_{2,0.975} \sqrt{3 \sum_{j=1}^{J} s_j^2 / S_v^2}, \qquad (6.2)$$

where $t_{2,0.975}$ is the 97.5th percentile of a t distribution with 2 degrees of freedom and s_j^2 is the sample variance based on three samples tested at the jth dilution level. The degrees of freedom of the t distribution was chosen to be 2 although there is no justification for it.

Applying the δ method and after some algebraic manipulations, it can be shown (Li and Yang 2012) that an approximately two-sided 95% CI for $\log_{10}T$ is given by

$$\log_{10} T_0 \pm t_{2,0.975} \times 0.434 \sqrt{3 \sum_{j=1}^{J} s_j^2/S_x} \,. \tag{6.3}$$

Using the data in Table 6.1, it can be calculated that $T_0 = 1.89 \times 10^5$ and $\sqrt{3 \sum_{j=1}^{J} s_j^2/S_x} = 0.0433$. Substituting these numbers into Equation 6.3, we obtained an approximate two-sided 95% CI (5.20, 5.36). It is worth reiterating that construction of the above CI relies on the assumption that the statistic $T_0/\sqrt{3 \sum_{j=1}^{J} s_j^2/S_v^2}$ approximately follows a t distribution with 2 degrees of freedom. This assumption is only true when $j = 1$, that is, when there is only one step dilution of the original sample. Potentially a more serious drawback of the method by Darling et al. (1998) is its dependence on the normality assumption. This issue becomes more pronounced particularly when there are no nonzero plaque counts observed. This is usually the case when the purification process is highly effective. Under such circumstances, the method by Darling becomes unreliable for either viral titer or RF estimation. The Poisson distribution is often used to describe count data that spread uniformly in space. On the basis of this distribution, Li and Yang (2012) proposed two alternative approaches, which are described as follows.

6.4.2 Estimation Method Based on Poisson Distribution

Let X denote the number of viruses in a sample of volume v. Assume that there are a total of n viruses in the overall volume V of material to be tested. Let y_i be a random variable such that $y_i = 1$ if virus i is contained in v; otherwise $y_i = 0$. Further, let p denote $P[y_i = 1]$, and assume that y_i are independently and identically distributed. Therefore, $X = \sum_{i=1}^{n} y_i$ follows a binomial distribution. When v is small when compared to V, the distribution of X can be approximated by a Poisson distribution with a density function:

$$f(x;T) = \frac{(vT)^x e^{-vT}}{x!},$$

where T is the titer of the original sample.

When the dilutions and aliquots are independely prepared, it is reasonable to assume that the X_{jk} in Equation 6.1 are independently distributed. Therefore, the total viral count S_x also follows a Poisson distribution, with mean TS_v.

6.4.2.1 Maximum Likelihood Estimate

The log likelihood function of $\{X_{jk}\}$ is given by

$$g(S_x; T) = S_x \log(vT) - \log(x!) - S_v T.$$

The maximum likelihood estimator (MLE) of T satisfies

$$\frac{\partial g(S_x; T)}{\partial T} = \frac{S_x}{T} - S_v = 0.$$

Solving the equation, we obtain the MLE of T:

$$T_0 = \frac{S_x}{S_v}.$$

Because

$$\mathrm{var}[T_0] = \mathrm{var}\left[\frac{S_x}{S_v}\right] = \frac{S_x}{S_v}\frac{\mathrm{var}[S_x]}{S_v^2} = \frac{TS_v}{S_v^2} = \frac{T}{S_v},$$

it can be estimated by

$$\hat{\mathrm{var}}[T_0] = \frac{T_0}{S_v}.$$

When the total virus count S_x is large, the MLE T_0 is approximately normally distributed. Consequently, a two-sided 95% CI for T can be obtained based on a normal approximation:

$$T_0 \pm z_{0.975}\sqrt{T_0/S_v}, \tag{6.4}$$

where $z_{0.975}$ is the 97.5th percentile of the standard normal distribution. Note that the variance of $\log_{10} T_0$ can be estimated by

$$\mathrm{var}[\log_{10} T_0] \approx \log_{10} e(1/T_0)\,\mathrm{var}[T_0]. \tag{6.5}$$

Combining Equations 6.4 and 6.5 and using the data from Table 6.1,

$$\hat{\text{var}}[\log_{10} T_0] = 0.434^2 / S_x,$$

where we use the fact that $\log_{10} e = 0.434$.

It is apparent that an approximate two-sided 95% CI for $\log_{10} T$ is given by

$$\log_{10} T_0 \pm z_{0.975} \times 0.434\sqrt{1/S_x}. \tag{6.6}$$

6.4.2.2 Exact Estimate for Poisson Method

The above approximation works well if the total viral count S_x is large. When S_x is small, the normal approximation is inaccurate, and applying it may result in an excessively wide 95% CI for the titer estimate, giving rise to an underestimate of the process capability. As a remedy, Li and Yang (2012) provided an exact method to construct the CI. The method is based on inverting an equal-tailed test for the hypothesis regarding the Poisson mean parameter λ, using a technique described by Casella and Berger (2002):

$$H_0: \lambda = \lambda_0. \tag{6.7}$$

Upon observing S_x, suppose we choose (S_L, S_U) such that S_L is the largest number satisfying

$$\sum_{s=0}^{S_x} \frac{S_L^s e^{-S_L}}{s!} \leq \alpha/2$$

and S_U is the largest number satisfying

$$\sum_{s=0}^{S_x} \frac{S_U^s e^{-S_U}}{s!} \geq 1 - \alpha/2;$$

the exact Poisson confidence limits for the viral titer T and $\log_{10} T$ are given by

$$\left(\frac{S_L}{S_v}, \frac{S_U}{S_v} \right) \tag{6.8}$$

TABLE 6.2

The Exact Poisson 95% Confidence Limits for $S_x \leq 5$

Total Observed PFUs	95% CI	
S_x	S_L	S_U
0	0	3.689
1	0.025	5.572
2	0.242	7.225
3	0.619	8.767
4	1.090	10.242
5	1.623	11.668

Source: Li, N. and Yang, H. (2012). Statistical evaluations of viral clearance studies for biological products. *Biologicals*, 40(6), 439–444.

and

$$\left(\log_{10} \frac{S_L}{S_v}, \ \log_{10} \frac{S_U}{S_v} \right), \tag{6.9}$$

respectively.

When $S_x = 0$, that is, there are no observable plaques, the lower limit $S_L = 0$ and the upper limit $S_U = -\log(\alpha/2)$. Standard software packages such as exact CI in R (Fay 2010) can be used to calculate the exact Poisson CI. For ease of application, the limits can be determined and provided in a look-up table such as Table 6.2.

6.4.2.3 Poisson Regression

Under the Poisson model introduced above, we can write a Poisson regression model with intercept only:

$$\log X_{jk} = \log v_{jk} + \alpha,$$

where X_{jk} is the plaque count and $\log v_{jk}$ is a fixed offset with v_{jk} being the sample aliquot volume. The intercept parameter $\alpha = \log T$ is the (natural) log titer. Thus, $\log_{10} T = 0.434\alpha$. This model can be fit using standard software such as the glm() function in R. This formula gives identical results to the large-sample Poisson model previously discussed. One potential advantage of the regression model is that it makes it possible to estimate overdispersion, which occurs when the variance of the plaque count is larger than what is expected under the Poisson model. Overdispersion may be present if the viral particles tend to cluster together in the solution or if there is correlation due to error in making dilutions, especially when the titer is high. More elaborate Poisson regression models have been proposed by Faddy and Smith (2008) to analyze serial dilution assays.

6.5 Reduction Factor Estimation

6.5.1 Approximate CI

Process capability is measured by log reduction of viral load (LRF, log reduction factor). For each process step, the reduction factor and associated variance can be estimated by

$$\text{LRF} = \log_{10} T_{01} - \log_{10} T_{02}$$

$$\text{var}[\text{LRF}] = \text{var}[\log_{10} T_{01}] + \text{var}[\log_{10} T_{02}] \approx \log_{10} e(1/S_{x1} + 1/S_{x2}).$$

When the total viral counts are relatively large, use of a normal approximation to estimate the LRF is appropriate. In such cases, an approximate two-sided 95% CI for LRF is given by

$$\log_{10} T_{01} - \log_{10} T_{02} \pm z_{0.975} \times 0.434\sqrt{1/S_{x1} + 1/S_{x2}}, \tag{6.10}$$

where T_{01} and T_{02} denote viral titers before and after the reduction process step, respectively.

When the normality assumption does not hold well, we could construct an approximate two-sided 95% CI for LRF by using the half-widths of the two-sided 95% CIs for the titers before and after process, as suggested in ICH Q5A (R1) (1999). That is, the interval is obtained as

$$\log_{10} T_{01} - \log_{10} T_{02} \pm \sqrt{\text{HW}_1^2 + \text{HW}_2^2}, \tag{6.11}$$

where HW_1 and HW_2 are the half-widths of the two-sided 95% CIs for the starting material titer and titer after the step, respectively.

When multiple viral clearance steps, say, n, are utilized, the overall process capability is estimated as the sum of capabilities from all the steps. That is,

$$\text{LRF} = \sum_{i=1}^{n} \text{LRF}_i.$$

An approximate two-sided 95% CI can also be obtained as

$$\text{LRF} \pm z_{0.975}\sqrt{\sum_{i=1}^{n} \text{HW}_i^2} \tag{6.12}$$

where HW_i represents the half-width of the two-sided 95% CI for the ith process step.

6.5.2 Exact CI

An exact CI for RF can be obtained by using the well-known fact that conditional on the sum of two independent Poisson variables, either variable has a binomial distribution (Lehmann and Romano 2005). Specifically, let $S_T = S_{x1} + S_{x2}$, where S_{x1} and S_{x2} are the total plaque counts in the before- and after-process samples, respectively. Let $\psi = T_1/T_2$. Thus,

$$S_{x1}|S_T = t \sim \text{Binomial } (p(\psi), t),$$

where

$$p(\psi) = \frac{S_{v_1}\psi}{S_{v_1}\psi + S_{v_2}}. \tag{6.13}$$

Similar to the construction of an exact CI for the Poisson mean parameter, exact $(1 - \alpha/2) \times 100\%$ confidence limits for $p(\psi)$ are obtained by finding p_L and p_U such that

$$\sum_{s=S_{x1}}^{S_T} \binom{S_T}{s} p_L^s (1-p_L)^{S_T-s} = \alpha/2$$

$$\sum_{s=0}^{S_{x1}} \binom{S_T}{s} p_U^s (1-p_U)^{S_T-s} = \alpha/2. \tag{6.14}$$

Note that (Johnson et al. 2005)

$$\sum_{s=S_{x1}}^{S_T} \binom{S_T}{s} p^s (1-p_L)^{S_T-s} = \int_0^p b(x, S_{x1}, S_T - S_{x1} + 1)dx, \tag{6.15}$$

where $b(x, S_{x1}, S_T - S_{x1} + 1)$ is the density function of a beta random variable. The lower and upper confidence limits can be obtained by numerically solving the following equations:

$$\int_0^p b(x, S_{x1}, S_T - S_{x1} + 1)dx = \alpha/2$$

$$\int_0^p b(x, S_{x1} + 1, S_T - S_{x1})dx = 1 - \alpha/2.$$

In other words,

$$(p_L, p_U) = \left(B_{S_{x1}, S_T - S_{x1} + 1}(\alpha/2), \ B_{S_{x1} + 1, S_T - S_{x1}}(1 - \alpha/2) \right),$$

where $B_{S_{x1}, S_T - S_{x1} + 1}(\alpha/2)$ and $B_{S_{x1} + 1, S_T - S_{x1}}(1 - \alpha/2)$ are the $100 \times (\alpha/2)$th and $100 \times (1 - \alpha/2)$th percentiles of two beta distributions with parameters $(S_{x1}, S_T - S_{x1} + 1)$ and $(S_{x1} + 1, S_T - S_{x1})$, respectively.
From Equation 6.13,

$$\psi = \frac{p(\psi) S_{v_2}}{[1 - p(\psi)] S_{v_1}}.$$

Because ψ is monotonically increasing in $P(\psi)$, the 95% CI for ψ is given by

$$\left(\frac{p_L}{1 - p_L} \frac{S_{v2}}{S_{v1}}, \ \frac{p_U}{1 - p_U} \frac{S_{v2}}{S_{v1}} \right). \tag{6.16}$$

6.6 Comparisons of Estimation Methods

6.6.1 Simulations

A simulation study was carried out by Li and Yang (2013) to compare the performance of the statistical methods to estimate viral clearance discussed in the previous sections. The performance of a statistical method to calculate a CI is characterized by how closely its coverage probability is to the nominal level. Coverage probability is the proportion of times the CI covers the true mean parameter. An interval estimate is considered accurate if its coverage probability is close to its nominal level. An interval with a coverage probability smaller than the nominal level is more conservative than the one that has a coverage probability greater or equal to the nominal level. In the context of process capability assessment, a conservative estimate is advantageous from a regulatory point of view, but inflates the producer risk.

PFU data were simulated based on a Poisson model with mean parameter ranging from 3.5 to 6.0 on the $\log_{10}$ scale, at 0.1 increments. The plaque assay involves three 10:1 dilutions. In total, 10,000 data sets were simulated for each mean viral titer. For each data set, all five methods previously introduced were used to estimate the titer, RF, or LRF, and its associated two-sided 95% CI. The results are shown in Figure 6.3.

It is evident that using 6 degrees of freedom renders a CI that is too narrow, resulting in coverages close to 90% as opposed to the nominal level 95%.

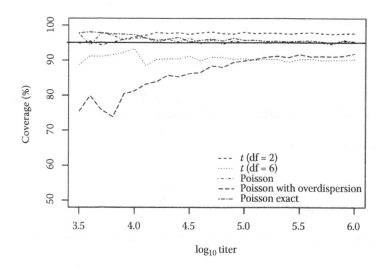

FIGURE 6.3
Coverage of titer CIs calculated by different methods. The horizontal line corresponds to the nominal 95% coverage. (From Li, N. and Yang, H. (2012). Statistical evaluations of viral clearance studies for biological products. *Biologicals*, 40(6), 439–444.)

Therefore, the method, consistently under covering the true titer values, is most imprecise. The t distribution with 2 degrees of freedom is second most imprecise at higher titers between 4.5 and 6.0 because its coverage probability consistently exceeds the nominal level 95% though it performs comparably well at low titers as the approximate and exact Poisson methods. The CIs based on either the approximate or exact Poisson method are slightly conservative at lower titers and approaches exact 95% coverage at higher titers. It is well known that exact CIs tend to be conservative because of the discreteness of the distribution but they do guarantee that the coverage is at least the nominal level. It should be noted that although the t distribution and approximate Poisson approaches work reasonably well at low titers, they are not applicable when the total PFU count is zero, which happened approximately 12% of the time in our simulation study. As shown in Table 6.3, when the total PFU count is less than 5, although the exact Poisson CI is conservative, the normal (t) distribution-based method may be too liberal (the interval is too narrow and the coverage percentage is less than the nominal 95%) at times. To ensure product safety, it might be better to use the conservative exact Poisson CI when the total PFU count is less than 5.

6.6.2 Example

Li and Yang (2012) applied the statistical methods for estimating viral titers discussed in this chapter to the results of a plaque assay presented in Table 6.1. The estimated virus titers along with associated two-sided 95% CIs are

TABLE 6.3

Estimates for Viral Titer before and after Processing (on Log_{10} Scale)

Sample	Method	Estimate	SE	95% CI HW	95% LCI	95% UCI
Before	Normal	5.277	0.019	0.081	5.195	5.358
	Poisson	5.277	0.039	0.076	5.201	5.352
	Poisson regression	5.277	0.026	0.052	5.225	5.328
	Poisson exact	5.277			5.197	5.352
After 1	Normal	1.357	0.087	0.374	0.983	1.730
	Poisson	1.357	0.112	0.220	1.137	1.576
	Poisson exact	1.357			1.104	1.574
After 2	Poisson exact	$-\infty$			$-\infty$	−0.256

Source: Li, N. and Yang, H. (2012). Statistical evaluations of viral clearance studies for biological products. *Biologicals*, 40(6), 439–444.

Note: The CIs are calculated based on t_2 distribution for the normal model.

listed in Table 6.3. It is apparent that results based on the normal model, the approximate Poisson model, and the exact Poisson intervals are comparable for the assay results of the starting material. This is primarily attributed to the relatively large total viral count (126 PFU/mL) in the starting material. However, for the "After 1" sample, as the total PFU count is reduced to 15, the normal-based CI is wider, thus overestimating viral titer after the process step(s). The approximate and exact Poisson methods continue to have comparable performance, giving rise to similar CIs to the normal method. When the total PFU count is 0, as in the "After 2" sample, only the exact Poisson CI can be calculated.

The RF and its two-sided 95% CI were also calculated, using the three methods discussed previously. The results on the log_{10} scale are summarized in Table 6.4. Similar observations can be made to the comparisons for the viral titer estimates: (1) the normal-based method is less accurate than either Poisson method, as evidenced by a wider CI; (2) the Poisson and exact Poisson methods have comparable performance; and (3) the exact Poisson is

TABLE 6.4

The LRF and Two-Sided 95% CIs for the Example Data in Table 6.1

Sample	Method	LRF	SE	Half-Width	Lower	Upper
Before–after 1	Normal	3.920	0.089	0.382	3.538	4.302
	Poisson	3.920	0.119	0.232	3.687	4.152
	Poisson regression	3.920	0.088	0.173	3.747	4.093
	Poisson exact	3.920			3.686	4.185
Before–after 2	Poisson exact	∞			5.527	∞

Source: Li, N. and Yang, H. (2012). Statistical evaluations of viral clearance studies for biological products. *Biologicals*, 40(6), 439–444.

the only method that can be used to estimate the RF when the postprocess total virus count is zero.

6.7 Concluding Remarks

Since most biological products are derived from cell lines, there is a potential risk of viral contamination. Such contamination may either arise from cell substrates themselves or adventitious introduction of virus during production. As viral contamination can have serious clinical consequences, its evaluation is required by regulatory guidelines. Statistical evaluation plays an important role in viral clearance study evaluation and is also recommended by regulatory guidance. In recent years, several statistical methods have been proposed for estimating viral titer and process capability for reducing viral load. The method by Darling et al. (1998) relies on a normality assumption. When the degrees of freedom is properly selected, it performs relatively well at the lower titer values. However, it underestimates process capability for higher titer values. Caution also needs to be exercised in applying Darling's method as its performance is strongly influenced by the choice of degrees of freedom. By contrast, the two Poisson-based methods consistently provide more accurate estimates of process capability than Darling's method when $\log_{10}$ titer exceeds 4. The exact Poisson method is the only approach that can be used to estimate process capability when there are no nonzero observations after the purification process.

7

Bioburden Testing and Control

7.1 Introduction

Bioburden is a measure of viable microbial contaminants associated with personnel, manufacturing environments (air and surfaces), product packaging, raw materials (including water), in-process materials, and finished products (Adley et al. 2015). Since drug substance manufacture is typically not sterile, bioburden can be introduced at any step of the manufacturing processes shown in Figure 7.1, from nonsterile raw materials, manual and mechanical handling of containers and closures, and the environment in which the product is processed. In addition, bioburden can contribute endotoxins and other impurities to the drug product, thus further compromising product quality.

Because of the public health implications of distributing a nonsterile product, bioburden control is subjected to a high level of regulatory scrutiny. In fact, issues related to bioburden control have been frequently cited in inspection findings by regulatory authorities, causing product recalls and shortages (Adley et al. 2015). Between 2004 and 2011, lack of sterility assurance topped the list of more than 600 microbiological-related FDA recalls (PDA 2015). Control of bioburden is not only a key component of quality systems but also a regulatory requirement (European Medicines Agency [EMA] 2012; Food and Drug Administration [FDA] 2004a,c). The Code of Federal Regulations (CFR) states that "Appropriate written procedures, designed to prevent microbiological contamination of drug products purporting to be sterile, shall be established and followed. Such procedures shall include validation of any sterilization process" (21 CFR 211.113(b)). The FDA Guidance for Industry: Sterile Drug Products Produced by Aseptic Processing (FDA 2004c) stipulates that all unit operations of aseptic processing must be designed, monitored, and controlled for bioburden to ensure production of sterile products. Figure 7.2 shows the quality system components related to aseptic unit operations. Each unit/responsible area should develop effective bioburden control strategies to ensure regulatory compliance and product quality. Key to achieving this objective are several critical steps: (1) understand the process and product, and associated bioburden risk at each unit

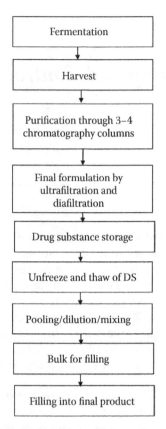

FIGURE 7.1
Process flow diagram for the manufacture of a sterile liquid drug product.

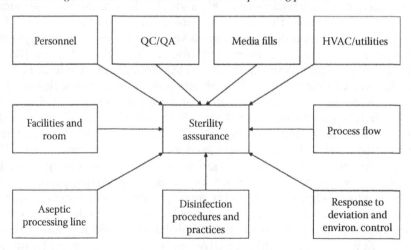

FIGURE 7.2
Quality system components in aseptic product manufacturing.

operation in the manufacturing process; (2) identify factors that affect the risk at each unit operation; (3) develop bioburden control strategies, including sampling plans microbiological testing, and so on; and (4) implement a quality risk management process. It is worth noting that bioburden risk and risk tolerance may vary from product to product. Therefore, risk control strategies need to be developed on a case-by-case basis, from a holistic perspective. Suffice it to say that it is essential to adopt a risk-based approach to establishing effective bioburden control strategies.

Development of a holistic approach to bioburden control has been discussed in the literature (Adley et al. 2015) and is not our primary focus. This chapter is intended to describe a risk-based approach to bioburden control in aseptic processing, emphasizing the importance of risk identification, statistical analysis, and control. This approach is centered on understanding the bioburden risk factors in aseptic processing, their relationships to bioburden risk, and the development of control strategies from a holistic perspective. By modeling bioburden in both the unfiltered and filtered drug solution, the relationships between prefiltration/postfiltration risk and the associated risk factors, such as test sample volume (batch size), are established. Such relationships allow for a quantitative evaluation of the impact of the risk factors on the risks and the development of effective risk control strategies, which include appropriate selections of sample test volume, maximum prefiltration bioburden level, batch size for final sterilizing filtration, and so on. It is shown that prefiltration bioburden test volumes and acceptance limits other than the regulatory requirement of 10 colony-forming units (CFU)/100 mL may be justified, without compromising sterility assurance.

7.2 Regulatory Guidelines

There are several regulatory guidelines concerning the production of sterile liquid products. In 2004, the FDA published a guidance entitled "Guidance for Industry: Sterile Drug Products Produced by Aseptic Processing—Current Good Manufacturing Practice." It discusses primarily current good manufacturing practice (cGMP) issues of finished drug product while providing limited information on upstream bulk processing steps. It dedicates an entire section to the validation of aseptic processing and sterilization. The EMA also issued several guidelines on the manufacture of bulk drug substance and finished dosage forms, including *Note for Guidance on Manufacture of the Finished Dosage Form* (EMA 1996) and *Guideline on the Requirements for Quality Document Concerning Biological Investigational Medicinal Products in Clinical Trials* (EMA 2012). Although the former does not pertain to biological drug products, like the latter, it discusses the use of sterilizing filters and related requirements. However, as pointed out by Jornitz et al. (2003), the guidelines issued by the FDA and EMA are not in full agreement on the requirements of sterile filtration. For example, the FDA guidance emphasizes the retention capability of sterilizing filters in bioburden control and validation of the filter using the microorganism *Brevundimonas diminuta* under worst-case conditions, whereas the EMA guidance focuses more on control of the bioburden level before the final filtration step, with no mention of organism species and worst-case conditions. In this section, we highlight key requirements of the FDA and EMA guidance documents regarding sterile filtration.

7.2.1 FDA Guidance

The bioburden risk control called for in the FDA guidance (FDA 2004c) relies on the retention capability of the final sterilizing filters. Therefore, the guidance specifically defines filters to be used for the final filtration and requires that the filters be validated. It states, "A sterilizing grade filter should be validated to reproducibly remove viable microorganisms from the process stream, producing a sterile effluent. Currently, such filters usually have a rated pore size of 0.2 μm or smaller." Filter validation usually includes microbiological challenges to the filter and an integrity test after the filtration. The guidance stresses the importance of conducting the validation experiment under worst-case production conditions. This includes the selection of a suitable challenge microorganism and setting factors that may potentially affect filter performance at their extremes. The guidance recommends the use of the microorganism *B. diminuta* at the concentration level of 10^7 CFU/cm^2 of effective filter area (EFA) for the validation experiments of 0.2/0.22-μm rated filters. It also lists nine factors that can be manipulated to simulate the worst-case condition. The factors include (1) viscosity and surface tension of the material to be filtered, (2) pH of the material to be filtered, (3) compatibility of the material or formulation components with the filter itself, (4) filtration pressures, (5) filtration flow rates, (6) maximum filter use time, (7) filtration temperature, (8) osmolality of the material, and (9) the effects of hydraulic shock. Noting that one sterilizing filter may not be sufficient, the guidance also suggests that the use of redundant sterilizing filters be considered and validated as well.

Furthermore, as bioburden can contribute endotoxin, metabolites, and other impurities to the drug product, causing additional safety concerns, the guidance stipulates "A prefiltration bioburden limit should be established." However, it does not prescribe any specific methods to establish an appropriate prefiltration bioburden limit.

7.2.2 EMA Perspective

By contrast, the EMA guidelines place less emphasis on the validation of sterilizing filters than FDA, although they do recommend the use of sterilizing filters for the final filtration step. As discussed above, there are factors other than the nominal pore size of the filter that may affect a filter performance; thus, it is critical to validate the retention capability of the filter through formal experiments. However, the EMA guidelines are very specific about their requirements for prefiltration bioburden testing and the associated acceptable limit(s). In both EMA CPMP *Notes for Guidance on Manufacture of Finished Dosage Form* and EMA *Guideline on the Requirements for Quality Documentation Concerning Biological Investigational Medicinal Products in Clinical Trials* (EMA 1996, 2012), it is stated, "[f]or sterilization by filtration the maximum acceptable bioburden prior to the filtration must be stated in the application. In most situations NMT 10 CFU/100 ml will be acceptable, depending on the volume to be filtered in relation to the diameter of the filter. If this requirement is not met, it is necessary to use a pre-filtration through a bacteria-retaining filter to obtain a sufficiently low bioburden." However, realizing that the batch size is likely small at an early stage of drug development, the EMA guideline further states, "Due to limited availability of the formulated medicinal product, a pre-filtration volume of less than 100 ml may be tested if justified" (EMA 2012).

7.2.3 Potential Limitations of Regulatory Standards

A critical review of regulatory requirements for sterile filtration was conducted by Jornitz et al. (2003). It was noted that there is no direct concordance between the FDA sterilizing filter requirement and the EMA maximum acceptable bioburden in the unfiltered drug solution. To highlight the incompatibility between the two regulatory requirements, several examples were provided by Jornitz et al. (2003). They noted that for a filter to achieve the FDA-required bioburden challenge of 10^7 CFU/cm^2 EFA using a suspension of no more than 10 CFU/100 mL, a batch size of 100,000 L would be needed. Alternatively, to exceed the retention capability, 10^7 CFU/cm^2 of a filter with EFA of 1000 cm^2, a 100-L bulk solution would need to contain 10^{10} CFU, which is equivalent to 10^7 CFU/100 mL. This is six orders of magnitude higher than the EMA limit. It is further noted in literature that the technical capability to accurately enumerate bioburden is limited (Adley et al. 2015). Because of the inherent variability of microbiological analyses, it is impossible to accurately enumerate bioburden at a level of 10 CFU/100 mL. While the true bioburden may be below 10 CFU/100 mL, the test outcome may exceed the limit. Given the sensitivity limitations of microbiological analyses, it is more reasonable to express the acceptance limit as 10 CFU plus a margin of error (Jornitz et al. 2003). Akers (2008) also argues that given the large variability of microbiological test methods, and considering that microorganisms are not homogeneously distributed in most environments or materials, it is not appropriate to set an acceptance limit without taking into account the inaccuracy of such assays. It is also true that a single CFU may correspond to a single or multiple viable microorganisms because of cell clumping. The variability and limited sensitivity of microbiological analyses, together with the large variation of microorganisms, constrain the precision of the prefiltration bioburden test result. As such, there is always a risk of rejecting a drug solution (due to a failing test result) with a true bioburden level below any prescribed acceptance limit, or likewise, of accepting a drug solution with an actual bioburden level above the limit. In fact, in Section 7.3.2.2.1, we demonstrate through modeling both assay variability and microorganism heterogeneity that if the true bioburden level is 9 CFU/100 mL, there is a 33.4% chance to reject the batch per the EMA-suggested acceptance limit. On the other hand, if the true bioburden level is 11 CFU/100 mL, the chance to accept the batch is 50%. Therefore, meeting or failing the 10 CFU/100 mL acceptance limit may not provide adequate assurance that the true bioburden level is below or above 10 CFU/100 mL. Most recently, recognizing the imprecision of microbiological analysis, USP Chapters <61> (USP 2004a), <62> (USP 2004b), and <1111> (USP 2003) concerning microbial limit tests state when an acceptance criterion for microbiological quality is prescribed, it is interpreted as follows: in case of an established level of 10 CFU/mL, the maximum acceptable count should be 20 CFU/mL. Here, the 20-CFU limit accounts for both a bioburden level of 10 CFU/mL, which is deemed acceptable, and microbiological analysis variability. In light of the above observations, the prefiltration acceptable limit should be chosen to ensure that batches that pass the acceptance criterion would have bioburden levels that would not exceed the retention capabilities of the final sterilizing grade filter. It is of great interest to determine such a limit with a prespecified probability of assurance.

7.3 Risk-Based Approach

As discussed in Chapter 1, the recent regulatory quality initiatives clearly encourage the use of modern pharmaceutical development concepts, quality risk management, and quality systems at all stages of the manufacturing process life cycle. The FDA process validation guidance recommends a risk-based process development paradigm, in which product quality is ensured through risk identification, analysis, and control, based on increased scientific understanding of both the process and product.

Likewise, management of bioburden in aseptic processes should also be driven by product and process knowledge. For example, for an antimicrobial product, the risk of microbial survival or proliferation may be low, even if there is breakthrough of bioburden. The risk may be low because the overall quality systems have been shown to be effective in controlling bioburden throughout the manufacturing process. As such, the EMA prefiltration bioburden limit of 10 CFU/100 mL may be relaxed when the overall bioburden control strategy, drug product attributes, and manufacturing process capabilities are considered together. It is in this spirit that a risk-based approach to setting sterile filtration bioburden limits was introduced by Yang et al. (2013a). Through modeling the relationship between bioburden risk and process parameters, such as sample test volume and batch size, they demonstrated that sterility assurance can be warranted by controlling various risk factors.

Expanding on this work, a comprehensive risk-based approach is introduced in this chapter. The essential components of the approach include (1) risk assessment based on an understanding of the product and aseptic processing, categorizing risk factors into low-, medium-, and high-risk categories; (2) establishment of direct links between bioburden risk and its associated risk factors; (3) development of control strategies, depending on risk severity; and (4) determination of a design space for risk factors to lend both quality assurance and regulatory flexibility.

7.3.1 Risk Assessment

7.3.1.1 Risk Factors

The identification of risk factors is dependent on understanding of both the process and product. Figure 7.3 displays process steps before and after the final sterilizing filtration, with factors that may affect the steps indicated.

As seen in Figure 7.3, there are two types of risk associated with the sterile filtration process: (1) a drug solution with an unacceptable bioburden level before sterile filtration passes the prefiltration bioburden test, due to either

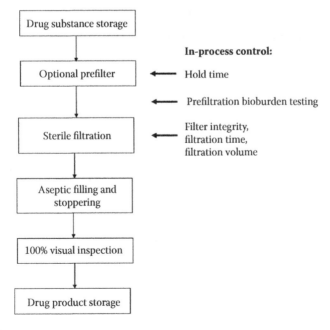

FIGURE 7.3
Sterlie filtration process and in-process control.

inherent test method variability or a sampling plan that does not have sufficient statistical power to detect drug solutions with unacceptable levels of
bioburden; and (2) breakthrough of bioburden through the final sterile filter.
These two risks are hereby referred to as the *prefiltration risk* and *postfiltration
risk*. They are interdependent, as high prefiltration risk would require more
stringent control of postfiltration risk, and vice versa. Therefore, an effective
overall control strategy should take into account this interdependency.

Bioburden risk assessment of the sterile filtration process starts with identifying risk factors. This includes examination of the above process steps and
understanding of the product characteristics. For example, if the product is
non-antimicrobial, it should be listed as a risk factor. Historical bioburden
trend data are often indicative of the effectiveness of the overall bioburden
control and need to be considered in identification of risk factors. Helpful
insights can also be gleaned from published regulatory guidance. It is useful to group risk factors by unit operation. For instance, for the risk factors
related to prefiltration, testing may include sample volume, number of samples to be tested, and acceptance criteria.

For aseptic processing, risk factors can be related to process, product, or
microbiological test methods. A useful tool called a fishbone or Ishikawa
diagram (1968) can be used to map out and organize potential risk factors in
a manner that facilitates risk assessment. Figure 7.4 presents a fishbone diagram. Potential causes of bioburden breakthrough in the sterilizing filtration

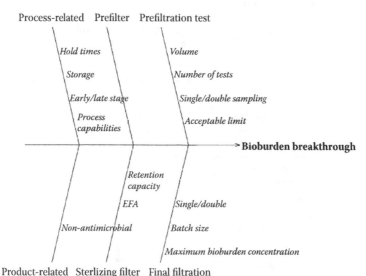

Cause-and-effect diagram

FIGURE 7.4
Fishbone (Ishikawa) diagram depicting relationships between potential bioburden risk factors
and bioburden breakthrough at the final sterile filtration step.

step are grouped into six categories: process related, product related, prefilter, prefiltration test, sterilizing filter, and final filtration, representing different sources/steps contributing to the total bioburden risk. In practice, factors within each group can be further grouped into smaller categories, to add more granularity in the cause–effect analysis.

7.3.1.2 Criticality Analysis of Risk Factors

After identification of risk factors, the criticality of these risk factors is assessed. This allows the team to focus on development of control strategies for risk factors that have high potential to cause bioburden breakthrough. A question-based process for criticality determination is outlined in the ICH Guidance for Industry Q9. It includes the following: (1) What might go wrong (potential risk factor)? (2) What are the consequences (severity)? and (3) What is the likelihood it will go wrong (probability)? After the severity ranking and probability of occurrence are determined, a risk score is calculated as the product of severity and probability of occurrence. By comparing the risk score of each risk factor to a cutoff for the risk score, factors that have high potential to cause bioburden breakthrough in the final filtration step are identified. Methods for criticality analysis, including assignment of severity score and probability of occurrence, have been well studied in literature. Commonly used approaches include Failure Mode and Effects Analysis (ICH 2007a), Cause and Effect Matrix, and Pareto analysis (Tague 2004; Yang et al. 2015c). Criticality analysis can also be conducted in a qualitative fashion based on expert opinion, published literature, and regulatory guidance. For example, process parameters that either have regulatory specifications or are required to be controlled by regulatory guidance should be viewed as high risk. However complex the factors affecting the sterile filtration bioburden are, a great deal has been learned about risk factors in aseptic processing, thanks to advances in filtration technology, science, and regulation. Therefore, here we categorize risk factors into high-, medium-, and low-risk categories, based on expert consensus, regulatory guidelines, and literature. The definitions of the three categories are given in Table 7.1.

TABLE 7.1

Risk Level Definitions

Risk Level	Definition
High	Factors known to have a direct impact on either prefiltration or postfiltration risks and required to be controlled within an acceptable range by regulatory guidelines
Medium	Factors known to have a direct impact on either prefiltration or postfiltration risks but that can be mitigated through control of the high-risk factors
Low	Factors that have an indirect effect on prefiltration and postfiltration risks and are routinely monitored through in-process testing and are known to be rare events

TABLE 7.2

Categorization of Risk Factors Related to Sterile Filtration

Unit Operation	Risk Factor	Risk Level
Process	Drug substance storage	Low
	Hold times	Low
	Early stage	Medium
	Capabilities	Medium
Product	Non-antimicrobial	Low
Prefilter	Prefilter	Low
Prefiltration test	Volume	High
	Number of tests	Medium
	Single/double sampling	Medium
	Bioburden level in unfiltered solution	High
	Acceptable limit	High
Sterilizing filter	Retention capability	High
	Effective filter area	High
Final filtration	Batch size	High
	Bioburden level in unfiltered solution	High
	Single/double filters	Medium
	Integrity test	High

Using the definitions in Table 7.1, we classify the risk factors in Figure 7.3 into the following categories in Table 7.2.

The categorization in Table 7.2 serves as a guide for developing risk control strategies. The method we adopt for mitigating bioburden risk is a tiered approach. Risk factors deemed to be of high risk, if out of control, are considered as first-tier factors for which acceptance limits need to be established, whereas risk factors categorized as having medium to low risk may be either controlled or monitored through standard bioburden sampling and monitoring programs such as microbial alert/action limits in a clean room. For example, prefilter is viewed as low risk because its capacity to reduce microbial concentration in the unfiltered solution can be assured through using effective sterilizing filter(s), whereas batch size of the product for the final filtration step is considered high risk because too large a batch may increase the overall mycobacterial load in the unfiltered solution, thus either overburdening the sterilizing filter and compromising its integrity or causing the solution to flow too slowly, rendering the filtration step impractical.

7.3.2 Statistical Risk Analysis

In this section, we present control strategies for risk factors deemed high risk in Table 7.2. This primarily involves establishing acceptable ranges for these risk factors. The key is to directly link risk factors to prefiltration and postfiltration bioburden risks, which allows for evaluation of the impact of these risk factors on the bioburden risks when the factors vary within their operating ranges. The acceptable ranges are determined such that, with high statistical confidence, movement of a risk factor within its acceptable range has little or no effect on the bioburden risks. This is in accordance with the quality by design (QbD) principles in ICH Q8 (R2) that enables manufacturers to define a manufacturing process design space that consistently produces high-quality drug substance and products through increased product and process knowledge.

In theory, the acceptable ranges can be determined through design of experiments (DOE), in which the impact of the risk factors is evaluated. Consider an experiment intended to assess the impact of sample volume on the acceptable bioburden limit prefiltration risk, which is the risk for a drug solution with a bioburden level exceeding the acceptable limit to pass the prefiltration bioburden test. The drug solutions may be simulated with bioburden levels above the acceptance limit and tested repeatedly using various sample volumes. At the conclusion of the experiment, the percentage of samples tested at each nominal volume that have bioburden levels determined to be below the acceptable limit is calculated. A statistical model such as four-parameter logistic regression can be fit to the data. This enables the determination of the test volume at which the probability of passing solutions with unacceptable levels of bioburden is below a small number. However, since there are other factors, such as the number of replicates to be tested at each nominal volume that may affect the prefiltration risk, a multifactorial DOE is needed to account for the interaction of these risk factors. As a result, the experiment may be too large to run. Yang et al. (2013a) provided a viable alternative based on statistical modeling to establish the relationships between risk factors and the prefiltration and postfiltration risks. The method they developed is presented here.

7.3.2.1 Modeling Prefiltration Bioburden

7.3.2.1.1 Poisson Model

The utility of using the Poisson distribution to describe biological phenomena is well recognized in the literature. Notable examples include modeling bacterial colonies in a Petri dish or the count of infected cells in cells for indirect bioassay. One way to describe the number of CFUs as a quantification of bioburden in the unfiltered solution is to use the Poisson distribution. However, the Poisson model has an implicit assumption that the bacteria in the drug solution are uniformly distributed. Let X denote the number of CFUs in a given volume V, say, 100 mL. If X follows a Poisson distribution, the probability for X to be equal to a number x is given by (Haight 1967)

$$P[X = x] = f(x|\lambda) = \frac{\lambda^x e^{-\lambda}}{x!}, \tag{7.1}$$

where $\lambda = DV$ is the mean bioburden level (average number of CFUs in a sample of test volume V), with D being the number of CFUs per unit (such as 1 mL). In statistics, there are methods that can be used to test if a particular model is fit to describe the data observed. For example, a χ^2 test is often used to test the goodness of fit of a data set to a specific distribution. In the following sections, a simulated data set is used to illustrate how this test is carried out. To ensure the validity of the model, it is important to perform such test.

7.3.2.1.2 Negative Binomial Model

As mentioned above, the use of a Poisson distribution to model CFU data is based on the assumption that the bacteria are distributed uniformly throughout the bulk volume; a χ^2 test can be used to assess the appropriateness of the model. The Poisson model only involves one parameter, λ, which is the mean CFUs per sample volume. Theoretically, the variance of a Poisson is equal to its mean, which is a direct consequence of the uniform distribution of bacteria in the bulk solution. In reality, this assumption often does not hold because 1 CFU may correspond to either one bacterium or a clump of bacteria differing in size. Therefore, it is conceivable that the CFUs may not be uniformly distributed in the container holding the bulk solution. As a result, the variability in the observed number of CFUs from a given sample is larger than that under the Poisson model assumption. Such a phenomenon is called overdispersion. To characterize the overdispersion, a negative binomial distribution is often used (DeGroot 1986). Its density function is given by

$$g(x \mid \lambda, k) = \frac{\Gamma(1/k + x)(k\lambda)^x}{x!\,\Gamma(1/k)(1 + k\lambda)^{1/k+x}} \qquad (7.2)$$

where $\lambda > 0$, and $k > 0$ is an overdispersion factor. The distribution of X has a mean λ and variance $\lambda(1 + k\lambda)$, which is greater than the mean. In the literature, the negative binomial distribution is also viewed as a mixture of Poisson distributions (Hilbe 2007). It is interesting to note that when $k \to 0$, $g(x \mid \lambda, k) \to \dfrac{\lambda^x e^{-\lambda}}{x!}$ (Cook 2009). This implies that X approximately follows a Poisson distribution with a mean microbial count of λ when the bioburden in the drug solution is approximately uniformly distributed. Therefore, the negative binomial model is more general than the Poisson model. However, ultimately which model to use depends on how well the two models fit the data. In the absence of empirical data, it is good practice to describe the bioburden distribution using a negative binomial model.

7.3.2.1.3 Model Selection

When bioburden data are available from historical testing of drug bulk solutions, they can be used to determine if a Poisson or negative binomial model should be used to describe bioburden. This can be accomplished through a χ^2 test. A general test procedure is described in many publications (Greenwood and Nikulin 1996). It consists of several steps: (1) choose a distribution, either Poisson or negative binomial, to describe the data; (2) use the observed data to estimate the model parameter(s); (3) determine the theoretical expected frequencies for observed CFU values; and (4) construct a χ^2 test statistic using the following formula:

$$\chi^2_{m-p-1} = \sum_{i=1}^{m} \frac{(\hat{f}_i - f_i)^2}{f_i}, \tag{7.3}$$

where m is the largest number of CFUs observed plus 1, p is the number of parameters in the model, $m - p - 1$ is the degrees of freedom for the χ^2 statistic in Equation 7.3, f_i is the theoretical frequency of observing i CFUs in a test, and $\hat{f}_i$ is the estimated frequency of observing i CFUs in a test. Let n denote the total number of samples tested. Thus, f_i can be calculated as $f_i = nf(X = i|\theta)$, where $f_i (X = i|\theta)$ is the probability that there are i CFUs in the sample, and θ is the model parameter equal to λ ($[\lambda, k]$) for the Poisson (negative binomial) distribution. The goodness-of-fit test is intended to test the null hypothesis that the number of CFUs follows a Poisson distribution. The null hypothesis is rejected if the test statistic in Equation 7.3 produces a P value less than 0.05, indicating that the data do not follow a Poisson distribution.

For illustration, a data set is simulated using a Poisson distribution with a mean bioburden concentration of 1 CFU/mL. The simulated data are presented in Table 7.3, along with the theoretical frequencies under the Poisson distribution.

Based on the data in Table 7.3, the mean CFU is estimated to be $\hat{\lambda} = 1.14$. The theoretical frequencies were calculated using the formula $f_i = n_f(X = i|\theta)$ with $n = 50$, $\theta = \hat{\lambda} = 1.14$, and degrees of freedom $7 - 1 - 1 = 5$. Using Equation 7.3, the χ^2 statistic χ^2_5 is determined to be 3.967, which corresponds to a P value of $0.446 > 0.05$. Therefore, the null hypothesis that the bioburden CFUs follow

TABLE 7.3

Data Set Based on 50 Simulated Samples from a Poisson Distribution with $\lambda = 1$

Observed CFUs	Observed Frequency	Theoretical Frequency
0	17	16.642
1	17	18.308
2	11	10.069
3	3	3.392
4	1	1.015
5	1	0.223
>5	0	0.949

a Poisson distribution is not rejected. In other words, the data can be considered from a Poisson distribution.

The same calculations can be carried out to test the null hypothesis that the bioburden (CFU) follows a negative binomial distribution. However, one needs first to estimate the two model parameters (λ, k). Using the fact that the mean and variance of the negative binomial distribution in Equation 7.2 are λ and $\lambda(1 + k\lambda)$, respectively, k can be estimated as $(\hat{\sigma}^2 - \hat{\lambda})/\hat{\lambda}$, where $\hat{\sigma}^2$ and $\hat{\lambda}$ are sample mean and variance, respectively. Overdispersion is a common phenomenon in Poisson modeling. It is conceivable that for a specific drug solution the answers to the questions, (1) whether or not the bioburden (CFU) is uniformly distributed, and (2) if not, how significant the overdispersion of the data is, may vary. However, testing approaches such as the Wald test, the likelihood ratio test, and the quasi-likelihood test for overdispersion are available, and the overdispersion factor k can also be estimated based on historical data (Agresti 1990; Haight 1967; Hilbe 2007). After a proper model is validated, the calculations done in Section 7.4 can be repeated to determine the maximum allowable batch size for the drug solution.

Regardless of whether the Poisson or negative binomial model is selected to describe bioburden distribution in the unfiltered drug solution, the prefiltration risk, which is defined as the probability of accepting a batch of drug substance for the final filtration when it has an undesirable level of bioburden, can be quantified as

$$R_{\text{Pre}} = \Pr[X \leq AL | D], \tag{7.4}$$

where X is the viral count in a test sample drawn from drug solution under evaluation, AL is the bioburden acceptance limit, and D is the bioburden concentration of the drug substance. The above probability is also dependent on the volume V of the test sample. As is shown in the following sections, all these factors have a direct impact on the probability in Equation 7.4, thus influencing the prefiltration risk.

7.3.2.2 Performance of Prefiltration Test Procedures

7.3.2.2.1 EMA Test

In this section, we evaluate the performance of the EMA-recommended prefiltration bioburden test scheme. It consists of testing a single sample of 100 mL in volume and declaring the batch acceptable if the observed bioburden is no more than 10 CFU/100 mL. For the purpose of illustration, we assume that the bioburden concentration in the drug solution can be described through a negative binomial distribution with a variance twice as large as its mean. It is also assumed that the true bioburden concentration of the solution is unknown. Of interest is the probability for a single test result not to exceed the acceptable limit 10 CFU/100 mL. Because the mean and variance of the negative binomial distribution in Equation 7.2 are λ and $\lambda(1 + k\lambda)$, respectively, we have

$$\lambda(1 + k\lambda) = 2\lambda.$$

Solving the above equation gives rise to

$$k = \frac{1}{\lambda}. \tag{7.5}$$

Substituting k in Equation 7.4, the probability that a single test result will not exceed the acceptable limit of 10 CFU/100 mL is given by

$$P[X \leq 10 \text{ CFU/mL}] = \sum_{x=0}^{10} g(x|\lambda, 1/\lambda), \tag{7.6}$$

where λ is the unknown mean bioburden concentration in the drug solution. A plot of the acceptance probability in Equation 7.6 against λ is given in Figure 7.5.

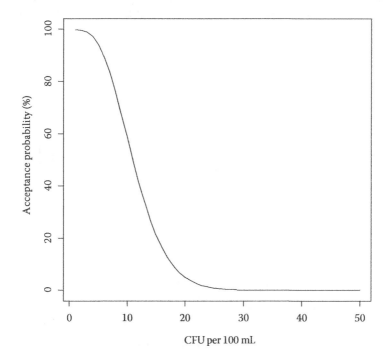

FIGURE 7.5
Plot of probability of acceptance based on the EMA-recommended test scheme using a negative binomial distribution with overdispersion parameter = 2.

From the plot, it can be seen that when the mean bioburden level is 9 CFU/100 mL, 10 CFU/100 mL, or 11 CFU/100 mL, the probability of accepting the drug solution is 66.6%, 58.8%, or 50%. In other words, if the true mean bioburden level is 9 CFU/100 mL, there is a 33.4% chance to reject the solution per the EMA test, whereas the chance to accept the solution is 50%, should the true mean bioburden level be 11 CFU/100 mL.

The results suggest that the EMA-recommended acceptance limit provides protection to neither the consumer's risk nor the producer's risk. Furthermore, for the test to have a high probability, say, 95%, of rejecting a batch of drug solution with an undesirable level of bioburden, the bioburden level of the batch needs to be at least 20 CFU/100 mL.

7.3.2.2.2 *Alternative Test Schemes*

We also evaluate two alternative schemes, which are often used in prefiltration testing. One consists of a test sample volume of 10 mL and an acceptable limit of 1 CFU/10 mL, and the other tests a sample volume of 30 mL and rejects the batch if the acceptable limit of 3 CFU/30 mL is exceeded. As before, a negative binomial distribution with variance being twice its mean is assumed for the bioburden in the solution in order to assess the performance of these two test schemes. The acceptance probabilities of the two test schemes are plotted in Figure 7.6 along with that of the EMA-recommended

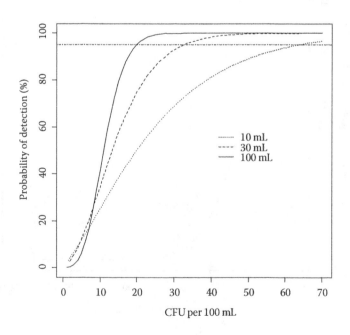

FIGURE 7.6
Performance characteristics of three different test schemes, based on a negative binomial distribution with an overdispersion factor of 2.

test scheme. The three test schemes are labeled as 10 mL, 30 mL, and 100 mL in the plot.

A couple of observations can be made from the plot: (1) None of the three test schemes is sensitive for detecting bioburden that is in between 10 CFU/100 mL and 15 CFU/100 mL. (2) To achieve a high level of detection such as 95% for unacceptable bioburden, smaller test volumes require higher true mean bioburden concentrations than larger test volumes do. For example, at a detection level of 95% (i.e., $P(\text{Accept}) \leq 5\%$), the bioburden concentrations required are 63, 32, and 20 CFU/mL, for the test volumes of 10, 30, and 100 mL, respectively.

7.3.2.3 Modeling Postfiltration Bioburden

In order to control the postfiltration bioburden risk, it is necessary to link it with associated risk factors, namely, batch size, maximum bioburden concentration before the final filtration, sterilizing filter retention capability, and EFA, which are all considered as high severity factors (see Table 7.2). This relationship can be established using the model suggested by Yang et al. (2013a). To facilitate the discussion of this model, we introduce some notation in Table 7.4.

According to the above definitions, it is apparent that

$$n = (S - V) \times D, \tag{7.7}$$

where $S - V$ is the total volume of the unfiltered batch after the prefiltration bioburden test. It is assumed that Y follows a binomial distribution:

$$\Pr[Y = y \mid X \leq AL] = \frac{n!}{(n-y)!y!} p_0^y (1 - p_0)^{n-y} \tag{7.8}$$

where $0 \leq y \leq n$. The above model is based on the assumption that all CFUs in the final filtered drug solution have an equal probability to penetrate the

TABLE 7.4

Notations for Postfiltration Bioburden

Notation	Definition
Y	Total number of CFUs in the drug solution after the final filtration
n	Total number of CFUs in the unfiltered drug solution that passes the prefiltration bioburden test
p_0	Probability for a single CFU to penetrate the final filter
V	Prefiltration test sample volume (mL)
AL	Acceptance limit of prefiltration bioburden (CFU/V mL)
D	Bioburden in the unfiltered solution (CFU/100 mL)
D_0	Maximum acceptable level of bioburden in the unfiltered solution (CFU/100 mL)
S	Batch size of unfiltered solution

sterilizing filter. However, in practice, accumulation of bioburden on the final filter may cause partial clogging. As a result, a CFU that reaches the filter early in the process may have a higher probability to penetrate the filter than those that reach the filter later. Therefore, it is conservative to assume that all CFUs in the solution have the same probability to go through the final filter as a single CFU, when it is the only CFU in a solution passing through the final filter. Since the postfiltration risk can be quantified by the probability of having bioburden break through the sterilizing filter, it can be readily calculated by

$$
\begin{aligned}
R_{Post} &= \Pr\left[Y \geq 1 \middle| X \leq AL\right] \\
&= 1 - \Pr\left[Y = 0 \middle| X \leq AL\right] \\
&= 1 - (1 - p_0)^{(S-V) \times D}.
\end{aligned}
\tag{7.9}
$$

Although Equation 7.9 establishes a relationship between the postfiltration risk and known risk factors V, D, and S, it also includes an unknown parameter p_0. However, this parameter can be estimated using data from a validation study of the sterilizing filter. In fact, a one-sided upper $(1 - \alpha)$ 100% confidence limit for p_0 was derived by Yang et al. (2013a). Let N be the total number of CFUs used in the filter validation study and n_1 be the number of CFUs that penetrate the filter. Because the FDA guidance requires that a challenge concentration of at least 10^7 CFU/cm^2 be used, resulting in no passage of the challenge microorganism, we have

$$
N \geq A \times 10^7 \quad \text{and} \quad n_1 = 0,
$$

where A is the area of the filter (cm^2). As a result, a one-sided upper $(1 - \alpha)$ 100% exact confidence limit for p_0 can be constructed, using the Clopper–Pearson method (Clopper and Pearson 1934):

$$
p_0 \leq \left[1 + \frac{N - n_1}{(n_1 + 1)F(\alpha, 2(n_1 + 1), 2(N - n_1))}\right]^{-1} = \frac{F(\alpha, 2, N)}{N + F(\alpha, 2, N)} \equiv p_1, \tag{7.10}
$$

where $F(\alpha, 2, N)$ is the $100(1 - \alpha)^{th}$ percentile of an F distribution with degrees of freedom of 2 and N.

Since the FDA guidance requires that a challenge concentration of at least 10^7 CFU/cm^2 be used, $N = A \times RC \geq A \times 10^7$ with RC and A being the retention capability and the EFA of the sterilizing filter, respectively. Combining Equations 7.9 and 7.10, a one-sided $(1 - \alpha)$ 100% upper limit on the probability of postfiltration bioburden risk is

$$
R_{Post} \leq 1 - (1 - p_1)^{(S-V) \times D}. \tag{7.11}
$$

The above relationship links prefiltration sample volume V, bioburden concentration of the drug solution at the point of final sterilizing filtration D, sterilizing filter retention capability RC, and area A. It becomes evident that the postfiltration risk can be controlled by confining the above-mentioned risk factors within their acceptable ranges.

7.3.3 Risk Control

As previously discussed in Section 7.3.1, a tiered approach is adopted to develop control strategies. Development of control strategies for the first-tier risk factors listed in Table 7.2 focuses on setting acceptance ranges for these factors. For the second-tier risk factors or factors of medium risk, control may or may not be needed depending on the effectiveness of the risk mitigation plans for the first-tier risk factors. Last, control strategies for the third-tier risk factors are usually a part of the overall bioburden control for aseptic processing and are not discussed in this article.

7.3.3.1 First-Tier Risk Factors

In the previous section, through modeling the processes of the prefiltration sampling test and the final sterilizing filtration, risk factors that are deemed to be of high risk are linked to the probabilities of occurrence of the prefiltration and final filtration risks. These relationships enable the establishment of effective control strategies and are summarized in Table 7.5, along with possible risk mitigation measures. As seen from the table, the probabilities of prefiltration and postfiltration risks are expressed as functions of the risk factors. These relationships account for the interdependencies among the

TABLE 7.5

Relationships between Bioburden Risk Factors and Associated Control Strategies

Risk	Risk Factor	Relationship	Control Strategies
Prefiltration	Volume (V) Acceptable limit (AL)	$R_{Pre} = \Pr[X \leq AL \mid D]$	Determine V and AL such that $R_{Pre} \leq \delta_0$, a very small number, e.g., 1%.
Final filtration	Retention capability (RC) Effective filter area (A) Batch size (S) Volume (V) Bioburden level in unfiltered solution (D)	$R_{Post} \leq 1 - (1 - p_1)^{(S-V) \times D}$ with $p_1 = \dfrac{F(\alpha, 2, N)}{N + F(\alpha, 2, N)}$ and $N = A \times RC$	Determine RC, A, S, and D such that $R_{Post} \leq \delta_1$, a very small number, e.g., 10^{-5}.
	Integrity test		Perform filter integrity test.

risk factors and make it possible to explore their joint effects on the risks. As noted by previous researchers (Yang 2013a; Yang et al. 2015c), setting the acceptance range for each risk factor in isolation may not render the same level of quality assurance as when the interdependencies of the risk factors are taken into account.

It is also worth pointing out that the probabilities R_{Pre} and R_{Post} are correlated. For example, they are both dependent on the sample volume V of the prefiltration bioburden test and bioburden concentration D in the unfiltered drug solution. Consideration should be given to this correlation when designing risk control strategies.

7.3.3.2 Prefiltration Risk Control

The primary purpose of the prefiltration bioburden test is to reject drug solution with undesirably high bioburden before the final sterilizing filtration. It is understandable that regardless of how stringent the test is, there is always solution with high bioburden that may pass the test. To minimize such risk, a small value δ_0 $(0 < \delta_0 < 1)$ is chosen to be the acceptable upper limit on the probability for the prefiltration risk to occur. Ideally, the acceptance ranges of the test sample volume V, acceptable limit AL, and bioburden concentration D are determined such that

$$R_{Pre} = \Pr\,[X \leq AL | D] \leq \delta_0. \tag{7.12}$$

For a given testing scheme, such as $V = 100$ mL and $AL = 10$ CFU/100 mL, the acceptable limit D_0 of D can be determined from Figure 7.6 by finding the bioburden concentration on the x axis that intersects the probability curve R_{Pre} at $\Pr[\text{Accept}] = \delta_0$ as illustrated in Figure 7.7.

Therefore, for this particular testing scheme, the probability of accepting a batch of solution with bioburden concentration greater than the acceptable limit D_0 is bounded by the preselected small value δ_0. It is true that D_0 may be greater than 10 CFU/100 mL. However, its impact on the final postfiltration risk will be mitigated through control strategies discussed in the next section.

7.3.3.3 Final Postfiltration Risk Control

When a batch of solution passes the prefiltration bioburden test, there is a high probability that its bioburden concentration is no greater than the acceptable limit D_0, as discussed in the previous section. Hence, the probability of bioburden breakthrough in the final filtration step R_{Post} is bounded by

$$R_{Post} \leq 1 - (1 - p_1)^{(S-V) \times D_0}. \tag{7.13}$$

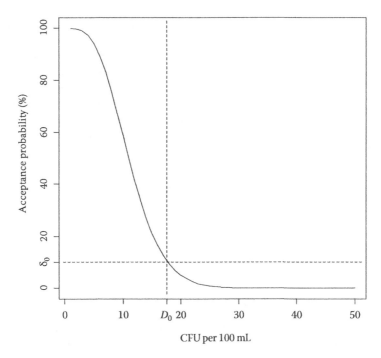

FIGURE 7.7
Determination of acceptable limit of bioburden concentration D_0 in unfiltered solution.

The acceptable ranges of risk factors (S, RC, A) associated with the final filtration listed in Table 7.5 are determined such that the upper bound on the probability of postfiltration bioburden risk satisfies

$$1-(1-p_1)^{(S-V)\times D_0} \le \delta. \tag{7.14}$$

Inequality (Equation 7.14) establishes a relationship between the maximum acceptable bioburden risk postfiltration (δ) and the one-sided 95% upper confidence bound on the probability of the postfiltration risk $1-(1-p_1)^{(S-V)\times D_0}$ (Equation 7.11). Because the influence of the batch size and prefiltration bioburden level are exerted on this upper bound through the maximum total bioburden $n = (S - V) \times D_0$ in the unfiltered drug solution, different combinations of batch size S and bioburden level D_0 may result in the same effect on R_{Post}. For example, two solutions with batch size and bioburden level $(S + V, D_0/2)$ and $((S + V)/2, D_0)$ have the same value of $1-(1-p_1)^{(S-V)\times D_0}$. The above observation renders manufacturers some flexibility in setting a prefiltration bioburden acceptance limit. In general, the relationship in Equation 7.14 can be used to explore the joint effect of the risk factors on the bioburden risk postfiltration. However, in practice, some of the risk factors might be fixed.

For example, for a drug that is in an early stage of clinical development, the batch size is usually small, and it is unlikely the sterilizing filter with an EFA greater than 1000 cm² would be used. Therefore, one might fix the filter size at 1000 cm² and determine acceptable ranges for other risk factors. As an illustration, consider the case where the sterilizing filter is selected (thus, the EFA is fixed) and where the final filtration risk is mitigated through restricting the batch size of the unfiltered drug solution. Solving the inequality in Equation 7.14 produces the acceptable limit for a batch size S_0:

$$S_0 = V + \frac{\ln(1-\delta)}{D_0 \ln\left[\dfrac{A \times RC}{A \times RC + F(\alpha, 2, A \times RC)}\right]}. \tag{7.15}$$

Likewise, if the batch size is fixed, one may explore acceptable ranges for sterilizing filter size and retention capability.

7.3.3.4 Control of Second-Tier Risk Factors

By definition, the second-tier risk factors are those that are known to have a direct impact on either prefiltration or postfiltration risks, but whose effect can be mitigated through control of the high-risk (first-tier) factors (see Table 7.1), for example, use of double sterilizing filters to mitigate the risk of bioburden passage of the first filter. In general, quality assurance for the final filtration can be achieved through the use of a single sterilizing filter, which has either a large EFA or a higher *RC*. However, there is an advantage to applying double filters, as the probability of bioburden breakthrough of both filters is bounded by the expression in Equation 7.16:

$$\left[1 - (1 - p_1)^{(S-V) \times D_0}\right]^2. \tag{7.16}$$

As is shown in the next section, to achieve this level of quality assurance with a single filter, a single filter of a much larger EFA would be needed. From a cost-saving standpoint, it might be preferable to use double filters, particularly when the batch sizes are small.

There are several risk factors for the prefiltration and final filtration in Table 7.2 that are listed as medium risk (second tier). They include the number of prefiltration tests, use of single/double sampling, and single or double filters. Double sampling is a technique conventionally used in product batch acceptance testing. The idea is that the disposition of the batch depends on the outcomes of both tests. The results of the first test lead to a decision to either accept the batch or perform the second test. At the end of the second test, the batch is either accepted or rejected. The benefit of this double sampling plan is that, on the average, it requires a smaller overall sample size than a single sampling plan, while maintaining the same levels of Type I and Type II error as a comparable single sampling plan (Schilling 1982). In the context of prefiltration bioburden testing, since it is desirable from the manufacturer's standpoint to test a smaller sample volume for the sake of cost saving, the double sampling plan may be potentially used to provide the same level of quality assurance as a single sampling plan, with the understanding that the double sampling plan does add some operational complexity. Figure 7.8 shows a diagram of a double sampling plan.

Similarly, a single sampling plan can be devised such that multiple tests are conducted using smaller sample volumes. Consider that the manufacturer intends to perform the prefiltration bioburden test, using a sample volume of 10 mL. One may split the 10-mL sample into two samples, each having a volume of 5 mL, and perform the prefiltration bioburden test in a sequential fashion. Specifically, a decision concerning the disposition of the batch is made using the following decision diagram: if both tests pass, the unfiltered solution is considered to have an acceptable level of bioburden; otherwise, the bioburden level of the solution is deemed to be unacceptable. For this particular test, the prefiltration risk is determined by

$$R_{Pre} = \Pr[X \le AL|D]^2. \tag{7.17}$$

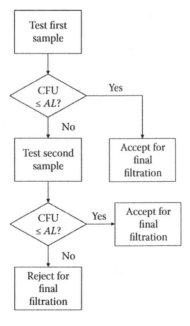

FIGURE 7.8
Diagram of a double sampling plan for prefiltration bioburden testing.

7.4 Applications of Risk-Based Methods

7.4.1 Justification of Alternative Sample Volumes and Decision Criteria

As there is no scientific rationale provided for the EMA recommendation of a single sample of 100 mL with an acceptance criterion of no more than 10 CFU/100 mL, it is very challenging to justify a sample volume smaller than 100 mL. In the previous sections, we demonstrated that bioburden risks can be mitigated through controlling associated risk factors, in addition to other controls in the quality systems for aseptic processing. Therefore, it is of interest to apply the methods in this paper to assess the feasibility of using the alternative test schemes previously introduced, namely, Scheme 1 and Scheme 2 corresponding to $(V, AL) = (10 \text{ mL}, 1 \text{ CFU}/10 \text{ mL})$ and $(30 \text{ mL}, 3 \text{ CFU}/30 \text{ mL})$, respectively, and compare them to the EMA-recommended scheme corresponding to $(V, AL) = (100 \text{ mL}, 10 \text{ CFU}/100 \text{ mL})$. For this assessment, the following assumptions are made: (1) the final filtration filter is of sterilizing grade, with an EFA of 1000 cm² and a microbial RC of $\geq 10^7$ CFU/cm²; (2) bioburden in the unfiltered drug solution follows a negative binomial distribution, with a variance twice as large as its mean. The primary focus is to determine the maximum acceptable batch size. The evaluation is done for several combinations of the risk bounds (defined in Sections 7.3.3.2 and 7.3.3.3), $\delta_0 = 5\%$ 1%, and 0.1%, and $\delta = 10^{-4}$ and 10^{-5}; δ_0 are the upper bounds for the risk of unacceptable prefiltration and postfiltration bioburden being accepted, respectively, typically referred to as consumer risk, and the values of 5%, 1%, and 0.1% are conventionally used. The bounds $\delta = 10^{-4}$ and 10^{-5} also have an intuitive interpretation: for example, the upper bound $\delta = 10^{-4}$ means that among 10,000 batches that go through the final filtration step, no more than 1 batch has bioburden breakthrough. For each choice of prefiltration bound, sample volume, and acceptance limit, the maximum bioburden concentration D_0 in the unfiltered drug solution is determined as a solution to Equation 7.13. This value, along with the postfiltration risk bound, is used to calculate the maximum batch size using Equation 7.16. The results are presented in Table 7.6.

It is evident that the maximum batch size is dependent on the test scheme, after the bounds on risks (i.e., risk tolerance) are selected. For example, when $\delta_0 = 5\%$ and $\delta = 10^{-4}$, the maximum batch sizes are 424, 826, and 1355 L for the test schemes $(V, AL) = (10 \text{ mL}, 1 \text{ CFU}/10 \text{ mL})$, $(30 \text{ mL}, 3 \text{ CFU}/30 \text{ mL})$, and $(100 \text{ mL}, 10 \text{ CFU}/100 \text{ mL})$, respectively. In general, the maximum allowable batch size decreases as the risk bounds decrease. As described previously, the risk bounds, δ_0 and δ, are upper limits on the probability for a solution of unacceptable level of bioburden to pass the prefiltration test, and the probability for at least 1 CFU to break through the final sterilizing filter, respectively. Smaller probability values offer a higher degree of confidence, that is, a lower tolerance for risk. By controlling the maximum batch size, Schemes 1

TABLE 7.6

Maximum Batch Sizes Based on Risk Bounds and Prefiltration Test Schemes

Risk Bound		Prefiltration Test Scheme		Maximum Bioburden[c] D_0 (CFU/100 mL)	Maximum Batch Size S_0 (L)
Prefiltration[a]	Postfiltration[b]	Sample Volume V (mL)	Acceptance Limit AL (CFU/V)		
5%	10^{-4}	10	1	63	424
		30	3	32	826
		100	10	20	1355
	10^{-5}	10	1	63	42
		30	3	32	82
		100	10	20	135
1%	10^{-4}	10	1	91	297
		30	3	43	620
		100	10	24	1106
	10^{-5}	10	1	91	29
		30	3	43	62
		100	10	24	110
0.10%	10^{-4}	10	1	128	210
		30	3	58	465
		100	10	30	897
	10^{-5}	10	1	128	21
		30	3	58	46
		100	10	30	89

[a] Prefiltration risk δ_0 = probability to pass a batch with a bioburden exceeding the maximum level D_0.

[b] Postfiltration risk δ = probability to have ≥ 1 CFU in the final filtered solution.

[c] Maximum bioburden D_0 = maximum acceptable level of bioburden in the unfiltered solution.

and 2 can achieve the same level of sterility quality assurance for any given δ or δ_0 as the EMA-recommended test plan.

7.4.2 Design Space

Based on the relationships in Equations 7.15 and 7.16, all acceptable values of the risk factors can be determined. These values represent a design space, within which the postfiltration risk is controlled to an acceptable level. As an example, consider an aseptic processing that has a risk tolerance of 5% prefiltration risk and 10^{-4} postfiltration. It is also assumed that the prefiltration bioburden test consists of testing a single sample, that one sterilizing filter of 10^7 CFU/cm^2 RC and an EFA of 1000 cm^2 is used for the final filtration. Furthermore, it is assumed that the prefiltration acceptance limit is set such that it is proportional to the volume of the test sample. Specifically,

$$AL = 10 \times V \text{ CFU/100 mL.}$$

In other words, for test volumes of 10, 30, and 100 mL, the corresponding acceptance limits are 1, 3, and 10 CFU, respectively. Under the above assumptions, the postfiltration risk probability is a function of sample volume and batch size. Figure 7.9 depicts this risk probability function in three-dimensional space. It is evident that as the risk increases, sample volume decreases and batch size increases.

The design space of sample volume and batch size is determined by identifying combinations of these two factors in Figure 7.8, which result in a risk probability no more than the prespecified risk bound 10^{-4}. Figure 7.10 displays the acceptable regions of sample volume and batch size.

The design space is a useful tool for determining appropriateness of a specific sample volume for the prefiltration bioburden test and batch size for the final sterilizing filtration. For example, from the plot, it can be determined that a test volume of 10 mL and a maximum batch volume of 424 L would be within stated risk tolerance. Therefore, this combination is deemed to be an acceptable alternative prefiltration and final filtration plan with the decision rule of ≤10 CFU/10 mL.

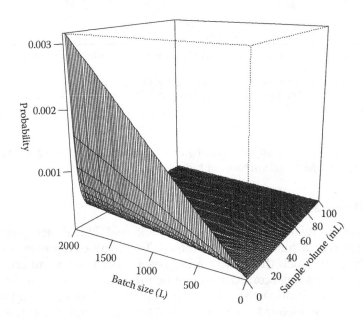

FIGURE 7.9
Response surface of postfiltration risk as a function of sample volume and batch size. The risk is defined as probability of having at least 1 CFU in filtered solution.

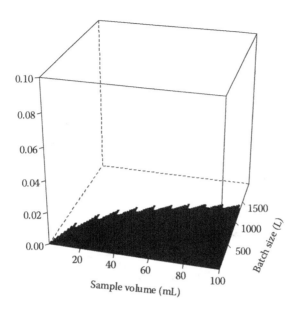

FIGURE 7.10
Design space of sample volume and batch size under the assumptions of no more than 5% probability of false negative and bioburden breakthrough in ≤1 in 10,000 batches. It is also assumed that a single sterilizing filter of 1000 cm² EFA is used and the retention capability of the filter is 10⁷ CFU/cm².

7.4.3 Effects of Risk Factors

7.4.3.1 EFA and Retention Capability

As previously discussed, the EFA of the sterilizing filter has a direct impact on postfiltration bioburden risk. This effect can be quantitatively evaluated. One way to assess the effect is to compare the design spaces for different filter sizes. Figures 7.11 and 7.12 display the design spaces for filter areas of 200 and 2000 cm², respectively, with the same risk tolerances described in the previous section. For the 200-cm² EFA filter, the maximum batch size for a given decision rule is approximately 300 L, whereas it is larger than 1500 L for the 2000-cm² EFA filter.

Similarly, the design space of sample volume and batch size is determined for a single filter with 200 cm² EFA but with an *RC* of 10⁸ CFU/cm² and plotted in Figure 7.12. Comparing the design space in Figure 7.12 with that in Figure 7.10, it is evident that the design space is much larger for the filter with higher retention capability. Additionally, the design space in Figure 7.13 is compared to that in Figure 7.11, which is created based on a single filter with 2000 cm² EFA but 10⁷ CFU/cm². In essence, the two filters result in the same design space. Factoring in the costs and availability of the filters and

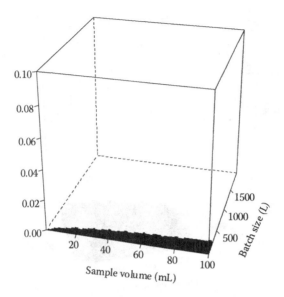

FIGURE 7.11
Design space of sample volume and batch size for the use of the 200-cm² EFA filter and no more than 5% probability of false negative and breach in 1 in 10,000 batches. It is also assumed that the retention capability of the filter is 10^7 CFU/cm².

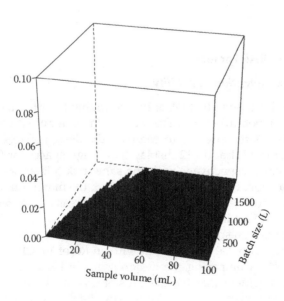

FIGURE 7.12
Design space of sample volume and batch size for the use of the 2000-cm² EFA filter and no more than 5% probability of false negative and breach in 1 in 10,000 batches. It is also assumed that the retention capability of the filter is 10^7 CFU/cm².

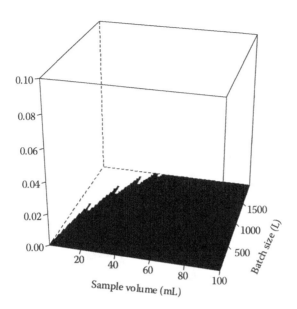

FIGURE 7.13

Design space of sample volume and batch size for the use of a single filter with 10^8 CFU/cm^2 retention capability and 200 cm^2 EFA and no more than 5% probability of false negative and breach in 1 in 10,000 batches.

operational complexity in implementing double filtration, one may make a better decision in choosing one filter over the other.

7.4.3.2 Effect of Risk Tolerance

Similarly, we evaluate the effect of different levels of postfiltration risk δ. Two design spaces are created for risk levels of 10^{-4} and 10^{-5} and shown in Figures 7.10 and 7.14, respectively, assuming the sterilizing filter has a size of retention capability of 1000 cm^2 EFA and 10^7 CFU/cm^2, respectively. The effect of the risk level on the design space is profound.

7.4.3.3 Double Filters

The impact of the use of double filters is also evaluated. The design space in Figure 7.15 is constructed for a double filter with an *RC* of 10^7 CFU/cm^2 and an EFA of 200 cm^2, and $\delta_0 \leq 5\%$ and $\delta \leq 10^{-6}$.

As shown in Figure 7.15, the double filters are very effective in mitigating the postfiltration risk as evidenced by the fact that any combination of the sample volume and batch size in the range of [1 mL, 100 mL] × [0, 2000 L] would result in an acceptable level of postfiltration risk.

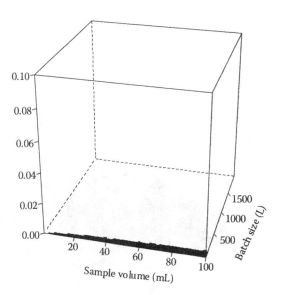

FIGURE 7.14
Design space of sample volume and batch size for the use of 1000 cm^2 EFA filter and no more than 5% probability of false negative and breach in 1 in 100,000 batches. It is also assumed that the retention capability of the filter is 10^7 CFU/cm^2.

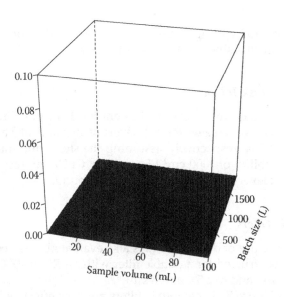

FIGURE 7.15
Design space of sample volume and batch size for the use of double filters with 10^7 CFU/cm^2 retention capability and 1000 cm^2 EFA and no more than 5% probability of false negative and breach in 1 in 1,000,000 batches.

7.5 Concluding Remarks

Sterile drug products are often manufactured through aseptic processing, which employs sterilizing filtration to remove microbial contaminants. High bioburden in unfiltered drug solution may increase the chance of breaching the sterilizing filter and causing safety and quality issues. As a result, a prefiltration bioburden test is recommended by regulatory guidelines. The EMA guidelines stipulate that a maximum acceptable bioburden level must be established before the sterile filtration step and that in general no more than 10 CFU/100 mL will be acceptable. However, a sample volume of 100 mL represents a significant proportion of the batch and a high cost for biotech products, particularly taking into account that an overage and reserve sample are often needed. Therefore, it is desirable to explore alternate sample volumes and test methods that warrant the same or higher level of quality assurance as the EMA-recommended method with smaller test volumes. Because the EMA guidelines do not provide scientific rationale for the limit 10 CFU/100 mL, it is difficult to justify a test volume smaller than 100 mL.

In this chapter, a risk-based approach was described for justifying alternate bioburden test volumes smaller than 100 mL, with associated decision criteria. By modeling bioburden in the unfiltered and final drug solution, the relationships between prefiltration/postfiltration risk and the associated risk factors, such as test sample volume and batch size, are established. Such relationships allow for a quantitative evaluation of the impact of the risk factors on the risks and development of effective risk control strategies, which include acceptable selections of sample test volume and maximum prefiltration bioburden level. The risk-based approach is in accordance with the QbD principles in ICH Q8 that enable manufacturers to define a manufacturing process design space that consistently produces high-quality products through increased understanding and knowledge of the product and process. It is also consistent with the ICH quality initiative, Quality Risk Management, which achieves greater product quality assurance through risk identification, analysis, and control.

Key results in this chapter include the following: (1) Prefiltration and postfiltration risks are intercorrelated. A holistic approach needs to be taken in developing risk mitigation strategies so that a high risk in one process step can be mitigated through controlling risk factors in the other step. (2) Risk factors are interdependent and should be considered jointly when evaluating their impact on the prefiltration and postfiltration risks. This includes selection of sample test volume, acceptable limits, sterilizing filters, and so on in a joint manner. (3) A bioburden level higher than 10 CFU/100 mL, which is a regulatory limit, in the unfiltered drug solution may not incur unnecessary risk as its impact can be mitigated through effective sterilizing filtration. (4) Sample volumes less than 100 mL and acceptance limits different from 10 CFU/100 mL can be justified, through controlling other risk factors such as batch size, without increasing the risk of bioburden breakthrough in the final filtration. (5) Adoption of either double sampling or double filters can lead to additional product quality assurance with smaller sample test volumes. (6) Increased understanding of process and product is key to successful bioburden risk management.

8

Process Validation

8.1 Introduction

Process validation is a regulatory requirement, and the traditional approach to process validation was a compliance-driven event. Success of process validation was characterized by a demonstration that the process is capable of producing three consecutive, commercial-scale batches that meet quality standards. This approach uses little product and process knowledge to identify critical quality attributes (CQAs). As a result, the process performance characteristics chosen for validation may not be truly indicative of product quality. In addition, even if the three-batch validation study is successful, the chance for future batches to meet acceptance limits remains unknown. In January 2011, the Food and Drug Administration (FDA) published updated guidance *FDA Guidance for Industry on Process Validation: General Principles and Practices* (FDA 2011). The guidance places a great deal of emphasis on process design and process control during commercial manufacturing. It stresses that process validation is not a one-time event, but an ongoing program. Process validation is defined as "the collection and evaluation of data, from the process design through commercial production, which establishes scientific evidence that a process is capable of consistently delivering quality." The guidance aligns process validation activities with a product life cycle and risk-based paradigm, as well as with other existing guidelines, including ICH Q8(R2) *Pharmaceutical Development* (ICH 2006), ICH Q9 *Quality Risk Management* (ICH 2007a), ICH Q10 *Pharmaceutical Quality Systems* (ICH 2007b), and ICH Q11 *Concept Paper* (ICH 2011). It represents a significant shift of regulatory requirements from the traditional "test to compliance" approach using one experiment to the "quality by design" approach throughout the life cycle of the product and process. It ushers in a science and risk-based development paradigm that yields product quality through process design and control. The new guidance approaches process validation in three stages:

- Stage 1—Process Design (PD): The commercial manufacturing process is defined during this stage based on knowledge gained through development and scale-up activities.

- Stage 2—Process Performance Qualification (PPQ): During this stage, the PD is evaluated to determine whether the process is capable of reproducible commercial manufacturing.
- Stage 3—Continued Process Verification: Ongoing assurance is gained during routine production that the process remains in a state of control.

The guidance emphasizes the use of information and knowledge from product and process developed as the basis for establishing control of the commercial manufacturing process and ensuring quality product. The alignment of the guidance with other ICH quality guidelines further promotes the use of modern pharmaceutical development concepts, quality risk management, and quality systems at all stages of the manufacturing process life cycle. The guidance also reiterates the importance of the use of statistical tools and analyses in understanding and controlling process variations. Specifically, areas where objective measures through well-designed studies and statistical thinking are needed include the following:

- Understand the sources of variation
- Detect the presence and quantify the degree of variation
- Understand the impact of variation on the process and ultimately on product attributes
- Control the variation in a manner commensurate with the risk it represents to the process and product

This chapter concerns statistical methods used for process validation. This includes identification of CQAs and associated control strategies, development of a design space based on understanding of process variations, selection of the number of PPQ batches for the second stage of process validation, and advancements in statistical control for continued process validation.

8.2 Process Design

Process design is the first stage of the life cycle approach to process validation. Various studies, mostly at small scale, are conducted to gain process knowledge and understanding. Process information, including different sources of variation and relationships between input variables and resulting outputs, serves as the basis of process design. Experiments need to be designed, using sound scientific and statistical principles and strategies, so that quality data can be generated with a minimum number of studies. Process design involves three critical components: identification of CQAs, development of design space, and establishment of process control. Determination of CQAs is an iterative process throughout the life cycle of the product. With new information, a CQA identified in an early stage of process design may become a non-CQA later, and vice versa. Well-defined CQAs enable the development of a manufacturing process that produces a product with the desired CQAs. Design spaces are results of experiments in which the impact of input process parameters and material attributes on product quality, safety, and efficacy characterized through CQAs is evaluated. A design space may be developed for each unit operation, but ultimately an overall design space is defined for the product. Operating within the design space should give rise to a product conforming to quality standards. Strategies for process control are aimed at reduction of or adjustment of input variation during manufacturing. Process knowledge and understanding is the basis for establishing effective control strategies. Specification testing, in-process testing, and characterization tests performed during process comparability studies and continuous process monitoring are elements of control strategies. More advanced control methods may include process analytical technology, which maintains constant output through adjustment of process conditions based on timely analysis of product quality attributes at various stages of processing.

8.2.1 Identification of CQAs

8.2.1.1 General Considerations

As previously discussed, knowledge used for CQA identification may include cumulative nonclinical and clinical experience of the product, the mechanism of action, data from molecules in the same class, and publications in literature. In addition, process understanding is another source of information useful for determination of CQAs. This may include understanding of process variability from early development, similar processes or platform technologies, data from unit operation development studies, and manufacturing experience.

Methods for criticality analysis, including assignment of severity scores and probabilities of occurrence, have been well studied in the literature. Commonly used approaches include Failure Mode and Effects Analysis (FMEA) (ICH 2007a), Cause and Effect Matrix, and Pareto analysis (Yang et al. 2015c). Criticality analysis can also be conducted in a qualitative fashion based on expert opinion, published literature, and regulatory guidance. A general method is described in Chapter 7 in the context of assessing criticality of risk factors for a prefiltration process to reduce bioburden. In the following sections, an example of how to assess the criticality of residual host cell DNA is discussed.

8.2.1.2 Example

As discussed in Chapter 5, it is inevitable that biological products contain residual host cell DNA. Although the actually oncogenic and infective risk attributed to the residual host DNA is unknown, it is theoretically possible that it could transmit oncogenes and infective agents to the product recipients. Of interest is the determination of the criticality of residual DNA, based on its impact on product safety and efficacy, in terms of bioactivity, PK/PD, immunogenicity, and adverse events. Data in the literature have suggested that DNA, being a process-related impurity, is not expected to affect product bioactivity (Schenerman et al. 2009). It is its potential for oncogenicity, infectivity, and immunomodulatory effects that is of concern (Dortant et al. 1997; Ishii et al. 2004; Petricciani and Loewer 2001; Rothenfusser et al. 2003; Sheng et al. 2008; Sheng-Fowler et al. 2009a,b, 2010).

8.2.1.2.1 Immunogenicity Risk

Immunostimulatory CpG motifs (i.e., unmethylated dinucleotides of cytosine and guanine) are normally not present in the human body. When introduced, they may result in immunogenic reactions. Klinman et al. (2006) showed that some DNA-based vaccines incorporate CpG motifs to increase immunogenicity. It has been reported that such vaccinations caused induction of anti-DNA antibodies (Arfaj et al. 2007). Interestingly, it has been shown in animal studies that the extent of immune response depends on several factors, including the source and type of DNA, the amount of CpG in a plasmid, and the ratio of CpG to all DNA present (Klinman et al. 1997; Kojima et al. 2002). Taken together, the published results suggest that residual DNA may have the potential to cause immunogenic reactions.

8.2.1.2.2 Oncogenicity and Infectivity Risk

It is theoretically possible that residual DNA may transmit either infectious viral genome or an activated oncogene to product recipients. This is particularly true when the biological product is manufactured in a cell line known to be tumorigenic (Peden et al. 2006). It is well recognized that the oncogenic and infective risk of residual DNA is related to both the size and amount of the DNA in the final dose. Guidance issued by both WHO (2007) and the FDA (2011) recommends mitigating such risk by reducing both the size and amount of residual DNA. The host cell DNA specification was set to 10 ng DNA/dose (WHO 2007), while fragments of DNA were recommended to be smaller than 200 base pairs to render substantial safety margins (FDA 2011).

8.2.1.2.3 Criticality and Control of Residual DNA

Residual DNA is of high safety risk. As regulatory guidelines require that both the amount and size of residual DNA be quantified to ensure conformance to specifications, residual DNA is considered a CQA. Since the size and amount of residual DNA are intercorrelated and may affect drug safety jointly, it is important to establish control strategies by taking into account the correlation. On the basis of the mechanistic model described in Chapter 5, Yang et al. (2015b) established the linkage between residual DNA and product safety, measured with respect to oncogenicity, infectivity, and immunogenicity. Such a link makes it possible to develop a joint acceptable range for these attributes of residual DNA.

8.2.2 Design Space

After the CQAs are identified, process characterization studies are carried out. These studies are based on multifactorial experiments, in which the effects of process parameters and input material attributes on the CQAs are evaluated. Typically, statistical designs of experiments are used to gain experimental efficiency. Before the characterization studies, a risk analysis is performed to select experimental (process or raw material) factors that are deemed to be of high or medium impact on CQAs. Knowledge gained from these studies, coupled with other historical data and manufacturing experience, serves as the basis for establishing a design space, product specifications, and manufacturing control strategies.

Per ICH Q8 (R2) (2007), a design space is "The multidimensional combination and interaction of input variables (e.g., material attributes) and process parameters that have been demonstrated to provide assurance of quality." For example, a design space for a cell culture system can be ranges of temperature, pH, feed volume, and culture duration that provide quality product. Design space is a key concept intimately tied with quality system risk management principles. By linking manufacturing variations with the variability of CQAs, it sets the stage for developing effective manufacturing controls. A design space also has regulatory implications for postapproval changes as "working within the design space is not considered as a change. Movement out of the design space is considered to be a change and would normally initiate a regulatory post-approval change process" (ICH Q8 (R2)). A well-developed design space enables the manufacturer to continuously improve the manufacturing process by adopting advanced technologies without incurring additional risk and creating more regulatory hurdles.

8.2.3 Statistical Methods for Design Space

Several statistical methods have been proposed to determine design space through multivariate regression analysis. Of note are two traditional approaches: overlapping mean response surfaces and the desirability function. The design space is determined to be either a multivariate region, in which the mean response values of CQAs are within specifications, or a region where the desirability function exceeds a prespecified threshold. The desirability function is the geometric mean of measures related to individual CQAs, each taking a value between 0 and 1. As pointed out by Peterson (2008), these traditional methods do not take into account correlations among CQAs, nor do they account for variability of the prediction. Recently, a Bayesian method was proposed (Peterson 2008). The method is based on the posterior predictive distributions of responses (CQAs) and determines the design space such that the product has high probability of conforming to specifications when process parameters are set within the space. The method was illustrated through practical applications by Stockdale and Cheng (2009). Extensions of the method to more complex experimental designs were discussed by Peterson (2009) and LeBrun (2012). In this section, we focus our discussion on the overlapping mean response surfaces and Bayesian methods.

8.2.3.1 Overlapping Mean Response Surfaces

In the appendix of ICH Q8(R2), an example of design space based on the overlapping mean response surfaces is provided. The design space consists of combinations of two process parameters that deliver satisfactory drug product characterized by dissolution and friability. Figures 8.1 and 8.2 depict the contour plots of dissolution and friability, respectively, as a function of two process parameters. It is desired that dissolution is greater than 80% and friability is less than 2%. The overlapping mean response surfaces method defines the design space as the combinations of the two parameters where the conditions dissolution >80% and friability <2% are both met. It is shown in Figure 8.3.

However, the design space as defined this way does not provide adequate assurance of product quality. For example, in the combination of parameters marked by the circle in Figure 8.3, there is only a 50% chance for the

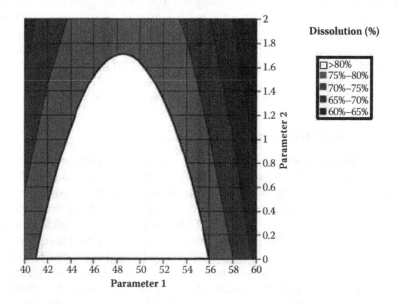

FIGURE 8.1
Contour plot of dissolution. (Adapted from ICH (2006). Q8(R2) Pharmaceutical Development. http://www.fda.gov/downloads/Drugs/.../Guidances/ucm073507.pdf.)

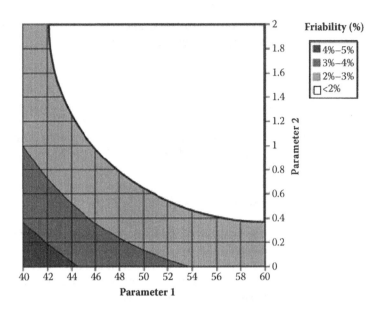

FIGURE 8.2
Contour plot of friability. (Adapted from ICH (2006). Q8(R2) Pharmaceutical Development. http://www.fda.gov/downloads/Drugs/.../Guidances/ucm073507.pdf.)

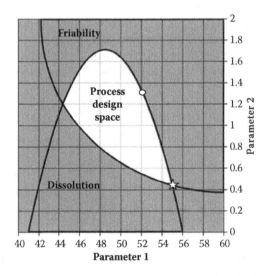

FIGURE 8.3
Overlapping mean contour plot with design space in the common region where both dissolution and friability meet their respective specifications. (Adapted from ICH (2006). Q8(R2) Pharmaceutical Development. http://www.fda.gov/downloads/Drugs/.../Guidances/ucm073507.pdf.)

conditions dissolution > 80% and friability < 2% to be met. The probability drops to 25% for the combination labeled by the star in Figure 8.3.

8.2.3.2 Bayesian Approach

A Bayesian approach to determining a design space was suggested by Peterson (2008). Application of the method was demonstrated by Stockdale and Cheng (2009) through two case studies. The Bayesian method and various extensions were also explored by LeBrun (2012). The Bayesian design space is defined as

$$\{x: \Pr[Y \in A|x, \text{data}] \geq R\}, \tag{8.1}$$

where $Y = (Y_1,...,Y_p)'$ is a $p \times 1$ vector of measures of p CQAs; A is the set of joint acceptable ranges of the CQAs; x is a $k \times 1$ vector of process parameters and other controllable inputs, such as material attributes; "Pr" stands for posterior predictive probability; "data" is the data set from a controlled experiment, which includes measured response values of CQAs and various settings of process parameters; and R is a preselected level of reliability.

Because the posterior predictive probability takes into account the uncertainty in model parameters and correlation among response variables, it overcomes the drawbacks of the overlapping mean response surface method. In addition, the Bayesian method can be easily extended to accommodate many different types of experiments such as split-plot and multibatch (Peterson 2007), as well as experiments involving mixed effects (LeBrun 2012). The Bayesian design space in Equation 8.1 can be determined by estimating the probability $\Pr[Y \in A|x, \text{data}]$ over a grid of x values. The posterior predictive probability can be estimated either through a closed-form solution or by Markov Chain Monte Carlo simulations. The concept of design (DS) is illustrated in Figure 8.4.

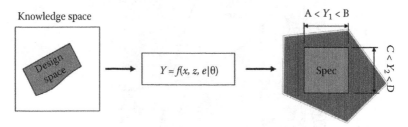

FIGURE 8.4
Design space (DS) based on Bayesian predictive modeling that links input process parameters *x* and material attribute *z* with CQAs *Y*. The DS is determined such that there is a high probability that the CQAs meet their acceptance criteria when the process parameters and material attributes are within DS.

8.2.3.2.1 Simple Regression Model

Following Peterson (2008) and Stockdale and Cheng (2009), we assume that the measured responses of CQAs (**Y**) can be described through a multivariate regression model:

$$Y = Bz(x) + e, \tag{8.2}$$

where **B** is a $p \times q$ matrix of regression coefficients, $z(x)$ is a $q \times 1$ vector function of **x**, and **e** is a $p \times 1$ vector of measurement errors having a multivariate normal distribution with mean **0** and covariance–variance matrix Σ.

It is assumed that $z(x)$ is the same for each CQA, although the method described in this section can be extended to the seemingly unrelated regressions (SUR) model (Peterson 2006), in which each response Y_i $(i = 1,...p)$ has a different set of covariates $Z_i(x)$.

8.2.3.2.2 Prior Information

Use of prior information is a critical step in statistical inference based on a posterior predictive distribution. Peterson (2008) discussed various ways in which prior information can be elicited. An informative prior distribution may be established from experiments done at the pilot scale, with the intent to be used for developing a design space for the commercial manufacturing. However, oftentimes data from pilot-scale experiments may not be sufficient for constructing informative priors. Peterson (2008) discussed three additional sources of information that can be potentially used. The first is the so-called first principles approach, which predicts process performance based on a combination of experimental data and mechanistic knowledge of the process. The second is to use a semiempirical approach to predict process performance at the manufacturing scale based on correlation among different scales. The third is to use subjective prior information from expert opinions. The prior information is expressed through a prior distribution and incorporated into the posterior predictive probability using Bayes' theorem.

8.2.3.2.3 Posterior Predictive Probability

Let $Y_{obs} = (Y_1,..., Y_n)'$ be an $n \times p$ matrix consisting of n observations of the $1 \times p$ response vector **Y**. Let $Z_{exp} = (Z_1,..., Z_n)'$ be an $n \times q$ matrix with $Z_i = z(x_i)$, $i = 1,...,n$, and let x_i be the ith condition of the controllable input variables and process parameters. Assuming that a noninformative prior is used to describe the parameters (B, Σ):

$$p(B, \Sigma) \propto |\Sigma|^{-(p+1)/2}. \tag{8.3}$$

It is well known (Press 1972) that posterior predictive distribution of a future observation $\tilde{\mathbf{Y}}$ is a multivariate t with degrees of freedom $v = n - p - q + 1$:

$$\tilde{\mathbf{Y}} \mid \mathbf{x}, \text{ data} \sim t_v\left(\hat{\mathbf{B}}\mathbf{z}(\mathbf{x}), \mathbf{H}\right) \tag{8.4}$$

where

$$\mathbf{D} = \sum_{i=1}^{n} \mathbf{Z}_i\mathbf{Z}_i' \quad \text{and} \quad \mathbf{H} = [1 + \mathbf{z}(\mathbf{x})'\mathbf{D}^{-1}\mathbf{z}(\mathbf{x})]\hat{\boldsymbol{\Sigma}}]$$

and $\hat{\mathbf{B}}$ and $\hat{\boldsymbol{\Sigma}}$ are the least square estimates of $\mathbf{B}$ and Σ given by

$$\hat{\mathbf{B}} = (\mathbf{Z}_{exp}'\mathbf{Z}_{exp})^{-1}\mathbf{Z}_{exp}'\mathbf{Y}_{obs}$$

$$\hat{\boldsymbol{\Sigma}} = [\mathbf{Y}_{obs} - (\hat{\mathbf{B}}\mathbf{Z})']'[\mathbf{Y}_{obs} - (\hat{\mathbf{B}}\mathbf{Z})']/v, \text{ with } v = n - p - q + 1.$$

8.2.3.2.4 Determination of Design Space

Because the posterior predictive distribution is a multivariate t distribution, it can be simulated as follows (Peterson 2007):

1. Draw $\mathbf{W}$ from the multivariate normal distribution $N(\mathbf{0}, \mathbf{H})$.
2. Draw U from the χ^2 distribution χ_v^2.
3. Calculate $Y_j = \sqrt{v}W_j/\sqrt{U} + \hat{\mu}_j$ for $j = 1,...,p$ where Y_j, W_j, and $\hat{\mu}_j$ are the jth elements of $\mathbf{Y}$, $\mathbf{W}$, and $\hat{\mathbf{B}}\mathbf{z}(\mathbf{x})$, respectively.

As suggested by Peterson (2009), the posterior predictive probability can be approximated using Monte Carlo simulation:

$$p(\mathbf{x}) = \Pr[\mathbf{Y} \in A \mid \mathbf{x}, \text{ data}]$$

$$\approx \frac{1}{N}\sum_{s=1}^{N} I(\mathbf{Y}^{(s)} \in A),$$

where $\mathbf{Y}^{(s)}$, $s = 1,...,N$, are independent random multivariate t variables simulated from the above-mentioned procedure, and $I(\cdot)$ is an indicator function taking values of either 0 or 1.

The design space defined in Equation 8.1 can be obtained by estimating the posterior predictive probability $p(\mathbf{x})$ over a grid of $\mathbf{x}$ and comparing it to the reliability threshold R.

8.2.3.2.5 Remarks

Alternatively, informative prior distributions may be used in the derivation of the posterior predictive probability. For example, one may use conjugate prior distributions for $p(\mathbf{B}|\Sigma)$ and $p(\Sigma)$ (LeBrun 2012):

$$\mathbf{B}|\Sigma \sim N_{p\times q}(\mathbf{B}_0, \Sigma, \Sigma_0)$$

$$\Sigma \sim W_1^{-1}(\Omega, v_0),$$

where $\mathbf{B}_0$ is the mean vector and Σ and Σ_0 are the covariance matrices of the columns and rows of $\mathbf{B}$, respectively; Σ follows an inverse-Wishart distribution with Ω being an a priori response scale matrix and v_0 being the degrees of freedom.

It was shown by LeBrun (2012) that the posterior predictive probability in this case is also a multivariate t distribution. Thus, using the Monte Carlo simulation procedure previously described, the Bayesian design space can be constructed.

In many cases, the standard multivariate regression model (Equation 8.2) cannot adequately describe different types of CQAs, as the model assumes the same regression model for each CQA. Under such circumstances, the SUR model provides greater flexibility and accuracy in modeling the CQAs (Peterson 2007). A SUR model takes the following form:

$$Y_j = \mathbf{z}_j(\mathbf{x})' \, \beta_j + e_j, \quad j = 1,...,p. \tag{8.5}$$

The SUR model includes the standard multivariate regression model as a special case where $\mathbf{z}_j(\mathbf{x}) = \mathbf{z}(\mathbf{x})$. Thus, a design space based on the SUR model and posterior predictive probability can be similarly obtained (Peterson 2007).

8.3 Process Performance Qualification

After process characterization studies are completed and design spaces are determined, PPQ activities commence. The goal of PPQ is to demonstrate through a formal study that the process is fit for commercial manufacturing. Data generated during PPQ are analyzed to confirm that the process is reproducible and capable of consistently delivering quality product. A formal study protocol is required. It details quality attributes to be tested, acceptance criteria, method(s) of statistical analysis, and, importantly, the number of PPQ batches. Traditionally, three batches produced from commercial-scale production were used for PPQ. However, there is little scientific basis for the three-batch-validation rule, nor was it determined based on statistical principles. Therefore, validation based on the three-batch method does not provide the necessary control over both consumer and producer risks, resulting in limited quality assurance. The new FDA guidance allows for a risk-based approach to the determination of the number of batches for PPQ. For instance, if the process was shown to be robust during the process design stage, it might not be necessary to have a large PPQ study. In contrast, for a process that had a history of inconsistent performance due to less controlled variations or product understanding, even if it passes three-batch PPQ acceptance criteria, it may not necessarily imply that it will provide a high level of assurance that batches produced in the future will consistently meet prespecified specifications. Therefore, consideration should be given to knowledge and understanding of the process gained from Stage 1 in determining number of batches for Stage 2 PPQ. This may include process capability, sources of variation, in-process control, and so on. The knowledge from the design stage may help determine the number of PPQ batches, which may be smaller or bigger than three batches. In the following section, we describe several methods for determining and justifying the number of batches for PPQ.

8.3.1 Risk-Based Approaches

A risk-based approach to determine the number of PPQ batches was proposed by Bryder et al. (2015). The general principle is that a high-risk process requires more PPQ batches successfully meeting acceptance criteria to demonstrate its capability of reproducibly producing quality product, whereas a low-risk process needs a fewer number of PPQ batches. The method provides a framework for determining overall residual risk based on product and process knowledge and understanding of control strategies. This residual risk serves as the basis for determining the number of PPQ batches.

8.3.1.1 Determination of Residual Risk Level

The residual risk level is determined based on risk assessment of product knowledge, process understanding, and control strategies. Product knowledge can be obtained through identification of CQAs and linking them to product safety and efficacy so as to determine the appropriate acceptable ranges. The risk related to product knowledge depends on how robust the acceptable ranges are. Acceptance ranges based on sound justifications mitigate safety and efficacy risk. Process understanding and associated risk can be established using data from the development phase, prior experience, studies conducted to develop unit operations, and scale-up activities using statistical modeling to predict commercial-scale performance based on small-scale data. The more understanding of variations that affect process performance, the more effectively can control strategies be devised;

TABLE 8.1

Residual Risk Levels

Residual Risk	Risk Level	Description
Severe	5	Multiple factors have high risk ratings
High	4	Few factors have high risk ratings or all have medium risk ratings
Moderate	3	Medium risk level for multiple factors or high risk level for one factor
Low	2	Medium risk level for a few factors and low risk for others
Minimal	1	Lower risk level for all factors

Source: Bryder, M., Etling, H., Fleming, J., Hu, Y., and Levy, P. (2015). Topic 1—Stage 2 process validation: Determining and justifying the number of process qualification batches, ISPE discussion paper: PV stage 2, number of batches (version 2). https://www.phar mamedtechbi.com/~/media/Supporting%20Documents/The%20Gold%20Sheet/47/2 /stage2processvalidation1.pdf

thus, less risk is associated with process variability. Product knowledge and process understanding culminate in the establishment of control strategies. Risks associated with control strategies directly correlate with how well the variability of critical material attributes and process parameters is understood and managed. In addition, consideration should be given to equipment qualification and manufacturing environmental controls, as they may contribute to risks associated with control strategies. For the aforesaid risk analysis, analytical tools such as FMEA can be utilized. The outcome of this risk assessment serves as the basis for determining the residual risk level of the process. Residual risk level is the level of remaining risk that the process will not produce a commercial-scale product that consistently meets quality standards. It should be assessed using quality risk management tools to provide a risk ranking of various factors, including CQAs. At the conclusion of this assessment, a residual risk level is assigned to the process. One example given by Bryder et al. (2015) categorizes residual risk into five levels: severe, high, moderate, low, and minimal, as shown in Table 8.1.

8.3.1.2 Determination of Number of PPQ Batches

The overall risk level of a process provides a basis for determining the number of PPQ batches. Three methods were suggested by Bryder et al. (2015).

8.3.1.2.1 Rationale-Based Approach

This method is based on the reasoning that increased residual risk should be overcome by an increased number of PPQ batches that are expected to meet acceptance criteria. When the process has a "Severe" residual risk level, it is deemed not ready for PPQ and more development efforts need to be made to improve the process and controls. For a process with a "High" residual risk level, 10 PPQ batches are recommended as a larger number of successful

PPQ batches than the traditional 3 are required to render confidence in the process. The number of PPQ batches is recommended to be 5, 3, and 1–2 for moderate, low, and minimal residual risk levels, respectively.

8.3.1.2.2 Approach Based on Target Process Confidence and Capability

This method determines the number of PPQ batches based on the process capability index C_{pk}. A process that produces a product that is highly likely to meet specifications is a capable process. How well a process meets specifications is assessed by comparing the variability of the process to the specifications. The process index C_{pk} defined below is one measure of capability:

$$C_{pk} = \min\left[\frac{USL - \mu}{3\sigma}, \frac{\mu - LSL}{3\sigma}\right], \tag{8.6}$$

where LSL and USL are the lower and upper specification limits, respectively, and μ and σ are the process mean and standard deviation, respectively.

When μ and σ are unknown, assuming the CQA is normally distributed, C_{pk} is often estimated by replacing μ and σ with the sample mean and standard deviation $\bar{X}$ and s, respectively:

$$\hat{C}_{pk} = \min\left[\frac{USL - \bar{X}}{3s}, \frac{\bar{X} - LSL}{3s}\right].$$

An approximate one-sided $(1 - \alpha) \times 100\%$ lower confidence limit for C_{pk} can be obtained (Bissell 1990):

$$\hat{C}_{pk} - z_{1-\alpha}\sqrt{\frac{1}{9n} + \frac{\hat{C}_{pk}^2}{2(n-1)}}, \tag{8.7}$$

where $z_{1-\alpha}$ is the $100(1 - \alpha)$th percentile of the standard normal distribution.

The method suggested by Bryder et al. (2015) chooses the number of PPQ batches n such that

$$\hat{C}_{pk} - z_{1-\alpha}\sqrt{\frac{1}{9n} + \frac{\hat{C}_{pk}^2}{2(n-1)}} \geq c_0, \tag{8.8}$$

where c_0 is a preselected cut point representing the smallest capability index a process needs to have in order to be deemed capable. It is referred to as target process performance by Bryder et al. (2015). $\hat{C}_{pk}$ is usually obtained based on data from Stage 1 of process validation.

TABLE 8.2

Target Confidence Level

Residual Risk Level	Severe	High	Moderate	Low	Minimal
Target confidence	N/A[a]	97%	95%	90%	N/A

Source: Bryder, M., Etling, H., Fleming, J., Hu, Y., and Levy, P. (2015). Topic 1—Stage 2 process validation: Determining and justifying the number of process qualification batches, ISPE discussion paper: PV stage 2, number of batches (version 2). https://www.pharmamedtechbi.com/~/media/Supporting%20Documents/The%20Gold%20Sheet/47/2/stage2processvalidation1.pdf

[a] NA, additional development studies are necessary and process is not ready for PPQ.

Bryder et al. (2015) argued that it is reasonable to choose $c_0 = 1$ as a process having a C_{pk} of 1.0 or greater and is a capable process. In order to solve the above inequality for n, one needs to specify the confidence level $1 - \alpha$, which is called target process confidence (Bryder et al. 2015). The number of PPQ batches should be chosen consummate with the residual risk level of the process previously discussed. In general, the higher the residual risk level is, the higher the target process confidence needs to be, in order to gain additional assurance during PPQ that the product produced by the process meets quality standards. A general guidance concerning how to determine the target confidence is provided in Bryder et al. (2015), and the recommended correlation of residual levels and target confidence levels is listed in Table 8.2.

From Equation 8.8 and Table 8.2, the minimum number of PPQ batches can be calculated. Bryder et al. (2015) provided an example for $\hat{C}_{pk} = 1.6$, which they referred to as the "Readily Pass" criterion. In other words, a process with a capability index of 1.6 is considered to have a high likelihood of passing PPQ.

8.3.1.2.3 Expected Coverage

This method is based on the properties of order statistics. That is, the expected probability for a future observation to fall within the minimum and maximum observed values $[x^{(1)}, x^{(n)}]$ is given by $\dfrac{n-1}{n+1}$. Considering this probability as the "coverage" of the future observations provided by the batch data used for PPQ, the number of PPQ batches n can be chosen to render the desired level of coverage. Consideration should be given to the residual risk of the process before PPQ. As noted above, the higher the residual risk, the more coverage is needed to provide sufficient quality assurance. Several examples were given by Bryder et al. (2015). For example, for a process with high residual risk, $n = 9$ is suggested to render 80% coverage; whereas $n = 3$ is recommended for a process with lower residual risk. These two scenarios are listed in Table 8.3, along with a few others.

TABLE 8.3

Number of Batches Needed to Achieve Expected Coverage Probability

Residual Risk	Expected Coverage	Number of PPQ Batches
Severe	N/A	Not ready for PPQ
High	80%	9
Moderate	70%	6
Low	50%	3
Minimal[a]	N/A	1–3

Source: Bryder, M., Etling, H., Fleming, J., Hu, Y., and Levy, P. (2015). Topic 1—Stage 2 process validation: Determining and justifying the number of process qualification batches, ISPE discussion paper: PV stage 2, number of batches (version 2). https://www.pharmamedtechbi.com/~/media/Supporting%20Documents/The%20Gold%20Sheet/47/2/stage2processvalidation1.pdf

[a] When a process has a severe residual risk level, it is deemed to be not ready for PPQ. Therefore, no number of PPQ batches is provided in the table.

8.3.2 Bayesian Alternative

The FDA guidance suggests that the approach to PPQ be based on sound science and the manufacturer's overall level of product and process understanding and demonstrable control. However, synthesizing information from both process design and quantification stages to confirm that the process performance meets quality standards can be a formidable task. Likewise, determining the number of PPQ batches using the combined data can be also challenging. Yang (2013c) proposed a Bayesian approach to this issue. A prominent feature of the Bayesian sample size calculation is that it uses prior information regarding process performance to fully account for the uncertainty in the predicted data. With this method, process performance data from Stage 1 are used to describe a prior distribution for process performance parameters. This distribution, coupled with expected outcomes of Stage 2 (PPQ), produces a posterior distribution for process performance parameters. Finally, the predictive probability for the future batches to meet acceptance criteria is calculated. Because this probability is dependent on the number of PPQ batches, the number can be determined to ensure that the predictive probability exceeds a prespecified threshold.

Now consider that n batches are intended to be used in the PPQ study. We further suppose for the purposes of illustration that the quality attribute is potency. Let x_i, $i = 1,..., n$ be random binary variables such that $x_i = 1$ if the potency of batch i is within specification; otherwise, $x_i = 0$. Therefore, x_i follows a Bernoulli distribution $B(p)$, that is,

$$P[x_i = 1|p] = p, \tag{8.9}$$

where $p(0 \leq p \leq 1)$ is the probability for a batch to pass the potency specification.

Hence, $\mathbf{x} = (x_1, \ldots x_n)$ represent the data from the PPQ study. Let $\tilde{x}$ be the potency test outcome of a future batch after PPQ is successfully concluded. The number of batches n is chosen such that

$$P[\tilde{x} = 1 \mid \mathbf{x}] \geq p_0, \tag{8.10}$$

where p_0 is prespecified to represent an appropriate level of statistical assurance. In other words, the sample size is chosen so that a future batch will meet specification with a high probability ($\geq p_0$) after the successful completion of PPQ. A prior distribution of the unknown parameter p is needed. Historical data can be used to construct the distribution of p. When there is little information available, a noninformative prior may be chosen. By contrast, the prior distribution can be estimated when a large amount of historical data are readily available. In Yang (2013c), it was assumed that the prior distribution of p is a beta distribution $B(\alpha, \beta)$. Various statistical methods, such as moment estimation, can be used to estimate the parameters (α, β) based on the historical data. Let $m = \sum_{i=1}^{n} x_i$ denote the total number of batches used in the PPQ study that are required to pass the potency specification. It is well known that the posterior probability of p given the observed data x follows a beta distribution $B(\alpha + m, \beta + n - m)$ (Spiegelhalter et al. 2004). Consequently,

$$\begin{aligned} P[\tilde{x} = 1 \mid \mathbf{x}] &= \int_0^1 P[\tilde{x} = 1 \mid p] P[p \mid x] dp \\ &= \int_0^1 p P[p \mid x] dp \\ &= \frac{\alpha + m}{\alpha + \beta + n}. \end{aligned} \tag{8.11}$$

As previously mentioned, a successful PPQ requires that all n validation batches pass the potency specification, which implies $m = n$. Certainly, alternative acceptance criteria can be used. For the purpose of illustration, we adopted the requirement that all batches pass. Under this requirement, we have

$$\Pr[\tilde{x} = 1 \mid x] = \frac{\alpha + n}{\alpha + \beta + n}. \tag{8.12}$$

As a direct consequence, the number of PPQ batches n satisfies

$$\frac{\alpha + n}{\alpha + \beta + n} \geq p_0. \tag{8.13}$$

This is equivalent to

$$n \geq \frac{p_0}{1-p_0} \beta - \alpha. \tag{8.14}$$

As an illustration, when $p_0 = 95\%$, the above inequality becomes

$$n \geq 19\beta - \alpha. \tag{8.15}$$

Using a moment method to estimate (α, β) can be estimated using historical data. For example, suppose there are J historical data sets, each providing an estimate, y_j, $j = 1,\ldots,J$, of the percentage of batches that meet the specification. It is also assumed that y_j follows a beta distribution $B(\alpha,\beta)$. Let $\bar{y}$ and s_{yy} be the sample mean and variance, respectively:

$$\bar{y} = \frac{1}{J}\sum_{i=1}^{J} y_i,$$

$$s_{yy} = \frac{1}{J-1}\sum_{i=1}^{J}[y_i - \bar{y}]^2 \tag{8.16}$$

Note that

$$E[y_j] = \frac{\alpha}{\alpha+\beta}$$

$$\mathrm{Var}[y_j] = \frac{\alpha\beta}{(\alpha+\beta)^2(\alpha+\beta+1)}. \tag{8.17}$$

The moment estimates $(\hat{\alpha},\hat{\beta})$ of (α, β) can be obtained as the solutions to the following equations:

$$\frac{\alpha}{\alpha+\beta} = \bar{y}$$

$$\frac{\alpha\beta}{(\alpha+\beta)^2(\alpha+\beta+1)} = s_{yy}.$$

Solving the above equations gives rise to

$$\hat{\alpha} = \frac{\bar{y}^2(1-\bar{y})}{s_{yy}} - \bar{y}$$

$$\hat{\beta} = \frac{\bar{y}(1-\bar{y})^2}{s_{yy}} + \bar{y} - 1. \tag{8.18}$$

As an illustration, assume that estimates of the prior beta distribution based on historical studies are given by $\hat{\alpha} = 28.4$ and $\hat{\beta} = 1.68$. By Equation 8.15, when $p_0 = 95\%$, the number of PPQ batches n satisfies

$$n \geq 19\hat{\beta} - \hat{\alpha} = 3.52. \tag{8.19}$$

Therefore, four PPQ batches are needed to provide adequate assurance for a future post-PPQ batch to meet the potency specification.

8.3.2.1 Generalization of Bayesian Method

The quality statement that leads to the sample size calculations such as those described above can be formulated in different ways. Particularly, for certain products, there are only a limited number of batches produced either annually or during the lifetime of the product. Under those circumstances, it may be more sensible to determine the number of PPQ batches such that with high confidence, at least k out of l ($1 \leq k \leq l$) future batches after PPQ will meet specifications. To determine the number of PPQ batches that will meet this requirement, we define

$$\tilde{p} = \Pr[\tilde{x} = 1 \mid \mathbf{x}] \quad \text{and} \quad \tilde{X} = \sum_{i=1}^{l} \tilde{x}_i, \tag{8.20}$$

where $(\tilde{x}_1, ... \tilde{x}_l)$ are the test outcomes of the future l batches produced after PPQ.

Because $\tilde{x}_i$, $i = 1, ..., l$, follow Bernoulli distribution $B(\tilde{p})$, it is apparent that $\tilde{X} \mid \mathbf{x} \sim \text{Binomial}(\tilde{p}, l)$. The number of PPQ batches n can be chosen such that the predictive probability $P[\tilde{X} \geq k \mid \mathbf{x}]$ satisfies

$$\Pr\left[\tilde{X} \geq k \mid \mathbf{x}\right] \geq p_0, \tag{8.21}$$

where k is the number of future batches that pass specification. It needs to be selected in accordance with quality standards.

8.3.3 Frequentist Method

Yang (2013c) also provided a Frequentist approach to determine the number of PPQ batches for the purpose of highlighting the advantages of the Bayesian method over the Frequentist solution. The Frequentist method determines the number of PPQ batches n based on the one-sided lower prediction interval of the total number of batches $\tilde{X}$ succeeding in passing specification, after l batches are produced after PPQ. An approximate method by Hahn and Nelson (1973) was used to construct the prediction interval.

Let k be the minimum number of batches out of l batches produced after PPQ that is required to pass specifications. Let $X = \sum_{i=1}^{n} x_i$, $\hat{p} = \dfrac{X}{n}$, $\hat{q} = 1 - \hat{p}$, and $\hat{Y} = l\hat{p}$. It can be calculated that $\sigma^2 = \mathrm{var}[\hat{Y} - \tilde{X}] = lp(1-p)\dfrac{n+l}{n}$.

Let $\hat{\sigma}^2 = l\hat{p}\hat{q}\dfrac{n+l}{n}$. The random variable $Y^* = \dfrac{\hat{Y} - \tilde{X}}{\hat{\sigma}}$ approximately follows a standard normal distribution. It can be shown that

$$Y^* = \frac{\hat{Y} - \tilde{X}}{\sqrt{\hat{Y}(l - \hat{Y})\left(\dfrac{1}{l} + \dfrac{1}{n}\right)}}. \tag{8.22}$$

This allows us to construct a one-sided lower p_0 100% prediction limit (PL) for $\tilde{X}$:

$$PL = \hat{Y} - z_{p_0}\sqrt{\hat{Y}(l - \hat{Y})\left(\frac{1}{l} + \frac{1}{n}\right)}, \tag{8.23}$$

where z_{p_0} is the p_0 100th percentile of the standard normal distribution.

When $X = n$, it is necessary to make a continuity correction to the estimate of $\hat{p}$. In such cases, $\hat{p}$ is estimated by $t\dfrac{n - 0.5}{n}$. As discussed above, the number of PPQ batches n is chosen such that

$$PL = \hat{Y} - z_{p_0}\sqrt{\hat{Y}(l - \hat{Y})\left(\frac{1}{l} + \frac{1}{n}\right)} \geq k. \tag{8.24}$$

The number of PPQ batches n can be determined by trial and error, using the above inequality.

8.3.4 Method Comparisons

8.3.4.1 Numerical Comparison

We determined the number of PPQ batches using both Bayesian and Frequentist methods. Three Beta(α, β) prior distributions $B(1.5, 25)$, $B(25, 1.5)$, and $B(1, 1)$, shown in Figure 8.5, are used to represent three processes with consistent, inconsistent, and poor performance, respectively.

Quality assurance is provided if at least 9 out of 10 future batches produced within a prespecified period, say, 1 year after PPQ, meet the potency specification. Applying the Bayesian and Frequentist methods, based on the above assumptions, the number of PPQ batches is determined for each scenario and presented in Table 8.4.

The Bayesian method resulted in drastically different estimates for n from the Frequentist method. For the poor process (Process 1), consistent process (Process 2), and inconsistent process (Process 3), the numbers of PPQ batches were determined to be >480, 15, and 26, respectively, using the Bayesian approach. It is apparent that the better the process performed historically, the fewer the number of PPQ batches needed. In this sense, the Bayesian approach is a risk-based method. The number of PPQ batches based on this method is

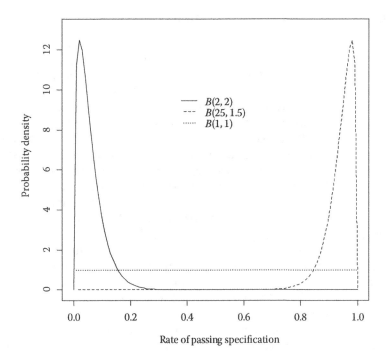

FIGURE 8.5

Probability densities of $B(2, 20)$, $B(20, 2)$, and $B(1, 1)$, representing three processes with consistent, inconsistent, and poor performance, respectively. (From Yang, H. (2013c). How many batches are needed for process validation under the new FDA guidance? *PDA J. Pharm. Sci. Technol.*, 67, 53–62.)

TABLE 8.4

Number of Validation Batches Needed to Ensure ≥9 out of 10 Future
Batches Will Pass Specification with ≥95% Probability

Process	Model Parameters (α, β)	Number of PPQ Batches (*n*)	
		Bayesian	Frequentist
1	(1.5, 25)	>480	29
2	(25, 1.5)	15	29
3	(1, 1)	26	29

Source: Yang, H. (2013c). How many batches are needed for process validation under the new FDA guidance? *PDA J. Pharm. Sci. Technol., 67,*
53–62.

consistent with the performance history of the process. However, by contrast,
the number of PPQ batches *n* based on the Frequentist method remains constant.

8.4 Continued Process Verification

Since experience of commercial production in Stages 1 and 2 is limited, not all
potential sources of variations in commercial manufacturing will have been
identified. It is expected that other sources of variation may be identified after
PPQ. These sources of information afford opportunities for process improvement. The continued process verification (CPV) stage is an integral part of the
life cycle approach to process validation as it is required by the 2011 FDA guidance to ensure that the process remains in a state of control after the successful
conclusion of the PPQ. Central to the fulfillment of this objective is a system
or systems for detecting unplanned departures from the process as designed.
It is also critical that data collection and analysis are performed in accordance
with current good manufacturing practice requirements to enable detection of
undesired process variability and that proper corrective and preventive action
be taken. To this end, an ongoing program for data collection and analysis is
required. As indicated in the guidance, the data should include relevant quality attributes and process parameters, quality of incoming materials or components, in-process materials, and finished products. The guidance also requires
that the data be evaluated and trended by trained personnel.

Statistical process control (SPC) is an effective tool for monitoring the performance of a process to ensure it is in a state of control. Traditionally, univariate
SPC charts such as Shewhart, cumulative sum (CUSUM), and exponentially
weighted moving average (EWMA) charts have been used (Montgomery 2009).
However, increasingly large and complex data concerning process parameters, quality attributes, properties of raw materials, and environmental factors of manufacturing rooms are collected. Application of univariate SPC often

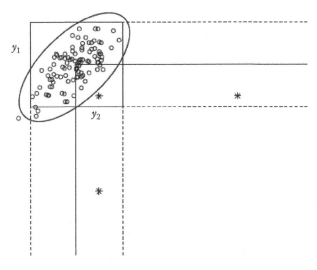

FIGURE 8.6
Performance of multivariate control chart versus univarite control charts. (From Kourti, T. and MacGregor, J.F. (1995). Process analysis, monitoring and diagnosis, using multivariate projection methods. *Chemom. Intell. Lab. Syst.*, 28, 3–21.)

assumes that the variables are independent. However, when interdependencies among responses exist, using independent univariate control charts may fail to identify out-of-control observations. The issue was illustrated by Kourti and MacGregor (1995), reproduced in Figure 8.6. The process data of two quality attributes (y_1, y_2) are plotted, with the confidence region of (y_1, y_2) indicated by the ellipse. It is clear that the out-of-control batch indicated by "*" would have been misidentified if only the univariate controls charts were used.

The example demonstrates the advantage of using multivariate control charts to identify departures from recent process performance. In the following sections, several multivariate control charts are described based on multivariate analysis, principal component (PC) model, and partial least squares (PLS).

8.4.1 Multivariate Control Chart

Because of the complexity of process data, advanced statistical techniques are needed to extract relevant information from the data to ensure manufacturing consistency. Assume that a response $\mathbf{X} = (X_1,\ldots,X_n)$ follows a multivariate normal distribution with mean vector and covariance matrix:

$$\boldsymbol{\mu} = (\mu_1,\ldots,\mu_n)$$

$$\Sigma = \begin{pmatrix} \sigma_1^2 & \cdots & \sigma_{1n} \\ \vdots & \ddots & \vdots \\ \sigma_{1n} & \cdots & \sigma_n^2 \end{pmatrix}.$$

When the covariance matrix Σ is known, the statistic below follows a χ^2 distribution with $n - 1$ degrees of freedom:

$$A = (X - \mu)' \Sigma^{-1} (X - \mu).$$

Therefore, an upper control limit is given by

$$UCL = \chi^2_{\alpha, n-1}, \tag{8.25}$$

where $\chi^2_{\alpha, n-1}$ is the $(1 - \alpha) \times 100$th percentile of the χ^2 distribution with $n - 1$ degrees of freedom.

A multivariate control chart can be set up by plotting the A values of all the samples versus sample number, along with the UCL in Equation 8.25. This control chart is analogous to the univariate Shewhart $\bar{x}$ chart. When Σ is unknown, we can estimate it using the sample covariance from a sample $X_1, \ldots, X_m$ collected when the process is in a state of control:

$$S = \frac{\sum_{i=1}^{m} (X_i - \bar{X})(X_i - \bar{X})}{m - 1}$$

with

$$\bar{X} = \frac{\sum_{i=1}^{m} X_i}{m}.$$

The statistic

$$T^2 = (X - \mu)' S^{-1} (X - \mu), \tag{8.26}$$

called the Hotelling T^2 statistic, satisfies $\frac{m-n}{n(m-1)} T^2 \sim F_{n, m-n}$. Therefore, a Hotelling T^2 control chart can be obtained by plotting $\frac{m-n}{n(m-1)} T^2$ against sequential sample number along with the upper control limit $\frac{m-n}{n(m-1)} F_{n, m-n}(1 - \alpha)$, where $F_{n, m-n}(1 - \alpha)$ is the $(1 - \alpha) \times 100$th percentile of the F distribution with degrees of freedom of n and $m - n$.

There are other types of multivariate control charts such as multivariate CUSUM and multivariate EWMA charts that can be used for process monitoring (Montgomery 1985). However, there are several issues with these traditional multivariate control charts. Most noticeable is that when the number of variables to monitor is large, they are usually correlated, resulting in near singular variance matrix Σ. This makes it challenging to invert the matrix. In addition, even if these control charts may detect disturbance owing to special causes, they do not provide an effective means to find the assignable causes. Both principal component analysis (PCA) and PLS analysis can overcome these challenges.

8.4.2 Principal Component Analysis

PCA provides a statistical procedure to reduce the dimensionality of a complex data set so that a small number of factors, or PCs, can explain the maximum variance of the data. PCA is most useful when understanding the variability of either process variables or quality attributes as opposed to their relationships of interest. Suppose that the original data consist of measurements of m variables $\mathbf{y} = (y_1, ..., y_m)$. PCs are obtained from the Singular Value Decomposition of the data matrix, such as the sample variance–covariance matrix $\mathbf{S}$:

$$\mathbf{S} = \frac{1}{n-1} \sum_{i=1}^{n} (\mathbf{y}_i - \bar{\mathbf{y}})'(\mathbf{y}_i - \bar{\mathbf{y}})$$

with $\bar{y} = \frac{1}{n} \sum_{i=1}^{n} \mathbf{y}_i$.

By the Singular Value Decomposition Theorem (Banerjee and Roy 2014), $\mathbf{S}$ can be decomposed as

$$\mathbf{S} = \mathbf{PDP}',$$

where $\mathbf{P}$ is an orthonormal matrix, consisting of eigenvectors $\mathbf{P} = (\mathbf{p}_1', ..., \mathbf{p}_m')$, with $\mathbf{p}_i = (p_{i1}, ..., p_{im})$. That is,

$$\mathbf{PP}' = \mathbf{P}'\mathbf{P} = \mathbf{I}_{m \times m},$$

and $\mathbf{D}$ is a diagonal matrix with elements being the square root of the eigenvalues such that $d_1 \geq d_2 \geq ... \geq d_k > 0$ and $d_{k+1} = d_{k+2} = ... = d_m = 0$.
The ith PC is obtained as

$$t_i = \mathbf{p}_i'(\mathbf{y} - \bar{\mathbf{y}}). \tag{8.27}$$

It can be verified that $\mathbf{p}_i^c$ has a mean of 0 and a variance of d_i. Note that

$$tr(\mathbf{S}) = tr(\mathbf{PDP}') = tr(\mathbf{DP}'\mathbf{P}) = tr(\mathbf{D}) = \sum_{i=1}^{k} d_i.$$

The quantity $d_i / \sum_{i=1}^{k} d_i$ is the amount of variability in the data set explained by the ith PC. Because d_i decreases with respect to i, the first PC explains the largest amount of variability in the data, the second explains the second largest amount of variability, and so on. Let $\mathbf{t} = (t_1,...,t_m)$. From Equation 8.27, we have

$$\mathbf{t} = \mathbf{P}'(\mathbf{y} - \bar{\mathbf{y}}).$$

Consequently,

$$\mathbf{y} - \bar{\mathbf{y}} = \mathbf{P}\mathbf{t}$$

$$= \sum_{i=1}^{k} t_i \mathbf{p}_i' \tag{8.28}$$

$$= \sum_{i=1}^{r} t_i \mathbf{p}_i' + \sum_{i=r+1}^{k-r} t_i \mathbf{p}_i'.$$

When most of the variability in $\mathbf{y}$ is explained by the first r PCs, the second term on the right-hand side of Equation 8.28 can be eliminated. Therefore, $\mathbf{y}$ can be approximated by

$$\mathbf{y} - \bar{\mathbf{y}} = \sum_{i=1}^{r} t_i \mathbf{p}_i'. \tag{8.29}$$

This expression indicates that the original observation $\mathbf{y}$, which has m elements, can be expressed as a point in the r dimension space Ω_r ($r < m$) spanned by the columns of $\mathbf{P}_r = (\mathbf{p}_1',...,\mathbf{p}_r')$, thus resulting in the reduction in the dimensionality of the original data $\mathbf{y}$. Figure 8.7 displays a process of multivariate parameters whose variability can be adequately explained by two PCs, which expand in the direction of the highest and second highest variability of the data.

After the PCs are extracted from historical data, for any future observation $\mathbf{y}_f$, centered on the mean, its projection onto the subspace Ω_r can be obtained by fitting the following regression model:

$$\mathbf{y}_f = \mathbf{P}_r \mathbf{t}_f + \mathbf{e}, \tag{8.30}$$

where $\mathbf{t}_f = (t_{1f},...,t_{rf})$ and $\mathbf{e}$ is a vector of random errors distributed according to a normal distribution.

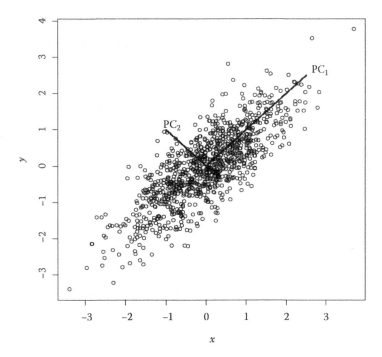

FIGURE 8.7
Principal component representation of a multivariate process with two PCs.

The estimate of $\mathbf{t}_f$ along with its variance estimate is given by

$$\hat{\mathbf{t}}_f = (\mathbf{P}_r'\mathbf{P}_r)^{-1}\mathbf{P}_r'\mathbf{y}_f = \mathbf{P}_r'\mathbf{y}_f \quad \text{and} \quad \hat{\text{var}}[\hat{\mathbf{t}}_f] = (\mathbf{P}_r'\mathbf{P}_r)^{-1}\mathbf{P}_r'\mathbf{y}_f = \mathbf{P}_r'\mathbf{y}_f, \quad (8.31)$$

where we used the fact that the columns of $\mathbf{P}_r$ are orthonormal.

A multivariate control chart can be constructed using the estimates in Equation 8.31. For example, the Hotelling T^2 statistic can be expressed as (Kourti and MacGregor 1995)

$$T^2 = \sum_{i=1}^{r} \hat{t}_{fi}^2 / d_i^2 + \sum_{i=r+1}^{k} \hat{t}_{fi}^2 / d_i^2. \quad (8.32)$$

When only the first r PCs are used to describe the data, the second term in Equation 8.32 can be dropped, and the new T^2 statistic, denoted $\hat{T}^2$, satisfies $\dfrac{m-n}{n(m-1)}\hat{T}^2 \sim F_{n,m-n}$. Therefore, a control chart based on $\hat{T}^2$ can be constructed along the same lines as described above to monitor the process.

As pointed out by Kourti and MacGregor (1995), irrespective of the amount of variance each PC explains, the contributions $\hat{t}_{fi}^2$ of all PCs to T^2 are weighted by their respective variances d_i^2. As a result, an insignificant deviation in PCs of small variances may cause a significant change in T^2, thus causing a false alarm. The control chart based on the first few PCs can adequately address this issue by focusing on PCs that have a major impact on the variability of the measured variables.

As with the traditional multivariate control charts, monitoring the process using PCA-based Hotelling T^2 is not adequate in dissecting the root cause of any out-of-control observations. However, this can be addressed by calculating and plotting the sum of squared residuals of a new observation, $\mathbf{y}_{new}$, which is often referred to as the Q statistic or squared predicted error (SPE) (Ahmed et al. 2012). The Q statistic is given as follows:

$$Q = \left\| \mathbf{y}_{new} - \hat{\mathbf{y}}_{new} \right\|^2 = \sum_{i=1}^{r} (y_{new,i} - \hat{y}_{new,i})^2. \tag{8.33}$$

The Q statistic measures the perpendicular squared distance between the new observation and the subspace Ω_r. The $100(1 - \alpha)\%$ upper control limit of Q is given by (Ahmed et al. 2012)

$$Q_{UCL} = \theta_1 \left[\frac{h_0 z_{1-\alpha} \sqrt{2\theta_2}}{\theta_1} + \frac{\theta_2 h_0 (h_0 - 1)}{\theta_1^2} \right]^{1/h_0}, \tag{8.34}$$

where $z_{1-\alpha}$ is the $100(1 - \alpha)$th percentile of the standard normal distribution,

$$\theta_l = \sum_{i=r+1}^{k} d_i^l \quad \text{and} \quad h_0 = 1 - \frac{2\theta_1 \theta_2}{3\theta_2^2}.$$

Taken together, the control charts based on $\hat{T}^2$ and Q are effective tools for detecting deviations caused by a new event. The Q plot is especially useful in diagnosing the root cause of a new out-of-control result by identifying the individual variables that make higher contributions to the Q statistic.

8.4.3 PLS Modeling

As discussed in the previous section, PCA is useful when the process control is focused solely on monitoring either process variables (hereafter denoted as X) or quality attributes (denoted as Y). However, process data typically include both measurements of process variables and quality parameters. It is conceivable that these variables are correlated. As a result, an out-of-control observation in the Y space may very well be caused by a change due to special cause in the X space. Therefore, understanding the relationship between the two sets of variables is very important in identifying the assignable cause. However, because of correlations among both process variables and quality measures, ordinary regression analysis is insufficient for analyzing these complex data.

PLS is a multivariate modeling technique that copes with both collinearity among variables and missing data through reduction in dimensionality. Assume X is an $n \times q$ data matrix of process variables and Y is an $n \times p$ data matrix of quality attributes. PLS analysis is carried out to determine the latent variables from both X and Y such that covariance among the extracted factors is maximized. This is accomplished through decomposing the covariance matrices $(X'Y)(Y'X)$ and $(Y'X)(X'Y)$. The final aim is to decompose the data matrices X and Y such that

$$X = T_x P_x + E_x$$
$$Y = T_y P_y + E_y, \tag{8.35}$$

where T_x (T_y), P_x (P_y), and E_x (E_y) are score, loading, and residual matrices of X (Y) data matrix, respectively.

The following procedure is performed to extract x scores (y scores), which are linear combinations of (X) and (Y). For instance, the first x score $t_{x,1}$ is a linear combination of X, $t_{x,1} = X p_{x,1}$, with $p_{x,1}$ being the first eigenvector of $(X'Y)(Y'X)$. Similarly, the first y score $t_{y,1} = Y p_{y,1}$, with $p_{y,1}$ being the first eigenvector of $(Y'X)(X'Y)$. After the first latent vector is determined, the original data matrices X and Y are deflated by regressing X and Y on $t_{x,1}$ and $t_{y,1}$, respectively, and calculating the residual matrices X_1 and Y_1. The above process is carried out using the residual matrices to determine the second latent vector, which represents the direction of the maximum variability of the residual X space and which is also most predictive of the residual Y space. Repeat the process until all latent variables are extracted and the score and loading matrices in Equation 8.35 obtained.

As with the PCA model, Model 8.35 can be simplified by using only the first few latent vectors to reduce the dimensions of both the X and Y spaces. The number of latent vectors used in the model is usually selected through cross-validation (Kourti and MacGregor 1995), in which a PLS model is developed based on $n - 1$ batches, and the response value of the left-out batch is predicted from the model and compared to its observed value. The number of latent vectors is chosen to optimize a cross-validation statistic such as predicted residual sum of squares.

8.5 Concluding Remarks

Drug product development has increasingly become more complex and challenging. Process validation based on the traditional three-batch method affords little assurance that future batches will meet quality standards. Adoption of risk management concepts and a life cycle approach to process validation entails the use of process and product knowledge to mitigate the risk engendered by the traditional method. This chapter discusses how advanced statistical methods can be used in the life cycle of process validation. Successful application of these statistical methods enables risk-based decision-making.

Section IV

Manufacturing

9

Specifications

9.1 Introduction

Specifications for drug products are an integral part of overall control strategies to ensure the quality of the products. The establishment of specification limits is accomplished based on desired product performance, supporting data, application of statistical methods, and, importantly, regulatory requirements. In ICH Guidelines Q6A and Q6B (ICH 1999a,b), it is stated that "A specification is defined as a list of tests, references to analytical procedures, and appropriate acceptance criteria, which are numerical limits, ranges or other criteria for the tests described. It establishes the set of criteria to which a drug substance, drug product should conform to be considered acceptable for its intended use. 'Conformance to specification' means that the drug substance and/or drug product, when tested according to the listed analytical procedures, will meet the acceptance criteria. Specifications are critical quality standards that are proposed and justified by the manufacturer and approved by regulatory authorities as conditions of approval." Developing specifications requires the synthesis of information from various sources, including data from preclinical and clinical trials, analytical method development, stability studies, and process validation. Special consideration should be given to process capability, variability of analytical methods, drug substance and drug product stability, specific regulatory and compendial requirements of drug identity, strength, quality, and purity, as well as data from preclinical and clinical studies and process validation. In recent years, there has been a shift in both industry practice and regulatory thinking toward the use of a life cycle risk-based approach for setting specifications. Such an approach begins with the identification of critical quality attributes (CQAs) that are critical to the safety, efficacy, and quality of the product. The initial specifications for CQAs can be made based on materials used in clinical development. Knowledge from nonclinical studies and similar products can be used to justify specifications wider than the clinically qualified range. Equally useful is consideration of analytical variability, process capability, and product stability. An understanding of product degradation is particularly important in setting the product release limits. Appropriate application of statistical methods is the key to robust specifications. It is also recommended by regulatory guidelines (ICH 1999b).

This chapter is aimed at discussion of several advanced statistical methods for setting specifications. While quality attributes may be correlated, specifications are often determined without taking into account the possible interdependencies. Such practice may potentially cause the resultant specifications to be narrower than the actual acceptable ranges of product performance, thus causing untoward out-of-specification investigations. Through multiple case studies, we discuss how this issue can be effectively coped with using multivariate statistical modeling and other advanced statistical techniques, such as generalized pivotal quantity (GPQ) analysis. The chapter also discusses statistical methods for setting product release limits.

9.2 Types of Specifications

In the literature, the terms *acceptance criteria* and *specifications* are often used interchangeably. Specifications can be defined either qualitatively or quantitatively. Selection of one over the other should be made to ensure proper control of the quality attribute(s) for which the specification is intended (European Biopharmaceutical Enterprise [EBE] 2003). Whenever possible, quantitative specifications are preferable as a certain amount of information is lost when a continuous measurement is dichotomized or discretized. In the following discussion, we primarily focus on the use of statistical methods for setting numerical limits.

9.2.1 Univariate Specifications

For a quantitative quality attribute, specification limits are conventionally set up as the mean plus and minus a multiple of the standard deviation of the available data. For such limits to make sense, the data need to be normally distributed. Should the data show nonnormal behavior, a transformation is warranted. The specification range derived from the transformed data is then back-transformed, resulting in a specification on the original scale. Alternatively, nonparametric methods can be used to determine the range. However, these methods usually require the data set to be sufficiently large.

One criticism of these methods is that specifications for quality attributes are usually established separately, without taking into account the interdependencies among them, which may have an important influence on the probability of meeting specifications (Peterson 2008; Yang 2013a). To illustrate this, suppose that the measurements of drug potency and impurity follow a bivariate normal distribution with a mean of (100, 10) and a variance of $(20^2, 2^2)$, and with the specification being (80, 120) and (0, 11) for potency and impurity, respectively.

It can be shown that the probabilities for both measurements to fall in their respective specifications are 0.5023 and 0.4736 when the correlation between the two CQAs is −0.75 or 0, respectively. Therefore, it is important to set specifications for quality attributes taking into account correlations with each other.

9.2.2 Multivariate Specifications

When product quality depends on the combined effect of related tests, the overall quality can be controlled by joint specifications. This idea was first suggested by Hotelling (1947, 1951) and further explored by Jackson (1956, 1959), Jackson and Bradley (1959, 1961a,b), and Shakun (1965) for product lot disposition. Over the years, multivariate testing and specifications have been applied broadly in many industries (Jenkins 1967; Shakun 1965), such as the chemical industry where the quality of petroleum products is warranted through simultaneous testing and control of organic chemicals in the products. Since correlated tests may result in redundant information and incur unnecessary costs, Jenkins (1967) applied a multivariate approach to identify a smaller set of "orthogonal" tests among a large number of tests. Interestingly, despite the advances in multivariate quality control methods, applications of multivariate analysis in quality control in the pharmaceutical industry have been relatively rare. It was only recently that several articles were published dealing with multivariate testing issues in the evaluation of drug dissolution profile similarity (Tsong et al. 1996). Zhang et al. (2010) suggested a generalized confidence interval method for setting acceptance criteria for the ratio of the test and reference sample in bioassay. Yang (2013a) derived multivariate specification for correlated quality attributes. These methods are discussed in the following sections.

9.3 Specifications for Correlated Quality Attributes

Yang (2013d) tackled a quality control issue concerning production of monoclonal antibodies (mAbs). It is well known that mAbs are heterogeneous because of the various posttranslational modifications. Since the variants of the product may have appreciable effects on the product safety, efficacy, and quality, it is important to assess the potential impact and establish control ranges for the variants. For instance, the variants may have different pharmacokinetic properties so that the half-life of one variant may differ from that of the others. In this case, too much of the variant with the longest half-life in the drug may increase a patient's drug exposure, thus causing potential safety issues. On the other hand, too much of the variant with the shortest half-life may result in a less effective dose. This demonstrates the need to control the overall composition of these active drug variants.

9.3.1 Linking Specifications to Drug Efficacy

Drug exposure is conventionally measured by the pharmacokinetic parameter area under the drug concentration curve (AUC). In general, AUC is a surrogate measure for drug efficacy. It is estimated from pharmacokinetic studies, in which blood samples from subjects receiving the drug are taken at various time points, and drug concentration is measured using analytical methods. The AUC can be directly estimated through a trapezoidal method (Hazewinkel 2001). For a marketed product, the AUC of the product, like the half-life, is usually well characterized. It is logical to assume that the composition of active variants in a product lot is deemed acceptable if the AUC of the lot is shown to be bioequivalent to the drug product AUC. This approach is described below.

For the sake of simplicity, we assume that the drug consists of three active variants. Let μ_i ($i = 0, 1, 2, 3$) be the true AUCs of the drug product ($i = 0$) and of three variants ($i = 1, 2,$ and 3) that take up $c_i \times 100\%$ of the drug ($0 \le c_i \le 1$). Thus, $c_1 + c_2 + c_3 = 1$, and the AUC of the lot is

$$\mu = \sum_{i=1}^{3} c_i \mu_i. \tag{9.1}$$

That is, the AUC of the lot is the sum of the AUCs of the three variants, weighted by the variant composition (distribution). Consequently, the relative AUC, that is, the ratio of the AUC of the lot to the AUC of the drug product, is given by

$$R(c_1, c_2, c_3) = \frac{\mu}{\mu_0}. \tag{9.2}$$

Specifications for c_1, c_2, and c_3 can be defined as

$$A = \{(c_1, c_2, c_3): \text{two-sided 90\% CI of } R(c_1, c_2, c_3) \in (0.8, 1.25)\}.$$

In other words, specification A consists of lots whose AUCs are bioequivalent to that of the product.

The two-sided 90% CI for $R(c_1, c_2, c_3)$ can be estimated using historical data. For instance, suppose that there were n lots used in the late-phase clinical trials. Let $\hat{\mu}_{ij}$ ($j = 1, \ldots, n$) be the sample mean AUC estimates of the true AUCs of the drug product ($i = 0$) and three active variants ($i = 1, 2,$ and 3), respectively, for lot j. Let σ_i^2 be the true variances of the AUCs of the drug product ($i = 0$) and active variant i ($i = 1, 2, 3$) and σ_{i0} be the true covariance between active variant i ($i = 1, 2, 3$) and the drug product. Then, the corresponding sample estimates of the true AUCs, variance, and covariance are obtained, respectively, as

$$\hat{\mu}_i = \frac{\sum_{j=1}^{n} \hat{\mu}_{ij}}{n}, \quad \hat{\sigma}_i^2 = \frac{\sum_{j=1}^{n}(\hat{\mu}_{ij} - \hat{\mu}_i)^2}{n-1}, \quad \text{and } \hat{\sigma}_{i0} = \frac{\sum_{j=1}^{n}(\hat{\mu}_{ij} - \hat{\mu}_i)(\hat{\mu}_{0j} - \hat{\mu}_0)}{n-1}. \quad (9.3)$$

Thus, an estimate of the relative AUC in Equation 9.2 is

$$\hat{R}(c_1, c_2, c_3) = \frac{\sum_{i=1}^{3} c_i \hat{\mu}_i}{\hat{\mu}_0}. \quad (9.4)$$

Applying the δ method, we have

$$\text{var}[\hat{R}(c_1, c_2, c_3)] \approx \left(\frac{\sum_{i=}^{3} c_i \mu_i}{\mu_0}\right)^2 \left[\frac{\sum_{i=1}^{3} c_i^2 \sigma_i^2}{\left(\sum_{i=1}^{3} c_i \mu_i\right)^2} - \frac{2\sum_{i=1}^{3} c_i \sigma_{i0}}{\left(\sum_{i=1}^{3} c_i \mu_i\right)\mu_0} + \frac{\sigma_0^2}{\mu_0^2}\right]/n, \quad (9.5)$$

where we use the assumption that $\hat{\mu}_i$ ($i = 1, 2, 3$) are independent. An estimate of var$[\hat{R}(c_1, c_2, c_3)]$ can be obtained using the sample estimates in Equation 9.3 for the parameters in Equation 9.5.

$$\hat{\text{var}}[\hat{R}(c_1, c_2, c_3)] \approx \left(\frac{\sum_{i=}^{3} c_i \hat{\mu}_i}{\hat{\mu}_0}\right)^2 \left[\frac{\sum_{i=1}^{3} c_i^2 \hat{\sigma}_i^2}{\left(\sum_{i=1}^{3} c_i \hat{\mu}_i\right)^2} - \frac{2\sum_{i=1}^{3} c_i \hat{\sigma}_{i0}}{\left(\sum_{i=1}^{3} c_i \hat{\mu}_i\right)\hat{\mu}_0} + \frac{\hat{\sigma}_0^2}{\hat{\mu}_0^2}\right]/n. \quad (9.6)$$

Note that $\hat{R}(c_1, c_2, c_3)$ in Equation 9.4 has an asymptotic normal distribution:

$$\hat{R}(c_1, c_2, c_3) \sim N\left(R(c_1, c_2, c_3), \text{var}[\hat{R}(c_1, c_2, c_3)]\right). \quad (9.7)$$

Thus, an approximate two-sided 90% confidence interval for $R(c_1, c_2, c_3)$ is

$$\hat{R}(c_1, c_2, c_3) \pm 1.65\sqrt{\hat{\text{var}}[\hat{R}(c_1, c_2, c_3)]}. \quad (9.8)$$

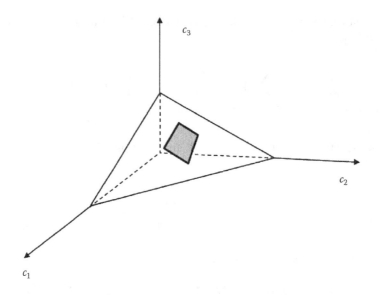

FIGURE 9.1
Specification for variant composition, represented by the irregular region, on the plane $c_1 + c_2 + c_3 = 1$, which contains compositions of three active variants of lots bioequivalent to the drug product. (From Yang, H. (2013d). Setting specifications of correlated quality attributes. *PDA J. Pharm. Sci. Technol.*, 67, 533–543.)

The specification depicted in Figure 9.1 can be re-expressed as

$$A = \{(c_1, c_2, c_3) : 0 \le c_1, c_2, c_3 \le 1, c_1 + c_2 + c_3 = 1,$$
$$\hat{R}(c_1, c_2, c_3) - 1.65\sqrt{\text{vâr}[\hat{R}(c_1, c_2, c_3)]} \ge 0.8, \text{ and} \qquad (9.9)$$
$$\hat{R}(c_1, c_2, c_3) + 1.65\sqrt{\text{vâr}[\hat{R}(c_1, c_2, c_3)]} \le 1.25\}.$$

9.3.2 Example

Through a simulated example, Yang (2013a) demonstrated the advantages of the above method when compared to the traditional mean ± constant × SD univariate approach. A simple exponential decay model is used to describe the kinetics of the drug and its three variants. That is,

$$y_{it} = A_{i0}e^{-\gamma_i t}, \qquad (9.10)$$

where y_{it} is the concentration of variant i ($i = 1, 2, 3$) at time t, A_{i0} is the concentration of variant i at time 0, and γ_i is the elimination rate of variant i. To simulate the data, it is was assumed that the three active variants have half-lives 15, 20, and 25 days, which correspond to the elimination rates of 0.0462, 0.0347, and 0.0277, respectively.

TABLE 9.1

Relative Compositions of Three Active Variants in Simulated Lots

Lot	Variant 1	Variant 2	Variant 3
1	0.33	0.33	0.33
2	0.33	0.17	0.50
3	0.33	0.50	0.17
4	0.17	0.33	0.50
5	0.50	0.33	0.17

Source: Yang, H. (2013d). Setting specifications of correlated quality attributes. *PDA J. Pharm. Sci. Technol.*, 67, 533–543.

Table 9.1 lists the relative compositions of the three variants in five lots used in a pharmacokinetic study in which a total of 50 subjects (10 per lot) were given the drug.

Serum concentrations (AUCs) were simulated using the model

$$y_{ijkt} = A_{i0}e^{-\gamma_i t} + \varepsilon_{ijkt}, \tag{9.11}$$

where the indices k, j, i, and t correspond to subject k ($k = 1, ..., 10$), lot j ($j = 1, ..., 5$), active variant i ($i = 1, 2, 3$), and time t ($t = 1, 2, 3, 4, 5, 7, 14, 21, 30, 37,$ and 60 days after dose), respectively, and ε_{ijkt} are measurement errors, following a normal distribution $N(0, \sigma_i^2)$. The model parameters used were set as $A_{i0} = 100$ and $\sigma_i = 15$.

For lot j with relative composition of active variants (c_{1j}, c_{2j}, c_{3j}), the serum drug concentration of subject k at time t who receives drug from lot j is estimated by

$$\hat{y}_{0jkt} = \sum_{i=1}^{3} c_{ij} y_{ijkt}. \tag{9.12}$$

Assuming the kinetics of lot j also follows the first-order decay mode, we obtain

$$\hat{y}_{0jkt} = A_{00}e^{-\gamma_0 t} + \varepsilon_{0jkt}, \tag{9.13}$$

where ε_{0jkt} follows a normal distribution $N(0, \sigma_0^2)$, and γ_0 is the elimination rate of the drug.

From Equation 9.11, the theoretical AUC of either the drug or its variants can be calculated:

$$\text{AUC} = \int_0^\infty A_0 e^{-\gamma t}\, dt = \frac{A_0}{\gamma}. \tag{9.14}$$

By replacing the parameters in Equation 9.14 with their corresponding estimates, an estimate of the AUC can be obtained. The AUCs of the five lots and their active variants in the simulated lots were estimated and are presented in Table 9.2, along with their mean and variance estimates.

Using the estimates in Table 9.2, the specification range was estimated as follows:

$$A = \{(c_1, c_2, c_3) : 0 \le c_1, c_2, c_3 \le 1, c_1 + c_2 + c_3 = 1,$$

$$\hat{R}(c_1, c_2, c_3) - 1.65\sqrt{\hat{\text{var}}[\hat{R}(c_1, c_2, c_3)]} \ge 0.8, \text{ and}$$

$$\hat{R}(c_1, c_2, c_3) + 1.65\sqrt{\hat{\text{var}}[\hat{R}(c_1, c_2, c_3)]} \le 1.25\},$$

where

$$\hat{R}(c_1, c_2, c_3) = 0.757c_1 + 1.026c_2 + 1.303c_3 \text{ and}$$

$$\hat{\text{var}}[\hat{R}(c_1, c_2, c_3)] = (0.757c_1 + 1.026c_2 + 1.303c_3)^2 \left[\frac{15,910c_1^2 + 2039c_2^2 + 28,593c_3^2}{(2147c_1 + 2910c_2 + 3696c_3)^2} \right.$$

$$\left. - \frac{2(10,672c_1 - 6715c_2 + 17,507c_3)}{2836(2147c_1 + 2910c_2 + 3696c_3)} + \frac{53,089}{2836^2} \right] / 5.$$

Figure 9.2 shows the specification region. It is a pentagon on the plane $c_1 + c_2 + c_3 = 1$ inside the unit cube.

TABLE 9.2

Estimates of AUC for Three Active Variants and Drug from Simulated Lots

Lot	Variant 1	Variant 2	Variant 3	Drug
1	1991	2964	3451	2703
2	2201	2860	3874	3025
3	2314	2888	3605	2781
4	2171	2886	3805	3114
5	2169	2900	3684	2906
Mean	2147	2910	3696	2836
Variance	15,910	2039	28,593	53,030
Covariance[a]	10,672	−6715	17,507	

Source: Yang, H. (2013d). Setting specifications of correlated quality attributes. *PDA J. Pharm. Sci. Technol.*, 67, 533–543.

[a] Covariance between variant i ($i = 1, 2, 3$) and the drug.

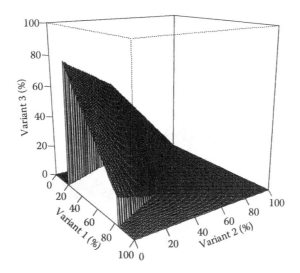

FIGURE 9.2
Specification region of three active variants, based on the multivariate method, is a pentagon on the plane $c_1 + c_2 + c_3 = 1$ inside the unit cube. (From Yang, H. (2013d). Setting specifications of correlated quality attributes. *PDA J. Pharm. Sci. Technol.*, 67, 533–543.)

9.3.3 Performance Evaluation

The univariate method based on a mean ± 1.96 SD range for each variant was used to determine the specifications for the three active variants. The ranges correspond to the intervals covering 95% of the corresponding active variant's measurements. The estimated specifications are presented in Table 9.3 and displayed in Figure 9.3.

To facilitate comparison of the two methods, the two specification regions are projected onto planes spanned by two of the three variants. It is apparent that the projections based on the univariate method are enclosed within those based on the multivariate method (Figures 9.4 through 9.6). Consequently, we can conclude that the specification region based on the univariate method is a subset of that derived from the latter. This finding reaffirms the advantage of accounting for correlations among quality attributes to develop joint specifications.

TABLE 9.3

Specifications of Three Active Variants Based on the Traditional Method for Simulated Lots

Specification	Variant 1	Variant 2	Variant 3
Lower limit	10.2%	10.2%	0.0%
Upper limit	56.4%	56.4%	66.0%

Source: Yang, H. (2013d). Setting specifications of correlated quality attributes. *PDA J. Pharm. Sci. Technol.*, 67, 533–543.
Note: Variant 1 + variant 2 + variant 3 = 100%.

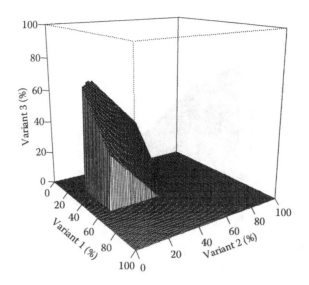

FIGURE 9.3
Specification region of three active variants based on univariate mean ± 1.96 SD method is a hexagon on the plane $c_1 + c_2 + c_3 = 1$ inside the unit cube. (From Yang, H. (2013d). Setting specifications of correlated quality attributes. *PDA J. Pharm. Sci. Technol.*, 67, 533–543.)

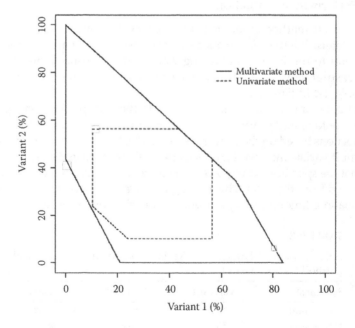

FIGURE 9.4
Specification regions of variants 1 and 2, based on the univariate and multivariate methods. (From Yang, H. (2013d). Setting specifications of correlated quality attributes. *PDA J. Pharm. Sci. Technol.*, 67, 533–543.)

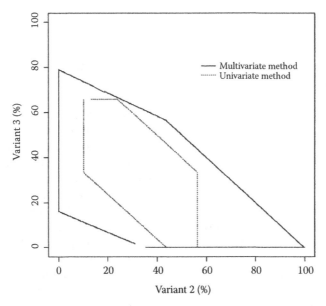

FIGURE 9.5
Specification regions of variants 2 and 3, based on univariate and multivariate methods. (From Yang, H. (2013d). Setting specifications of correlated quality attributes. *PDA J. Pharm. Sci. Technol.*, 67, 533–543.)

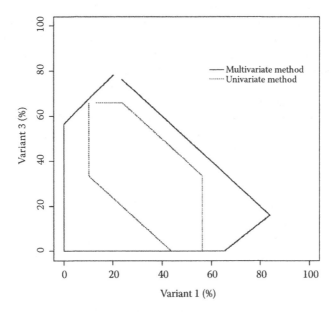

FIGURE 9.6
Specification regions of variants 1 and 3, based on the univariate and multivariate methods. (From Yang, H. (2013d). Setting specifications of correlated quality attributes. *PDA J. Pharm. Sci. Technol.*, 67, 533–543.)

9.4 Specification of Ratio

Often, there is a need to set specifications or acceptance criteria for the ratio of two measurements. For example, a bioassay may determine the potency of a test sample relative to a reference standard to offset the impact of large assay variability. The result is reported as "relative potency," calculated as the ratio of EC_{50} values estimated from the test sample and reference standard. The estimate is compared to a specification to evaluate if the lot from which the sample was taken is deemed acceptable. Although the construction of a confidence interval for the ratio of two model parameters has been well studied, little attention has been given to the computation of a plausible range for the ratio of two random measurements or estimates.

The same problem was encountered by Zhang et al. (2010) in the context of setting acceptance criteria for a reverse transcriptase (RT) assay. The method is a standard technique for screening potential retroviral contamination in the raw materials used for production of biological products. It can also be used as a sterility test to determine if retroviruses are present in bulk or finished products. Since most retroviruses do not produce pathological changes in cell substrates, direct detection of these viruses through pathological changes is challenging. RT relies on the detection of a particular enzyme as an indicator for the presence of retrovirus in a test sample (Baltimore 1970). The amount of the enzyme, which is characterized through radioactivity counts, is correlated with the presence of the retroviruses. To ensure the reliability of the assay, a negative control is usually included in the assay to calibrate the radioactivity count resulting from the cell culture itself. A sample is classified as negative if the ratio of radioactivity count between the sample and the negative control is below a prespecified limit. Such a limit needs to be established to ensure that a given proportion of future assay results of either raw materials or products of acceptable quality will fall within the limit with certain confidence. Several approaches for constructing the limit were proposed by Zhang et al. (2010) and are described in the following sections.

9.4.1 One-Sided Upper Tolerance Interval

Let X be a random variable and θ be the parameter(s) associated with the distribution of X. We further let $\hat{\theta}$ be an estimator of θ based on a random sample. A function $g(\hat{\theta})$ is called the upper tolerance limit with content β and confidence level $1 - \alpha$ if it satisfies

$$P_{\hat{\theta}}[P_X[X \leq g(\hat{\theta}) \mid \hat{\theta}] \geq \beta] = 1 - \alpha. \tag{9.15}$$

Zhang et al. (2010) described a method to determine the one-sided tolerance limit $g(\hat{\theta})$. It is summarized in the following theorem.

Theorem 9.1

Let $h(\hat{\theta}, t)$ be the lower $100(1 - \alpha)\%$ confidence limit of the cumulative probability function of $P_X[X \le t]$. There exists $g^*(\hat{\theta})$ such that

$$h(\hat{\theta}, g^*(\hat{\theta})) = \beta. \tag{9.16}$$

Furthermore, $g^*(\hat{\theta})$ is an upper tolerance limit of X with content β and confidence level $1 - \alpha$. ∎

Proof

Note that $h(\hat{\theta}, t)$ is a monotonic continuous function of t with $h(\hat{\theta}, t) \to 0$ as $t \to -\infty t$ and $h(\hat{\theta}, t) \to 1$ as $t \to \infty$. By the Intermediate Value Theorem, for $0 < \beta < 1$, there exists t_0 satisfying $h(\hat{\theta}, t_0) = \beta$. Because t_0 is dependent on $\hat{\theta}$, it can be denoted as $g^*(\hat{\theta})$. It is evident that an upper tolerance limit of X with content β and confidence level $1 - \alpha$ exists and is a solution to Equation 9.16.

$$P_{\hat{\theta}}[P_X[X \le g^*(\hat{\theta}) \mid \hat{\theta}] \ge \beta] = P_{\hat{\theta}}[P_X[X \le g^*(\hat{\theta}) \mid \hat{\theta}] \ge h(\hat{\theta}, g^*(\hat{\theta}))] = 1 - \alpha.$$

9.4.2 Upper Tolerance Limit for X_1/X_2

In this section, we introduce two methods to construct an upper tolerance limit for the ratio of two random variables. The first is an approximate method, while the second solution is exact.

9.4.2.1 Approximate Method

We assume that the two measurements $(X_1, X_2)'$ follow a bivariate normal distribution $N(\mu, \Sigma)$ with $\mu = (\mu_1, \mu_2)'$ and $\Sigma = \begin{pmatrix} \sigma_{11} & \sigma_{12} \\ \sigma_{21} & \sigma_{22} \end{pmatrix}$. Consider the case where the mean of the second measurement X_2 is positive; that is, $\mu_2 > 0$ and coefficient of variation is sufficiently small. Under these assumptions, the cumulative density function (cdf) of the ratio X_1/X_2 can be approximated as follows (Hinkley 1969; Zhang et al. 2010):

$$P\left(\frac{X_1}{X_2} \le t\right) = P\left(\frac{X_1}{X_2} \le t, X_2 > 0\right) + P\left(\frac{X_1}{X_2} \le t, X_2 \le 0\right)$$

$$\approx P(X_1 \le tX_2) \tag{9.17}$$

$$= \Phi(-u(t; \mu, \Sigma)),$$

where

$$-u(t;\mu,\Sigma) = \frac{T\mu}{T\Sigma},$$

$$T = (1,-t)',$$

(9.18)

and $\Phi(\cdot)$ is the cdf of the standard normal distribution.

According to Theorem 9.1, to obtain the upper tolerance limit of X_1/X_2, it is necessary to find a lower confidence limit of $P(X_1/X_2 \leq t)$. This can be accomplished using the GPQs of the parameters (μ, Σ) (Krishnamoorthy and Mathew 2004). Let $X_i = (X_{1i}, X_{2i})'(1 \leq i \leq n)$ be a random sample from the bivariate normal distribution $N(\mu, \Sigma)$ with $\bar{X} = \sum_{i=1}^{n} X_i/n$. Define $A = \sum_{i=1}^{n} (X_i - \bar{X})(X_i - \bar{X})'$. It is well known that $\bar{X}$ follows a bivariate normal distribution with mean μ and variance–covariance matrix Σ/n, and A has a bivariate Wishart distribution with scale matrix Σ and degree of freedom $n - 1$. That is, $\bar{X} \sim N(\mu, \Sigma/n)$ and $A \sim W(\Sigma, n - 1)$. Following Krishnamoorthy and Mathew (2009), let $\bar{x}$ and $\bar{a}$ denote the observed values of $\bar{X}$ and A, respectively. Since for any $r \times 2$ matrix, $BAB' \sim W(B\Sigma B', n - 1)$, it can be verified that

$$H(a, A, \mu, \Sigma) = a^{-\frac{1}{2}}(a\Sigma a^{-\frac{1}{2}})(aAa)(a\Sigma a)^{-\frac{1}{2}}a^{-\frac{1}{2}} \sim W(a^{-1}, n-2). \qquad (9.19)$$

Note that $H(a, a, \mu, \Sigma) = \Sigma^{-1}$. $H^{-1}(a, A, \mu, \Sigma)$ is a GPQ for Σ. Let

$$Z = (\Sigma/n))^{-\frac{1}{2}}(\bar{X} - \mu).$$

Thus, $Z \sim N(0, I_2)$ with $0 = (0, 0)'$ and I_2 being the 2×2 identify matrix. Consider

$$K(\bar{x}, \bar{X}, \mu, \Sigma) = \bar{x} - [H^{-1}(a, A, \mu, \Sigma)/n]^{-\frac{1}{2}}Z. \qquad (9.20)$$

It can be shown that $K(\bar{x}, \bar{X}, \mu, \Sigma)$ is a GPQ for μ. By Equation 9.17, a GQP for $P(X_1/X_2 \leq t)$ is obtained:

$$R(\bar{x}, \bar{X}, a, A, t, \mu, \Sigma) = \Phi(-u(t; H^{-1}, K)). \qquad (9.21)$$

This enables us to obtain the lower $100(1 - \alpha)\%$ confidence limit of the cumulative probability function of $P(X_1/X_2 \leq t)$. Let $h(\bar{x}, a, t)$ denote this limit. By

Theorem 9.1, an upper tolerance limit of X_1/X_2 with content β and confidence level $1 - \alpha$ is a solution to

$$h(\overline{x}, \mathbf{a}, t) = \beta, \qquad (9.22)$$

which can be obtained using the bisection method (for details, see Krishnamoorthy and Mathew 2004; Zhang et al. 2010).

9.4.2.2 Exact Methods

Two exact methods for constructing the upper tolerance limit of the ratio of two normally distributed random variables were also developed by Zhang et al. (2010). The first method makes use of the representation of the cdf of X_1/X_2 by Hinkley (1969). The second method expresses the cdf of X_1/X_2 in terms of integration of the conditional probability of X_1 given X_2. In both cases, the GPQs in Equations 9.19 and 9.20 for $(\boldsymbol{\mu}, \boldsymbol{\Sigma})$ are used to construct a GPQ for the cdf of X_1/X_2.

Let $F(t) = P(X_1/X_2 \le t)$. Per Hinkley (1969),

$$F(t) = L(d_1, d_2; d_3) + L(-d_1, -d_2; -d_3), \qquad (9.23)$$

where

$$L(d_1, d_2; d_3) = \frac{1}{2\pi\sqrt{1-d_3^2}} \int_{d_1}^{\infty} \int_{d_2}^{\infty} e^{-\frac{x^2 - 2d_3 xy + y^2}{2(1-\rho^2)}} \, dx \, dy$$

$$d_1 = \frac{\mu_1 - t\mu_2}{\sqrt{\sigma_{11}\sigma_{22}}\, b(t)}$$

$$d_2 = -\frac{\mu_2}{\sqrt{\sigma_{22}}}$$

$$d_3 = \frac{t\sigma_{22} - \sigma_{12}}{\sqrt{\sigma_{11}\sigma_{22}}\, b(t)}$$

$$b(t) = \sqrt{\frac{t^2}{\sigma_{11}} - \frac{2t\sigma_{12}}{\sigma_{11}\sigma_{22}} + \frac{1}{\sigma_{22}}}. \qquad (9.24)$$

From Equations 9.23 and 9.24, $F(t)$ is a function of $(t, \boldsymbol{\mu}, \boldsymbol{\Sigma})$. We denote it as $F(t) = g(t, \boldsymbol{\mu}, \boldsymbol{\Sigma})$. Thus, $g(t, \mathbf{H}^{-1}, \mathbf{K})$ is a GPQ for $F(t)$.

Zhang et al. (2010) suggested an alternative representation of $F(t)$, using the well-known fact that

$$X_1 | X_2 = x_2 \sim N\left(\mu_1 + \sigma_{12}\sigma_{22}^{-1}(x_2 - \mu_2), \sigma_{11.2}\right),$$

where $\sigma_{11.2} = \sigma_{11} - \sigma_{12}^2\sigma_{22}^{-1}$.

Consequently,

$$
\begin{aligned}
F(t) = {} & \int_0^\infty \Phi\left(\frac{x_2 t - \mu_1 - \sigma_{12}\sigma_{22}^{-1}(x2 - \mu_2)}{\sqrt{\sigma_{11.2}}}\right) f(x_2; \mu_2, \sigma_{22}) dx_2 \\
& + \int_{-\infty}^0 \left[1 - \Phi\left(\frac{x_2 t - \mu_1 - \sigma_{12}\sigma_{22}^{-1}(x2 - \mu_2)}{\sqrt{\sigma_{11.2}}}\right)\right] f(x_2; \mu_2, \sigma_{22}) dx_2 \\
= {} & \Phi\left(-\frac{\mu_2}{\sqrt{\sigma_{22}}}\right) + \int_{-\frac{\mu_2}{\sqrt{\sigma_{22}}}}^\infty \Phi\left(\frac{(\mu_2 + z\sqrt{\sigma_{22}})t - (\mu_1 + z\sigma_{12}/\sqrt{\sigma_{22}})}{\sqrt{\sigma_{11.2}}}\right) \varphi(z) dz \\
& - \int_{-\infty}^{-\frac{\mu_2}{\sqrt{\sigma_{22}}}} \Phi\left(\frac{(\mu_2 + z\sqrt{\sigma_{22}})t - (\mu_1 + z\sigma_{12}/\sqrt{\sigma_{22}})}{\sqrt{\sigma_{11.2}}}\right) \varphi(z) dz, \quad (9.25)
\end{aligned}
$$

where $f(x_2; \mu_2, \sigma_{22})$ is the density function of the normal distribution with mean μ_2 and variance σ_{22}, and $\varphi(z)$ is the density function of the standard normal distribution. The transformation $z = (x_2 - \mu_2)/\sqrt{\sigma_{22}}$ was performed to obtain the simplified expression.

Since this representation of $F(t)$ is also a function of $(\boldsymbol{\mu}, \boldsymbol{\Sigma})$, a GPQ of $F(t)$ can be easily obtained using the GPQs of $(\boldsymbol{\mu}, \boldsymbol{\Sigma})$.

9.4.2.3 Method Performance

The performance of the above three methods was evaluated by Zhang et al. (2010). Because of the one-to-one correspondence between the upper tolerance limit of the ratio of X_1/X_2 and the lower confidence limit of its cdf $F(t)$, the performance was assessed with respect to the coverage probability of the lower confidence limit. It was carried out through a simulation study. The results showed that the approximate method maintains satisfactory coverage probability when the CV of X_2 is no more than 30%. To evaluate the performance of the exact methods, numerical approximations are needed to estimate the integrals in Equation 9.25. This was accomplished using a subroutine by Drezner and Wesolowsky (1989). It turned out that the coverage probability is more satisfactory for a larger sample size than $n = 60$ (see Zhang et al. 2010 for detailed discussion).

9.4.2.4 Application

The approximate method was used to set the acceptance limit for RT assay previously described. Forty-five historical test results were available. The normality of the data was tested and confirmed, based on the Shapiro–Wilk test. The observed values $\bar{x} = (\bar{x}_1, \bar{x}_2)'$ and **a** are

$$\bar{x} = (38.1, 38.9)'$$

$$\mathbf{a} = \begin{pmatrix} 56.3 & 36.0 \\ 36.0 & 35.1 \end{pmatrix} / 44$$

Because the estimated CV of X_2 is 15.2%, it is appropriate to apply the approximate method. The tolerance limits corresponding to $(\beta, 1 - \alpha) = (0.95, 0.95)$ and $(0.99, 0.95)$ were constructed. In each case, the generalized lower confidence limit for $P(X_1/X_2 \leq t)$ was constructed. The upper tolerance limit was obtained by solving Equation 9.22. For $\beta = 0.95$ and 0.99, the corresponding upper tolerance limits were estimated to be 1.230 and 1.239, respectively.

9.5 Release Limits

Release limits are bounds placed on product quality attributes at the time when a lot of products are tested for release. These bounds, narrower than specifications, are determined to ensure a greater chance for the lot to meet the specification at the end of its shelf life than if no narrower bounds were placed on the attributes at release as shown in Figure 9.7. Although the Food and Drug Administration views release limits as in-house limits, the European Medicines Agency requires that the limits be part of the regulatory dossier. To set appropriate release limits, consideration should be given to all sources of variation such as batch-to-batch and within-batch variability, product degradation profile, and level of quality assurance. In the literature, several statistical methods have been proposed for this purpose. The most

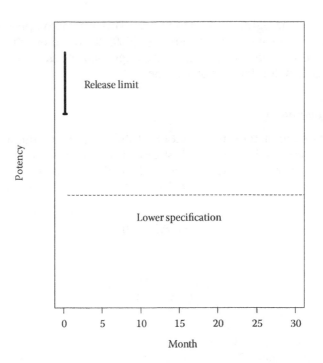

FIGURE 9.7
Release limit is determined to ensure that the potency of the product is above the lower specification limit within the 24-month shelf life.

simplistic is the method by Allen et al. (1991). Applying decision theory, Shao
and Chow (1991) suggested a Bayesian approach to determine the release
limits that warrant the minimum loss. Wei (1998, 2003) proposed two alternative methods in which the chance for out-of-specification results at the end
of shelf life is controlled at a prespecified level. More recently, Manola (2012)
evaluated the impact of release limits in the context of Bayesian analysis,
suggesting the use of the operating characteristic (OC) curve to select release
limit. In this section, we briefly describe these methods.

9.5.1 Random Batch Model

We assume that the stability characteristic y_{ij} of a batch of product is described
through a linear mixed-effects model:

$$y_{ij} = \alpha + u_0 + \beta x_i + u_1 x_i + \varepsilon_{ij}, \tag{9.26}$$

where y_{ij} is the jth ($j = 1, \ldots, m$) measured value at time point x_i ($i = 1, \ldots, n$),
with $x_1 = 0$ and $x_n = T$ corresponding to time zero and the end of shelf life,
respectively, α and β are the intercept and slope parameters, $\mathbf{u} = (u_0, u_1)$ are

deviations of the batch from the overall intercept and slope, respectively, following a bivariate distribution, $\mathbf{u} \sim MVN(\mathbf{0}, \mathbf{D})$, with

$$\mathbf{D} = \begin{pmatrix} \sigma_\alpha^2 & 0 \\ 0 & \sigma_\beta^2 \end{pmatrix}, \tag{9.27}$$

and ε_{ij} are measurement errors that are assumed to be independently and identically distributed according to a normal distribution $N(0, \sigma_e^2)$. Without loss of generality, we suppose that y_{ij} are potency values and that an equal number of samples is tested at each time point, that is, $j = 1, ..., m$. It is also assumed that potency degrades over time so that we concentrate our discussion on shelf life estimation based on one-sided interval approaches. Let $\mathbf{Y}_i =$

$(y_{i1}, ..., y_{im})'$, $\mathbf{Y} = (\mathbf{Y}_1', ..., \mathbf{Y}_n')'$, $\mathbf{b} = (\alpha, \beta)^T$, $\mathbf{X}_i = \begin{pmatrix} 1 & \cdots & 1 \\ x_i & \cdots & x_i \end{pmatrix}'_{m \times 2}$, $\mathbf{X} = (\mathbf{X}_1', ..., \mathbf{X}_n')'$, $\mathbf{e}_i =$

$(\varepsilon_{i1}, ..., \varepsilon_{im})^T$, and $\mathbf{e} = (\mathbf{e}_1', ..., \mathbf{e}_n')'$. Hence, Model 9.26 can be expressed as

$$\mathbf{Y} = \mathbf{Xb} + \mathbf{Zu} + \mathbf{e}, \tag{9.28}$$

with $\mathbf{Y} \sim MVN(\mathbf{Xb}, \mathbf{V})$, $\mathbf{V} = \mathbf{X'DX} + \sigma_e^2 \mathbf{I}_{(mn) \times (mn)}$.

9.5.2 Estimation of Release Limits

9.5.2.1 Method by Allen et al.

Allen et al. (1991) considered setting release limits, taking into account the degradation rate of the product and variability associated with both the degradation rate estimate and the analytical method. To be consistent, let RL and LRL stand for release limit and lower registered limit, respectively, that is, the lower specification limit. The general idea is to set the RL to be equal to the LRL plus a maximum amount of change that is expected over the course of the product shelf life. Specifically,

$$LR = LRL + bT + rT + t_{1-\alpha, df} \sqrt{S_T^2 + S_R^2 + \frac{S^2}{n}}, \tag{9.29}$$

where T is the shelf life, b and r are average degradation rates due to product degradation and reconstitution, respectively, S_T and S_R are the associated standard errors of b and r, S is the assay variability, and $t_{1-\alpha, df}$ is the $100(1 - \alpha)$th percentile of the central t distribution with degrees of freedom that can be estimated using the Satterthwaite approximation.

When use of the product does not require reconstitution, the RL is obtained by setting r and S_R in Equation 9.29 equal to zero. Although the method is intuitive and simple to implement, it lacks in statistical rigor (Wei 2009). For example, it does not quantify the risk for a good batch to be out of specification before the end of the product shelf life. Wei (1998, 2009) suggested two alternate methods to address this issue, which are described in Section 9.5.2.2.

9.5.2.2 Wei's Methods

Wei et al. (2009) used the model in Equation 9.26 to describe test results from a batch. Given the average t_0 value $y_0 = \sum_{j=1}^{n} y_{0j}/n$, two decision rules for estimating the RL were proposed:

Conditional Rule

RL is determined such that for $y_0 \geq RL$, $f_1(RL, y_0) = P$(Lower 95% confidence interval of the true potency at time $T < LRL|y_0) \leq \alpha$.

Unconditional Rule

The RL is determined such that $f_2(RL) = P$(Lower 95% confidence interval of the true potency at time $T < LRL|RL \leq y_0 \leq M) \leq \alpha$.

To facilitate the discussion, as above, we assume that the quality attribute of interest is potency. Based on the model in Equation 9.28, the predicted mean potency value $\hat{Y}_T$ at the end of the shelf life (T) is given by

$$\hat{Y}_T = (1, T)\hat{\mathbf{b}}, \tag{9.30}$$

with

$$\hat{\mathbf{b}} = (\mathbf{X}'\mathbf{V}^{-1}\mathbf{X})^{-1}\mathbf{X}'\mathbf{V}^{-1}\mathbf{Y},$$

$$E[\hat{\mathbf{b}}] = (\alpha, \beta), \text{ and}$$

$$\text{var}[\hat{\mathbf{b}}] = (\mathbf{X}'\mathbf{V}^{-1}\mathbf{X})^{-1}.$$

Let μ and σ^2 be the mean and variance of $\hat{Y}_T$, respectively. Combining Equations 9.28 and 9.30, it can be verified that

$$\mu = \alpha + \beta T \quad \text{and} \quad \sigma^2 = (1, T)(\mathbf{X}'\mathbf{V}^{-1}\mathbf{X})^{-1}(1, T)'. \tag{9.31}$$

9.5.2.2.1 *Conditional Release Limit*

Wei (2009) considered the case where the parameters α, β, σ_α^2, σ_β^2, and σ_β^2 are well characterized and known. Under such circumstances, the lower 95% confidence interval for the true mean potency at time T is given by

$$\hat{Y}_T - z_{0.95}\sigma_{11}, \tag{9.32}$$

where $z_{0.95}$ is the 95th percentile of the standard normal distribution.

Through reparameterization of Model 9.26, Wei (2009) derived an expression for $P[\hat{Y}_T - z_{0.95}\sigma_{11} \leq \text{LRL}|y_0]$. The release limit, RL, is chosen such that when $y_0 \geq \text{RL}$, $P[\hat{Y}_T - z_{0.95}\sigma_{11}|\leq \text{LRL}|y_0] \leq 5\%$. However, Wei's derivations are very complicated and hard to follow. In the following, we directly derive an expression for $P[\hat{Y}_T - z_{0.95}\sigma_{11}|\leq \text{LRL}|y_0]$ based on conditional distribution arguments.

Because

$$y_0 \sim N\left(\alpha, \sigma_\alpha^2 + \sigma_\beta^2/n_0\right) \quad \text{and} \quad \hat{Y}_T \sim N(\alpha+\beta T, \sigma^2), \tag{9.33}$$

we have

$$\hat{Y}_T|y_0 \sim N(\alpha+\beta T + \sigma_{12}\sigma_{22}^{-1}(y_0-\alpha), \sigma_{11} - \sigma_{12}^2/\sigma_{22}), \tag{9.34}$$

where

$$\begin{pmatrix} \sigma_{11} & \sigma_{12} \\ \sigma_{12} & \sigma_{22} \end{pmatrix} = \begin{pmatrix} \text{var}[\hat{Y}_T] & \text{cov}[y_0,\hat{Y}_T] \\ \text{cov}[y_0,\hat{Y}_T] & \text{var}[y_0] \end{pmatrix}.$$

Note that we can re-express $y_0 = \sum_{j=1}^{n} y_{0j}/n$ as $y_0 = (1'_{n_0}, 0'_{n_1}, ..., 0'_{n_T})Y/n_0$. It is obvious that

$$\text{cov}[y_0,\hat{Y}_T] = \left(1'_{n_0}, 0'_{n_1}, ..., 0'_{n_T}\right)(X'V^{-1}X)^{-1}(1,T)'/n_0. \tag{9.35}$$

Therefore,

$$\hat{Y}_T - z_{0.95}\sigma_{11}|y_0 \sim N\left(\alpha + \beta T - z_{0.95}\sigma_{11} + \sigma_{12}\sigma_{22}^{-1}(y_0 - \alpha), \ \sigma_{11} - \sigma_{12}^2/\sigma_{22}\right) \quad (9.36)$$

As a result,

$$f_1(RL, y_0) = P[\hat{Y}_T - z_{0.95}\sigma_{11} \le LRL|y_0]$$

$$= \Phi\left(\frac{LRL - [\alpha + \beta T - z_{0.95}\sigma_{11} + \sigma_{12}\sigma_{22}^{-1}(y_0 - \alpha)]}{\sigma_{11} - \sigma_{12}^2/\sigma_{22}}\right).$$

In order for it to be true that $f_1(RL, y_0) \le 0.05$, the mean potency value at time 0 must satisfy

$$\Phi\left(\frac{LRL - [\alpha + \beta T - z_{0.95}\sigma_{11} + \sigma_{12}\sigma_{22}^{-1}(y_0 - \alpha)]}{\sigma_{11} - \sigma_{12}^2/\sigma_{22}}\right) \le 0.05,$$

or, equivalently,

$$\frac{LRL - [\alpha + \beta T - z_{0.95}\sigma_{11} + \sigma_{12}\sigma_{22}^{-1}(y_0 - \alpha)]}{\sigma_{11} - \sigma_{12}^2/\sigma_{22}} \le z_{0.05}.$$

This implies that

$$y_0 \ge \alpha + \frac{LRL - \alpha - \beta T + z_{0.95}\left(2\sigma_{11} - \sigma_{12}\sigma_{22}^{-1}\right)}{\sigma_{12}\sigma_{22}^{-1}}. \quad (9.37)$$

Therefore, the release limit can be chosen to be equal to the right-hand side of inequality (Equation 9.37).

9.5.2.2.2 Unconditional Release Limit

Using Equation 9.36, we get the following representation:

$$f_2(\text{RL}) = P\left[\hat{Y}_T - z_{0.95}\sigma_{11} \le \text{LRL} \middle| \text{RL} \le y_0 \le M \right]$$

$$= \frac{P[\hat{Y}_T - z_{0.95}\sigma_{11}| \le \text{LRL} \cap \text{RL} \le y_0 \le M]}{P[\text{RL} \le y_0 \le M]}$$

$$= \frac{\displaystyle\int_{\text{RL}}^{M} \Phi\left(\frac{\text{LRL} - \left[\alpha + \beta T - z_{0.95}\sigma_{11} + \sigma_{12}\sigma_{22}^{-1}(x - \alpha)\right]}{\sigma_{11} - \sigma_{12}^2/\sigma_{22}} \right) f(x;\alpha,\sigma_{22})\,dx}{\displaystyle\int_{\text{RL}}^{M} f(x;\alpha,\sigma_{22})\,dx}$$

$$= \frac{\displaystyle\int_{(\text{RL}-\alpha)/\sqrt{\sigma_{22}}}^{(M-\alpha)/\sqrt{\sigma_{22}}} \Phi\left(\frac{\text{LRL} - \left(\alpha + \beta T - z_{0.95}\sigma_{11} + \sigma_{12}\sigma_{22}^{-1/2}z\right)}{\sigma_{11} - \sigma_{12}^2/\sigma_{22}} \right) \varphi(z)\,dz}{\displaystyle\int_{(\text{RL}-\alpha)/\sqrt{\sigma_{22}}}^{(M-\alpha)/\sqrt{\sigma_{22}}} \varphi(z)\,dz}$$

$$= \frac{\displaystyle\int_{(\text{RL}-\alpha)/\sqrt{\sigma_{22}}}^{(M-\alpha)/\sqrt{\sigma_{22}}} \Phi\left(\frac{\text{LRL} - \left(\alpha + \beta T - z_{0.95}\sigma_{11} + \sigma_{12}\sigma_{22}^{-1/2}z\right)}{\sigma_{11} - \sigma_{12}^2/\sigma_{22}} \right) \varphi(z)\,dz}{\Phi\left[(M - \alpha)/\sqrt{\sigma_{22}}\right] - \Phi\left[(\text{RL} - \alpha)/\sqrt{\sigma_{22}}\right]},$$

where $f(x_2; \alpha, \sigma_{22})$ is the density function of the normal distribution with mean α and variance σ_{22}, and $\varphi(z)$ is the density function of the standard normal distribution. The transformation $z = (x - \alpha)/\sqrt{\sigma_{22}}$ was performed to obtain the simplified expression.

Therefore, an unconditional RL can be obtained by solving the equation

$$\frac{\displaystyle\int_{(\text{RL}-\alpha)/\sqrt{\sigma_{22}}}^{(M-\alpha)/\sqrt{\sigma_{22}}} \Phi\left(\frac{\text{LRL} - \left(\alpha + \beta T - z_{0.95}\sigma_{11} + \sigma_{12}\sigma_{22}^{-1/2}z\right)}{\sigma_{11} - \sigma_{12}^2/\sigma_{22}} \right) \varphi(z)\,dz}{\Phi[(M - \alpha)/\sqrt{\sigma_{22}}] - \Phi[(\text{RL} - \alpha)/\sqrt{\sigma_{22}}]} = 0.05. \quad (9.38)$$

This equation can be solved using routine algorithms for numerical integration. Alternatively, the RL can be estimated through simulation. Define

$$g(\text{RL}, z) = \frac{\Phi\left(\dfrac{\text{LRL} - \left(\alpha + \beta T - z_{0.95}\sigma_{11} + \sigma_{12}\sigma_{22}^{-1/2}z\right)}{\sigma_{11} - \sigma_{12}^2/\sigma_{22}}\right)}{\Phi\left[(M-\alpha)/\sqrt{\sigma_{22}}\right] - \Phi\left[(\text{RL}-\alpha)/\sqrt{\sigma_{22}}\right]} I_{[(\text{RL}-\alpha)/\sqrt{\sigma_{22}},(M-\alpha)/\sqrt{\sigma_{22}}]}(z),$$

where $I_{[(\text{RL}-\alpha)/\sqrt{\sigma_{22}},(M-\alpha)/\sqrt{\sigma_{22}}]}(z)$ is an indicator function that assumes 1 when $z \in \left[(\text{RL}-\alpha)/\sqrt{\sigma_{22}},(\text{RL}-\alpha)/\sqrt{\sigma_{22}}\right]$ and 0 when z is elsewhere.

Let Z be a random variable following the standard normal distribution. The left-hand side of Equation 9.38 can be rewritten as $E[g(\text{RL}, Z)]$. We take a random sample Z_i, $i = 1, \ldots, N$, from $N(0, 1)$. Thus, $g(\text{RL}, Z_i)$ are independently identically distributed with mean $E[g(\text{RL}, Z)]$. By the Large Number Theorem,

$$\bar{g}(\text{RL}) = \frac{\sum\limits_{i=1}^{N} g(\text{RL}, Z_i)}{N} \rightarrow E[g(\text{RL}, Z)].$$

Therefore, the left-hand side of Equation 9.38 can be approximated by $\bar{g}(\text{RL})$. The approximation can be carried out over a grid of RL. The final RL is selected such that it meets the condition in Equation 9.38.

9.5.2.3 Bayesian Methods

Although the methods discussed in Section 9.5.2.2 control failure rate at the end of the product shelf life, the consumer risk, they do not take into account the producer risk, that is, the loss due to rejecting a lot at release even though the lot has the desired shelf life. To address this issue, Shao and Chow (1991) suggested an alternate approach based on Bayesian decision theory. Consider k release tests with specification limits of $[L_i, U_i]$, $i = 1,\ldots,k$. It is assumed that for each attribute, two-sided release limits are needed. Thus, each selection of potential limits $d_i = [a_i, b_i]$ represents a decision made or action taken for the ith test. The entire action space D is given by

$$D = \{\mathbf{d} = (d_1,\ldots,d_k): L_i \le a_i \le b_i \le U_i, i = 1,\ldots,k\}. \tag{9.39}$$

Let y, μ, and s be the measurements, average values, and stability losses, respectively, of k stability characteristics such as potency and impurity. Both μ and s are considered to be random to account for batch-to-batch variability.

Let $l(s, \mu, y, d)$ be a loss function. The expected loss caused by action d is given by the expected value of $l(s, \mu, y, d)$:

$$\rho(\mathbf{d}) = E^{(s, \mu, y)} [l(\mathbf{s}, \mu, \mathbf{y}, \mathbf{d})]. \tag{9.40}$$

The release limits are the optimal actions $\mathbf{d}^*$ that minimize $\rho(\mathbf{d})$. They can be obtained by numerically finding $\mathbf{d}^* \in D$ such that

$$\rho(\mathbf{d}^*) = \min \{\rho(\mathbf{d}): \mathbf{d} \in D\}. \tag{9.41}$$

Shao and Chow (1991) discussed how to determine an appropriate loss function $l(s, \mu, y, d)$ using utility analysis. In addition, they also suggested a Monte Carlo method for solving the above minimization problem.

While conceptually appealing, Shao and Chow's method is statistically involved. An alternative method was proposed by Wei (1998). The release limit is determined such that it minimizes the expected loss defined as

$$\text{Expected Loss} = L_0 P[\text{A batch failed at time 0}]$$
$$+ L_T P[\text{A batch failed at time } T],$$

where L_0 and L_T are costs associated with the failed batch at time 0 and T, respectively.

However, this formulation is incomplete as it does not take into account all possible outcomes of disposing of the batch. More recently, Manola (2012) suggested a Bayesian approach to the determination of the release limit. One way to accomplish this is to determine the release limit, RL, such that the best trade-off between the consumer risk (CR) and producer (risk) can be achieved:

$$CR = P(y_{SL} < LRL | y_0 \geq LR)$$

$$PR = P(y_0 < LRL | y_{SL} \geq LRL), \tag{9.42}$$

where y_0 and y_{SL} are measured values of the stability characteristic of a future lot at time 0 and the product shelf life, respectively, and can be simulated from the method described below.

There are many ways such a trade-off can be made. For example, the trade-off can be determined based on (1) both CR and PR meet preselected acceptance criteria, (2) the minimum or maximum of CR and PR is below a prespecified limit, or (3) the total cost associated with the two types of risk is minimized.

The selection of RL can be achieved through simulation. It is assumed that the stability characteristic following the mixed-effects model (Equation 9.26), with uniform priors for the intercept and slope (α, β) and Jeffreys' priors for variances $\left(\sigma_\alpha^2, \sigma_\beta^2, \sigma_e^2\right)$:

$$P(\alpha) \sim \text{Uniform}$$

$$P(\beta) \sim \text{Uniform}$$

$$P\left(\sigma_\alpha^2\right) \propto \frac{1}{\sigma_\alpha^2},$$

$$P\left(\sigma_\beta^2\right) \propto \frac{1}{\sigma_\beta^2},$$

$$P\left(\sigma_e^2\right) \propto \frac{1}{\sigma_e^2}. \tag{9.43}$$

Note that the posterior distribution of the model parameters at a sampling time t satisfies

$$p\left(\alpha, \beta, u_0, u_1, \sigma_\alpha^2, \sigma_\beta^2, \sigma_e^2 | Y_t\right)$$
$$\propto p\left(\alpha, \beta, u_0, u_1, \sigma_\alpha^2, \sigma_\beta^2, \sigma_e^2\right) p\left(Y_t | \alpha, \beta, u_0, u_1, \sigma_\alpha^2, \sigma_\beta^2, \sigma_e^2\right),$$

with $p\left(Y_t | \alpha, \beta, \sigma_\alpha^2, \sigma_\beta^2, \sigma_e^2\right)$ being a likelihood function of Y_t. From Equations 9.26 and 9.43, the posterior distribution, after some algebraic simplification, is given by

$$p\left(\alpha, \beta, u_0, u_1, \sigma_\alpha^2, \sigma_\beta^2, \sigma_e^2 | Y_t\right) \propto \frac{e^{-\left\{\frac{1}{2\sigma_e^2}\sum_{j=1}^{m}\left[y_{tj}-(\alpha+u_0+\beta x_t+u_1 x_t)\right]^2 - \frac{\alpha^2}{2\sigma_\alpha^2} - \frac{\beta^2}{2\sigma_\beta^2}\right\}}}{\left(\sqrt{\sigma_\alpha^2 \sigma_\beta^2}\right)^3 \sqrt{\sigma_e^2}}. \tag{9.44}$$

Manola (2012) suggested that the following Monte Carlo simulation procedure be used to determine RL such that it provides the best trade-off between CR and PR:

1. Generate a random sample of the fixed effects and variability $\left(\alpha, \beta, \sigma_\alpha^2, \sigma_\beta^2, \sigma_e^2\right)$ from the posterior distribution (Equation 9.32) and denote them as $\left(\alpha_i, \beta_i, \sigma_{\alpha i}^2, \sigma_{\beta i}^2, \sigma_{ei}^2\right)$, $i = 1, \ldots, m$.

2. For each i, simulate the random effect $\mathbf{u} = (u_0, u_1)$ based on $\left(\sigma_{\alpha i}^2, \sigma_{\beta i}^2\right)$ and denote them as $\mathbf{u}_k = (u_{k0}, u_{k1})$. Calculate the posterior expected value of the kth random lot at time t ($t = 0$ or shelf life), $E[y_{k(i)t}|(\alpha_i, \beta_i)] = \alpha_i + u_{k0} + \beta_i t + u_{k1}$.

3. For each of the future lot k ($k = 1, ..., K$), simulate the analytical assay error $\varepsilon_{k(i)t} \sim N\left(0, \sigma_{ei}^2\right)$ to obtain $y_{k(i)t} = E = [y_{k(i)t}|(\alpha_i, \beta_i)] = \varepsilon_{k(i)t1}$.

4. Repeat steps 1–3 for sufficient number of times, for example, $N = 10,000$.

5. For each choice of RL, estimate CR and PR in Equation 9.42. Finally, choose RL per the trade-off criteria.

9.6 Concluding Remarks

Specifications are acceptance criteria for the suitability of either drug substance or drug product for its intended use. Before a drug substance or drug product lot is released for use, quality attributes of the lot, including identity, strength, and purity, are tested to ensure that they meet their specifications. Traditionally, specifications for a quality attribute are established independent of other quality attributes. This potentially could result in ranges that are narrower than the acceptable performance of the product. This issue can be effectively coped with using multivariate statistical modeling and other advanced statistical techniques, such as GPQ analysis. The chapter also discusses statistical methods for setting product release limits.

10

Environmental Monitoring

10.1 Introduction

Sterile drug products are manufactured in facilities where airborne particles are controlled. Although a sterile manufacturing environment consists of rooms that are designed, maintained, and controlled to minimize the introduction and retention of airborne particles and microbial excursions, opportunistic contaminations are unavoidable. Therefore, it is essential to establish an environmental monitoring (EM) program to assess the cleanliness of the manufacturing areas and to ensure a state of environmental control. In fact, establishment of an EM program is required by both regulatory guidance and law (Food and Drug Administration [FDA] 2004c; 21 CFR 211). The FDA 2004 Guidance for Industry: Sterile Drug Products Produced by Aseptic Processing—Current Good Manufacturing Practice and the Code of Federal Regulations governing the manufacture of pharmaceutical products clearly state the need to establish and follow procedures to prevent microbiological contamination of sterile drug products. Rooms where sterile products are manufactured are termed cleanrooms. Each of these rooms has a class designation and associated action limit for the maximum acceptable microbiological level. For example, in Class 100 (ISO 5) cleanrooms and isolation systems, it is expected that the normal microbial recovery is zero. The performance of the cleanrooms is monitored and corrective steps are taken if an unacceptable microbial level is identified. To this end, an EM program should specify sampling frequency and location, types of samples, and culture media. Before specifying these, alert and action limits should be defined. Data from real-time monitoring are compared to these limits so as to detect any microbial excursion that might put the product at risk. This chapter discusses statistical methods for trending environmental data from cleanrooms and setting alert and action limits.

10.2 Alert and Action Levels

Alert and action levels are quality indicators used to gauge if the microbial system is in control. USP <1231> (USP 1997) provides the following definitions of alert and action levels:

> **Alert levels** are events or levels that, when they occur or are exceeded, indicate that a process may have drifted from its normal operation condition.
>
> **Action levels** are events or higher levels that, when they occur or are exceeded, indicate that a process is probably drifting from its normal operation range.

USP <1231> further states "Alert level excursions constitute a warning and do not necessarily require corrective actions. Alert level excursions may also lead to additional monitoring with more intense scrutiny of resulting and neighboring data as well as other process indicators." By contrast, exceeding an action level triggers immediate investigation to identify the root cause and take corrective measures so as to bring the process to its normal operating range. Historically, data collected when the process was in control are usually used to establish the alert and action limits. To minimize false alarms and false negatives, the alert and action limits should be derived based on robust statistical methods that characterize the historical data well. Before any statistical analysis is performed, it is important to remove "out of control" data to avoid overestimation of the alert and action limits.

10.3 Statistical Methods

10.3.1 Historical Practice

10.3.1.1 Normal Distribution

Historically, it was a common practice to use the mean ± 2 or 3 standard deviations (SDs) as alert and action limits, respectively (Wilson 1997). When the microbial data are normally distributed, these limits have a probabilistic interpretation. That is, they cover fixed proportions of all possible observations. However, in reality, the normality assumption rarely holds. For example, in Class 100 cleanrooms, there is usually zero microbial recovery. As a result, the data distribution is usually skewed. Although transformation of the data may help "normalize" the distribution, there are other distributions such as the Poisson that are better suited for describing count data.

10.3.1.2 Nonparameter Intervals

Alternatively, nonparametric methods can be used to set alert and action limits. These methods do not rely on an underlying assumption of the distribution of the data. Rather, they make use of the empirical distribution of the data. For example, the alert and action levels can be set as the 95th and 99th percentiles of the empirical distribution, estimated as follows:

$$F(x) = \frac{\# \text{ of observations} \leq x}{N},$$

where $x \geq 0$ and N is the total number of observations in the data set. The alert and action levels based on the empirical distribution are observed microbial counts that cover prespecified proportions of the historical data.

A more rigorous approach is to use the nonparametric tolerance interval suggested by Conover (1999). Consider $X_1 \ldots X_n$ to be a random sample of microbial counts and $X_{(1)}, \ldots, X_{(n)}$ to be the ranked values. Let q and $1 - \alpha$ be the percentage of population covered by the tolerance interval and the confidence level, respectively. Further, we let m be an integer such that

$$q = \frac{4n - 2(m-1) - \chi^2_{2m}(1-\alpha)}{4n - 2(m-1) + \chi^2_{2m}(1-\alpha)},$$

where $\chi^2_{2m}(1-\alpha)$ is the $(1-\alpha)$th percentile of a χ^2 distribution with $2m$ degrees of freedom. Thus, with probability of at least $(1-\alpha)$, the one-sided tolerance limit $X^{(n-m)}$ covers $100q\%$ of the population (Conover 1999).

However, there are several drawbacks to the nonparametric methods. First of all, as pointed out by several researchers (Christensen et al. 2003; Yang et al. 2013b), the reliability of these nonparametric approaches depends heavily on the amount of data available. In the absence of large data sets, these approaches produce alert and action levels that far exceed the nominal significance levels, thus artificially creating wider ranges. Second, they run the risk of selecting as the alert/action limits the outlying data points caused by out-of-control conditions. This again results in inflated estimates of alert and action limits. In addition, there is also no optimality criterion, such as the shortest interval width, for selecting these intervals. As a result, there is a risk that the chosen intervals may be much larger than what is needed to cover a certain percentage of the future observations. Therefore, recent efforts have been centered on setting alert and action levels using parametric model-based methods.

10.3.2 Poisson Distribution

The Poisson distribution has been widely applied to model count data. If X follows a Poisson distribution, the probability for X to be equal to a number x is given by (Haight 1967)

$$f(x \mid \lambda) = \frac{\lambda^x e^{-\lambda}}{x!},$$

where λ is the mean count in a unit sample. One unique characteristic of the Poisson distribution is that the mean of the distribution is equal to the variance. The parameter λ can be estimated using maximum likelihood. Let $\hat{\lambda}$ be such an estimator.

In general, a one-sided upper confidence limit (UCL) can be obtained, using either of the following two methods, one of which is based on normal approximation and the other is deemed to be exact. Using the approximate method, the one-sided UCL is given by

$$\hat{\text{UCL}}^P_{\text{Approximate}} = \hat{\lambda} + z_{1-\alpha} \sqrt{\hat{\lambda}/n}, \tag{10.1}$$

and the exact one-sided UCL is given by

$$\hat{\text{UCL}}^P_{\text{Exact}} = \min \left\{ n : \sum_{x=0}^{n} f(x \mid \hat{\lambda}) \geq 1 - \alpha \right\}, \tag{10.2}$$

where $z_{1-\alpha}$ is the upper $(1 - \alpha) \times 100$th percentile of the standard normal distribution.

However, when applied to environmental data, the Poisson model is often inadequate as the actual variability in the data is often larger than that expected under the Poisson assumption as discussed in Chapter 7. This phenomenon is often referred to as overdispersion. For microbial count data, several factors may contribute to overdispersion. Chief among these is that measurements are taken at different times and various locations. Conceivably, the mean count may differ from time to time and location to location because of various factors. Although the microbial count may exhibit behavior that can be described through a Poisson distribution at each fixed time or location, the collective data as a whole may not follow any Poisson distribution. Blindly applying a single-parameter Poisson model to environmental data consisting of several subpopulations may underestimate the variability of the data, leading to lower alert and action limits, and thus causing more frequent false alarms of microbial excursion.

10.3.3 Negative Binomial

The negative binomial distribution is a variant of Poisson distribution that has increased flexibility to address the issue of overdispersion. It can be viewed as either a generalization of the geometric distribution or a mixture of Poisson distributions (Hoffman 2004). Hoffman (2004) and Christensen et al. (2003) suggest using the negative binomial distribution to correct for the effect of overdispersion. Assume X follows a negative binomial distribution $NB(\mu, \kappa)$, with density function given by

$$g(x_i \mid \mu, k) = \frac{\Gamma(1/k + x_i)(k\mu)^{x_i}}{x_i! \Gamma(1/k)(1 + k\mu)^{1/k + x_i}},$$

where $\mu > 0$ and $k > 0$. The distribution of X has a mean μ and variance $\mu(1 + k\mu)$. It is evident that the variance is greater than the mean, whereas they are equal for the Poisson distribution. As a consequence, the negative binomial distribution is useful for modeling overdispersed data as previously discussed in Chapter 7.

10.3.3.1 Direct Approximation

Hoffman (2004) suggested two methods to set alert and action limits using the negative binomial distribution. The first is based on the cumulative density function (CDF) of the negative binomial distribution with the parameters being estimated by their maximum likelihood estimators (MLEs). The second method determines the limits based on a χ^2 approximation to the negative binomial distribution. Both methods are briefly described below.

Let $1 - \alpha$ be the confidence level for a one-sided UCL and $(\hat{\mu}, \hat{k})$ be the MLEs of the distribution parameters. The UCL is determined such that

$$\hat{UCL}_{Exact}^{NB} = \min\left\{ n : \sum_{x=0}^{n} \hat{g}(x \mid \hat{\mu}, \hat{k}) \geq 1 - \alpha \right\}. \tag{10.3}$$

Because of the discrete nature of the data and approximation of the true model parameters, the above limit might not be truly exact (Hoffman 2004).

The second method by Hoffman (2004) uses the following approximation suggested by Guenther (1972):

$$P[X \leq \text{UCL}] = P\left[\chi_v^2 \leq \frac{2\text{UCL}+1}{1+\mu k} \right] = 1-\alpha, \qquad (10.4)$$

where χ_v^2 is a random variable following a χ^2 distribution with v degrees of freedom $v = 2\hat{\mu}/(1+\hat{k}\hat{\mu})$. Solving the above equation with parameters (μ, k) being replaced by their MLEs gives rise to an estimate of the UCL:

$$\text{UCL}^{\text{NB}}_{\text{Approximate}} = \left[\chi_v^2(1-\alpha)(1+\hat{\mu}\hat{k}) - 1 \right]/2, \qquad (10.5)$$

where $\chi_v^2(1-\alpha)$ is the $100(1-\alpha)$th percentile of the χ^2 distribution with v degrees of freedom.

10.3.3.2 Model Comparison

Hoffman (2004) compared the Poisson and negative binomial methods for calculating alert and action limits using a real-world example. The data consisting of 18 water bacteria count (per milliliter), 20, 5, 23, 19, 13, 12, 14, 17, 2, 7, 30, 4, 16, 2, 4, 1, 2, and 0, were collected from a water purification system when it was in a state of control.

Both the Poisson model and the negative binomial model were fit to the data. The parameter λ of the Poisson model was estimated to be $\hat{\lambda} = 10.611$. In the case of the negative binomial model, the estimated model parameters are $\hat{\mu} = 10.611$ (the same mean estimate as under Poisson) and $\hat{k} = 0.7902$. Applying Equation 10.2 and assuming that $\alpha = 0.001$, the approximate and exact upper control limits were estimated to be $\text{UCL}^P_{\text{Approximate}} = 21.4$ and $\text{UCL}^P_{\text{Exact}} = 22$, respectively. Note that 2 out of 18 samples have bacteria counts above both $\text{UCL}^P_{\text{Approximate}}$ and $\text{UCL}^P_{\text{Exact}}$, which represents a Type I error estimate of 11.1%. A similar analysis was carried out, using the negative binomial model, resulting in $\text{UCL}^{\text{NB}}_{\text{Approximate}} = 67.5$ and $\text{UCL}^{\text{NB}}_{\text{Exact}} = 67$, respectively. All the observed counts are well below the limits. The results suggest that the Poisson model renders an inflated Type I error estimate. If used in practice, it may cause more false alarms. The fits of the two models were further compared through visual inspection. Hoffman (2004) illustrated, through a plot, the difference among the estimated CDFs of the Poisson and negative binomial models, with the parameters estimated from the example data and the empirical CDF based on the observed data. The data are replotted in Figure 10.1. It is evident that the negative binomial model provides a better estimate of the distribution from which the data were generated.

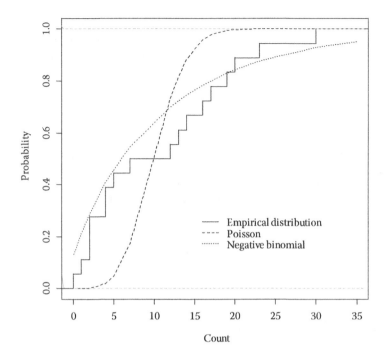

FIGURE 10.1
Estimated CDFs based on empirical data and from Poisson and negative binomial fits. (From Hoffman, D. (2004). Negative binomial control limits for count data with extra-Poisson variation. *Pharm. Stat.*, 2, 127–132.)

The advantages of the negative binomial model may be better demonstrated through a simulation study, in which the true distribution of the data being analyzed is known.

10.3.4 Hierarchical Poisson–Gamma Modeling

Independent of Hoffman (2004), Christensen et al. (2003) also proposed the use of the negative binomial distribution to set alert and action levels for EM programs in cleanrooms, in order to model both overdispersion and an excess of zeros. As pointed by Christensen et al. (2013), using the negative binomial distribution to model overdispersed count data does not provide insight into variability due to time and location, particularly when sample sizes are different at different times/locations. They proposed that the microbial data be modeled using a hierarchical Poisson–Gamma model, which is a variant of the Poisson distribution. In this model, the count from each group (time point or sampling location) is viewed as a random variable from a Poisson distribution. However, the parameter of the Poisson distribution may vary from group to group to account for potential between-group variations. Apart from accounting for the observed overdispersion, the model has two additional benefits: (1) the model can be fit with different sample sizes at different time points or locations, and (2) it quantifies both within- and between-time (or location) variability. Such insights can help guide the decision concerning whether or not group-specific alert and action levels are necessary.

10.3.4.1 Hierarchical Model

It is assumed that there are m sampling groups (locations or time points) and that the count data from each group follow a Poisson distribution. Let X_{ij} be the count data obtained from sample j in group i, $i = 1, ..., m$, and $j = 1, 2, ..., n_i$. Christensen et al. (2003) described X_{ij} using the following hierarchical model:

$$X_{ij}|W_i \sim \text{Poisson}(n_i W_i)$$

$$Z_i \sim \text{Gamma}(1/\gamma, \mu\gamma), \tag{10.6}$$

where X_{ij} follows a Poisson distribution with mean W_i, W_i being a random variable following a gamma distribution with shape parameter $1/\gamma$ and scale parameter $\mu\gamma$.

Let $Z_i = \sum_{j=1}^{n_i} X_{ij}$. Then,

$$Z_i|W_i \sim \text{Poisson}(n_i W_i). \tag{10.7}$$

$$Z_i = \sum_{j=1}^{n_i} X_{ij}.$$

Because of Equations 10.6 and 10.7, the marginal distribution of Z_i follows negative binomial distribution with a density function given by

$$h(z_i|\mu,\gamma) = \frac{\Gamma(1/\gamma + z_i)}{z_i!\,\Gamma(1/\gamma)}\left(\frac{1}{1+n_i\gamma\mu}\right)^{1/\gamma}\left(\frac{n_i\gamma\mu}{1+n_i\gamma\mu}\right)^{z_i} \quad \text{for } x_i = 0, 1, ...$$

The mean and variance of Z_i are

$$E[Z_i] = n_i\mu$$

$$\text{Var}[Z_i] = n_i\mu(1 + n_i\gamma\mu).$$

Therefore, the parameter γ is associated with the overdispersion of X_{ij}. Following Thyregod (1998), Christensen et al. (2003) suggested a likelihood ratio test based on X_{ij} to test the null hypothesis:

$$H_0 : \gamma = 0 \quad \text{versus} \quad H_1 : \gamma > 0. \tag{10.8}$$

Using the fact that $\Gamma(x) = (x - 1)\Gamma(x - 1)$, it follows that

$$\frac{\Gamma(1/\gamma + x_i)}{x_i!\,\Gamma(1/\gamma)} = \prod_{j=0}^{x_i-1} (1/\gamma + j).$$

After algebraic manipulations, the log-likelihood function of $\{Z_i\}$, by disregarding some constant, is

$$l(\mu, \gamma) = \ln(\mu) \sum_{i=1}^{k} z_i + \sum_{i=1}^{k} \sum_{j=0}^{z_i-1} \ln(1 + n_i j\gamma) - \sum_{i=1}^{k} (1/\gamma + z_i)\ln(1 + n_i \gamma \mu). \tag{10.9}$$

When $\gamma = 0$, the log-likelihood function in Equation 10.9 achieves its maximum at

$$\tilde{\mu} = \sum_{i=1}^{k} z_i \bigg/ \sum_{i=1}^{k} n_i. \tag{10.10}$$

The MLEs $(\hat{\mu}, \hat{\gamma})$ of (μ, γ) are solutions to the equations

$$\frac{\partial l(\mu, \gamma)}{\partial \mu} = \frac{\sum_{i=1}^{k} z_i}{\mu} - \frac{\sum_{i=1}^{k} (1/\gamma + z_i)n_i \gamma}{1 + n_i \gamma \mu} = 0$$

$$\frac{\partial l(\mu, \gamma)}{\partial \gamma} = \sum_{i=1}^{k} \sum_{j=0}^{z_i-1} \frac{j}{1 + j\gamma} - \frac{\sum_{i=1}^{k} (1/\gamma + z_i)n_i \mu}{1 + n_i \gamma \mu} + \frac{1}{\gamma^2} \sum_{i=1}^{j} \ln(1 + n_i \gamma \mu) = 0. \tag{10.11}$$

The $(\hat{\mu}, \hat{\gamma})$ can be obtained by numerically solving the above equations. As discussed in Christensen et al. (2003), the MLEs $(\hat{\mu}, \hat{\gamma})$ for various scenarios were explored by several authors. For example, when the same number of samples is taken in each group, $\hat{\mu} = \tilde{\mu}$, which is given in Equation 10.10.

In general, the log-likelihood ratio test statistic for the null hypothesis in Equation 10.8 is

$$Q = 2[l(\hat{\mu}, \hat{\gamma}) - l(\tilde{\mu}, 0)], \tag{10.12}$$

which approximately follows a χ^2 distribution with one degree of freedom.

Therefore, the null hypothesis at the significance level of α is rejected if $Q > \chi^2_{1,1-\alpha}$, with $\chi^2_{1,1-\alpha}$ being the upper $(1 - \alpha) \times 100$th percentile of the χ^2 distribution with one degree of freedom. If the null hypothesis is rejected, the alert and action limits can be obtained through the exact method in Equation 10.3. If the null hypothesis is not rejected, the negative binomial distribution parameterized μ, $\gamma = 0$, and n_i degenerates to a Poisson distribution. Consequently, the alert and action limits can be determined, following the method described in Section 10.3.2.

10.3.4.2 Method Comparison

Through a real example, Christensen et al. (2003) compared their hierarchical model to several other methods in determining alert and action limits. These methods include limits based on (1) an empirical method based on percentiles, (2) the Poisson distribution, (3) the exponential distribution, (4) a normal approximation after either a log or a square root transformation, and (5) the Weibull distribution. The data were taken from one sampling location at different time points, with a total of 325 observations in the data set.

Applying the above methods, alert and action limits were determined and presented in Table 10.1. Overdispersion of the data was investigated using the likelihood ratio test in Equation 10.12, which resulted in a P value of 0.001. Consequently, the null hypothesis (Equation 10.8) was rejected. Using Equation 10.4, the alert and action limits defined as the 95th and 99th percentiles of the negative binomial distribution were estimated to be 34 and 62, respectively. As seen from the table, the alert and action limits based on the hierarchical model are comparable to those from the direct empirical estimate. The Poisson,

TABLE 10.1

Alert and Action Limits Determined from Various Methods

Method	Alert Limit	Action Limit
Empirical	29	55
Poisson	13	18
Exponential	25	39
Weibull	18	22
Normal (log-transformation)	34	81
Normal (square-root transformation)	29	45
Hierarchical model	34	62

Source: Christensen, A., Melgaard, H., and Iwersen, J. (2003). Environmental monitoring based on a hierarchical Poisson–Gamma model. *J. Qual. Technol.*, 35(3), 275–285.

exponential, and Weibull distribution approaches all underestimate the alert and action limits, due to failing to account for the overdispersion in the data. The normal approximation approach after log and square-root transformations results in alert limit estimates that are comparable to those of the empirical distribution, but the log-transformation approach overestimates the action limit and the square root transformation approach underestimates it.

10.3.5 Modeling Excess Zero Counts

Environmental data often exhibit an excess of zeros. This is especially true for microbial count data collected from cleanrooms and isolation systems (Caputo and Huffman 2004). The high occurrence of zero observations often invalidates the assumption that the data follow an underlying distribution such as normal or Poisson distribution. Although a negative binomial model can account for variability due to location or sampling time, it is insufficient to model data with frequent zero values. Caputo and Huffman (2004) argued that greater importance should be given to directional trend than to individual microbial counts, as observations below alert and action limits may not indicate a state of control. A metric that measures the frequency of nonzero observations is defined as

$$\Phi_i = \frac{365}{N_i},$$ (10.13)

where N_i $(1 \leq i \leq n)$ is the number of days since the last nonzero observation.

Therefore, Φ_i represents the frequency of nonzero observations on an annual basis that corresponds to N_i. As a continuous variable, Φ_i may be described through a continuous distribution such as the normal distribution, possibly after a transformation. Alert and action limits can be accordingly determined using the techniques described in Section 10.3.1.1.

10.3.5.1 Zero-Inflated Models

As pointed out by Yang et al. (2013b), although the level of microbial count is most indicative of a potential excursion, it is not considered in the Caputo and Huffman (2004) method described above. As a result, unacceptable excursions may go undetected. Furthermore, the method does not account for heterogeneity of the subpopulations, such as due to location to location variability. An alternative method based on a zero-inflated negative binomial model was suggested (Yang et al. 2013b). A zero-inflated model is a mixture model having two populations, where the first population places all its mass at zero (Erdman et al. 2008; Lambert 1992). For microbial count data from a cleanroom, the data may be viewed as being generated from a mixture model. The two subpopulations correspond to sterile and nonsterile populations. A sample comes from one of the two populations with probabilities p and $1 - p$, respectively.

Let $X = \{X_i, i = 1,...,n\}$ denote the microbial counts of n samples taken in a monitoring cycle. X_i is modeled through the following zero-inflated negative binomial (ZINB) model (Erdman et al. 2008):

$$X_i = WY + (1 - W)Z, \tag{10.14}$$

where W is the Bernoulli random variable with $\Pr[W = 1] = p$, Y is a degenerated random variable with $\Pr(Y = 0) = 1$, and Z follows a negative binomial distribution $NB(\mu, \kappa)$, with density function given in Section 10.3.3.

Assuming that W, Y, and Z are independent, the density function of the observed microbial count X_i is

$$h(x_i \mid p, \mu, k) = \begin{cases} p + (1-p)g(x_i \mid \mu, k) & \text{if } x_i = 0 \\ (1-p)g(x_i \mid \mu, k) & \text{if } x_i > 0. \end{cases} \tag{10.15}$$

Clearly, when $p = 0$, $h(x_i|p, \mu, k) = g(x_i|\mu, k)$, which implies that X_i follows a negative binomial distribution. When $p = 0$, $k \to 0$, and $k\mu \to \lambda$, $h(x_i|0, \mu, k) = g(x_i|\mu, k) \to \dfrac{\lambda^{x_i} e^{-x_i}}{x_i!}$. That is, X_i has an asymptotic Poisson distribution. Because when the mean λ of a Poisson distribution is large, the distribution is approximately normal, the zero-inflated model is also approximately normal for $p = 0$ and large λ. These observations suggest that a zero-inflated model intuitively would describe microbial count data well, even if the underlying distribution is either normal, Poisson, or negative binomial. As test methods are readily available for determining which model is most appropriate, a general strategy for model selection was recommended by Yang et al. (2013b) and is discussed in Section 7.3 of Chapter 7.

10.3.5.2 Parameter Estimation

The parameters in Equation 10.15 can be estimated through the maximum likelihood method. Let $n_x(0 < x \le m)$ denote the number of observations out of n samples $X = \{X_i, i = 1, ..., n\}$ that take value x. Thus, n_0 is the number of zeros in the sample. The log-likelihood function of X is given by

$$L(p, \mu, k) = n_0 \log\left[p + (1-p) \frac{1}{(1+k\mu)^{1/k}} \right] + \sum_{x=1}^{m} n_x \log[(1-p)g(x \mid \mu, k)]. \tag{10.16}$$

The MLEs $(\hat{p}, \hat{\mu}, \hat{k})$, being solutions of the partial derivatives of the log-likelihood in Equation 10.16, can be found through a numerical algorithm. Both SAS and R provide such algorithms.

10.3.5.3 Alert and Action Limits

As before, the alert and action limits can be obtained using the estimated probability function $\hat{h}(x \mid \hat{p}, \hat{\mu}, \hat{k})$. Let $1 - \alpha_1$ and $1 - \alpha_2$ be the confidence levels for alert and action limits, respectively. The alert limit (ALL) and action limit (ACL) are determined as

$$\hat{ALL} = \min\left\{ n : \sum_{x=0}^{n} \hat{f}(x \mid \hat{p}, \hat{\mu}, \hat{k}) \geq 1 - \alpha_1 \right\}$$

$$\hat{ACL} = \min\left\{ n : \sum_{x=0}^{n} \hat{f}(x \mid \hat{p}, \hat{\mu}, \hat{k}) \geq 1 - \alpha_2 \right\}. \tag{10.17}$$

10.3.5.4 Simulation Study

Yang et al. (2013b) evaluated the performance of the zero-inflated negative binomial model against the normal, Poisson, and negative binomial models. The true values of the parameters used to generate random samples from the mixture model in Equation 10.15 were $(p, \mu, k) = (0.5, 2.8, 0.04)$. The confidence levels for the alert and action limits were set at 0.05 and 0.01, respectively. The simulation was done for sample sizes of 100, 1000, and 10,000. For each scenario, 1000 data sets were simulated.

For each data set, normal, Poisson, negative binomial, and ZINB models were fit to the data to obtain estimated model parameters. For the normal distribution, mean ± 2SD and mean ± 3SD were used to determine the alert and action limits, respectively. The estimated probability functions in Equations 10.2, 10.5, and 10.17 were used to estimate the respective alert and action limits for the other three models. The mean estimates (over all 1000 simulations) are given by, along with their SD estimates,

$$\hat{ALL}(n) = \frac{\sum_{m=1}^{1000} \hat{ALL}(m, n)}{1000} \quad \text{and} \quad SD_{ALL}(n) = \sqrt{\frac{\sum_{m=1}^{1000} [\hat{ALL}(m, n) - \hat{ALL}(n)]^2}{1000 - 1}}, \tag{10.18}$$

$$\hat{ACL}(n) = \frac{\sum_{m=1}^{1000} \hat{ACL}(m, n)}{1000} \quad \text{and} \quad SD_{ACL}(n) = \sqrt{\frac{\sum_{m=1}^{1000} [\hat{ACL}(m, n) - \hat{ACL}(n)]^2}{1000 - 1}}. \tag{10.19}$$

The true ALL and ACL are determined to be 5 and 7, respectively, based on Equation 10.15 with parameters (p, μ, k) being replaced by their true values

TABLE 10.2

Mean Estimates of Alert and Action Limits Based on 1000 Simulated Data Sets

Sample Size	Limit	True Limit	Mean Estimate (SD)			
			ZINB	Normal	Poisson	Negative Binomial
100	Alert	5	5.1 (0.49)	4.5 (0.53)	3.6 (0.50)	5.9 (0.64)
	Action	7	7.1 (0.70)	5.7 (0.60)	4.8 (0.46)	10.2 (1.12)
1000	Alert	5	5.0 (0.04)	4.4 (0.48)	3.6 (0.48)	6.0 (0.16)
	Action	7	7.0 (0.19)	5.9 (0.30)	5.0 (0.17)	10.1 (0.40)
10,000	Alert	5	5.0 (0.00)	4.1 (0.35)	3.9 (0.31)	6.0 (0.00)
	Action	7	7.0 (0.00)	6.0 (0.00)	5.0 (0.00)	10.0 (0.04)

Source: Yang, H., Zhao, W., O'Day, T., and Fleming, W. (2013b). Environmental monitoring: Setting alert and action limits based on a zero-inflated model. *PDA J. Pharm. Sci. Technol.*, 67(1), 1–9.

Note: SD, standard deviation.

(0.5, 2.8, 0.04). The mean estimates of alert and action limits are presented in Table 10.2, along with their associated SDs.

It can be seen from the table that the normal and Poisson models underestimate the dispersion of the data, while the negative binomial overestimates the dispersion. As a result, the former generate alert and action limits narrower than the actual ALL and ACL, whereas the latter results in wider ALL and ACL. The ZINB model appropriately models the dispersion of the data and affords the most accurate estimates of ALL and ACL. In short, the ZINB model outperforms the other methods because it adequately models the excess of zeros and overdispersion in the data, thus resulting in decreased risk of both false alarms and underdetection of microbial excursions. The superiority of the ZINB model over the other three models is further demonstrated through visual inspection of the estimated density functions of the four models imposed on a histogram of the microbial data, shown in Figure 10.2. The data were simulated from Model 10.14 with parameters $(p, \mu, k) = (0.5, 2.8, 0.04)$.

10.3.6 Holistic Solution

Various models for setting alert and action limits have been discussed. The zero-inflated negative binomial model appears to be particularly advantageous in the presence of excess zeros and overdispersion in the data. Even if the data do not show an excess of zeros or overdispersion, it is expected that the ZINB model provides comparable performance as other methods. However, simple models are easier to estimate and interpret than more complex ones; thus, it is sensible to use simple models when the model assumptions are approximately met. This requires decision rules through which a particular model is chosen for establishing alert and action limits. Figure 10.3

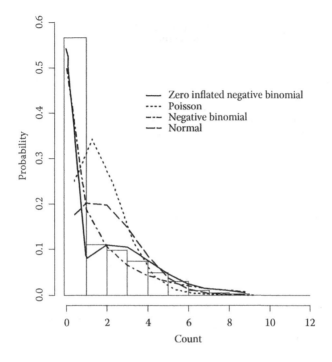

FIGURE 10.2
Plots of estimated density functions of ZINB, normal, negative binomial, and Poisson models against the empirical histogram of the simulated data. (From Yang, H., Zhao, W., O'Day, T., and Fleming, W. (2013b). Environmental monitoring: Setting alert and action limits based on a zero-inflated model. *PDA J. Pharm. Sci. Technol.*, 67(1), 1–9.)

depicts such a procedure for model selection. The decision process begins with evaluation of the fitness of the simplest model, followed by assessments of incrementally more complicated models. As shown in the diagram, data are first tested for normality. For this, either the Shapiro–Wilk test or a normal probability plot can be used. The former tests for deviation from normality through a nonparametric rank test. A P value less than 0.05 is indicative of nonnormality. The latter assesses if the empirical quantiles of the standardized data closely mimic those of the standard normal distribution through visual inspection. If the data pass the normality test, alert and action limits are determined based on mean ± 2SD and 3SD; otherwise, the above test is repeated after the data are log-transformed. In the event that neither the raw data nor the log-transformed data are normally distributed, and if there is no excess of zeros, a Poisson model is fit to the data. A goodness-of-fit test is performed to evaluate if the data follow Poisson distribution or not. The goal is to select the most simplistic and appropriate model to describe the data and set alert and action limits. One should bear in mind that the procedure is only one among many that potentially can be used for model selection.

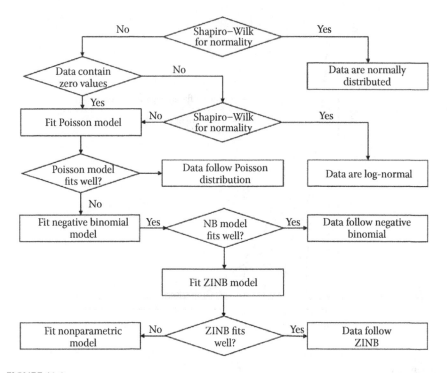

FIGURE 10.3
Procedure used for determining data distribution and appropriate model for estimating alert and action limits. (From Yang, H., Zhao, W., O'Day, T., and Fleming, W. (2013b). Environmental monitoring: Setting alert and action limits based on a zero-inflated model. *PDA J. Pharm. Sci. Technol.*, 67(1), 1–9.)

10.4 Trending EM Data

10.4.1 Univariate Control Chart

Control charts are important and effective graphical tools for monitoring environmental data and evaluating if the manufacturing environment is in a state of control. There are many types of control charts, such as Shewhart individual control charts, also known as individual/moving range (I-MR) control charts. I-MR charts consist of two plots. The first plots individual observations against time or order in which the samples were collected, whereas the second chart displays the moving range defined as the absolute difference between two consecutive measurements. A typical control chart of a quality attribute includes a centerline and lower and upper controls limits, which are usually estimated from historical data collected when the process is in a state of control. However, for microbial data, it is the upper trend that is of concern. Therefore, an appropriate control chart consists of measured observations along with alert and action limits. As microbial recoveries in cleanroom monitoring are rare, Caputo and Huffman (2004) argued that it makes more sense to construct the control charts for the frequency of non-zero observations Φ_i (see Section 10.3.1.2). They suggested the use of both I-MR and exponentially weighted moving average (EWMA) control charts (Montgomery 2009). The latter is presumably more sensitive in detecting small shifts in the microbial data.

10.4.1.1 I-MR Charts

Construction of I-MR charts is relatively straightforward. The underlying assumption is that Φ_i is normally distributed. If the data are skewed, they need to be transformed to approximate normality. For the sake of discussion, we assume $\Phi_i \sim N(\Phi, \sigma^2)$. Thus, the mean and SD of Φ_i can be estimated as

$$\hat{\Phi} = \frac{\sum_{t=1}^{n} \Phi_t}{n}$$

$$\hat{\sigma} = \sqrt{\frac{\sum_{i=1}^{n} (\Phi_i - \hat{\Phi})^2}{n-1}}.$$

Therefore, the alert and action limits can be estimated by

$$\text{Alert limit} = \hat{\Phi} + 2\hat{\sigma}$$

$$\text{Action limit} = \hat{\Phi} + 3\hat{\sigma}. \tag{10.20}$$

The I-MR control chart is obtained by plotting Φ_i against the sample number i, along with the alert and action limits being estimated from Equation 10.20. The chart allows for detection of a shift that is characterized by one or more points above either the alert or action limit.

To set up the MR chart, we first calculate the moving range, $M_i = |\Phi_i - \Phi_{i-1}|$, $i = 1, \ldots, n$. The average of M_i is given below:

$$\bar{M} = \frac{\sum_{t=2}^{n} M_t}{n-1}.$$

Accordingly, the alert and action limits are determined to be

$$d_1 \bar{M}$$

$$d_2 \bar{M}, \tag{10.21}$$

where d_1 and d_2 are constants listed in standard tables (DeVor et al. 1992).

Similarly, the MR control chart is obtained by plotting M_i versus i, with its alert and action limits.

10.4.1.2 EWMA Control Chart

The EWMA control chart was first introduced by Roberts (1959). It is defined as

$$z_i = \lambda x_i + (1 - \lambda)x_{i-1},$$

where z_i, $i = 1, \ldots, n$, is a value calculated as a weighted average of two adjacent observations, x_{i-1} and x_i, and λ is a constant between 0 and 1. The initial value z_0 is defined as either the target value or the average of historical data.

It can be shown that z_i is a weighted average of previous sample means (Montgomery 2009). Because of this property, it is not sensitive to the normality assumption and is thus suitable to use when the underlying distribution of the data is not normal. Assuming that x_i are independent observations, with variance of σ^2, it can be verified that the variance of z_i is

$$\sigma^2 \left(\frac{\lambda}{2 - \lambda} \right)[1 - (1 - \lambda)^{2i}].$$

Thus, the alert and action limits are given by

$$\text{Alert limit} = z_0 + 2\hat{\sigma}\sqrt{\left(\frac{\lambda}{2 - \lambda} \right)[1 - (1 - \lambda)^{2i}]}$$

$$\text{Action limit} = z_0 + 3\hat{\sigma}\sqrt{\left(\frac{\lambda}{2 - \lambda} \right)[1 - (1 - \lambda)^{2i}]}. \tag{10.22}$$

There is no theoretical guidance concerning the choice of the weighting parameter λ. As a rule of thumb, the smaller is the magnitude of the shift to be detected, the smaller λ should be. In practice, λ is typically chosen to be between 0.05 and 0.25 (Montgomery 1991). Through a simulated data set, Caputo and Huffman (2003) demonstrated the utility of the I-MR and EWMA control charts.

10.4.2 Multivariate Control Chart

As previously discussed, for EM, both the frequency of zero observations and the magnitude of nonzero microbial recoveries are important measures to assess if the environment is in a state of control. As they are quality attributes characterizing the same system, estimates or measures of these attributes are correlated.

Although univariate control charts can be used to monitor these two attributes, they do not take into account the correlation between the two quantities. As a result, the univariate control charts may not detect out-of-control data, which will become obvious when the two attributes are evaluated together based on their joint statistical distribution. In addition, if each control chart is established to warrant a Type I error rate of α, the overall Type I error rate of n control charts is $1 - (1 - \alpha)^n$, which is bigger than α. For example, for the bivariate case, assuming $\alpha = 0.05$, the overall Type I error is 0.0975. These potential drawbacks make it necessary to control quality attributes jointly.

Multivariate control charts, originally proposed by Hotelling (1947), and researched and popularized by other authors (Montgomery 2009), provide a way to resolve the above issues. Central to this method is to define the joint distribution of the quality attribute measurements of interest and a quality metric that describes the joint behavior of the above measurements. For example, construction of the Hotelling T^2 control chart relies on the assumption that $\mathbf{X} = (X_1,\ldots,X_n)$ follows a multivariate normal distribution with mean and covariance matrix:

$$\boldsymbol{\mu} = (\mu_1,\ldots,\mu_n)$$

$$\boldsymbol{\Sigma} = \begin{pmatrix} \sigma_1^2 & \cdots & \sigma_{1n} \\ \vdots & \ddots & \vdots \\ \sigma_{1n} & \cdots & \sigma_n^2 \end{pmatrix}.$$

The quality metric is defined as

$$A = (\mathbf{X} - \boldsymbol{\mu})' \boldsymbol{\Sigma}^{-1} (\mathbf{X} - \boldsymbol{\mu}).$$

Because A has a χ^2 distribution with $n - 1$ degrees of freedom, an upper control limit can be obtained as

$$UCL = \chi_{\alpha,n-1}^2, \tag{10.23}$$

where $\chi^2_{\alpha,n-1}$ is the $(1 - \alpha) \times 100$th percentile of the χ^2 distribution with $n - 1$ degrees of freedom.

A multivariate control chart can be set up by plotting the A values of all the samples versus sample number, along with the UCL in Equation 10.23. This control chart is analogous to the univariate Shewhart $\bar{x}$ chart.

10.4.2.1 Bivariate Control Chart

Note that a random variable X has the same mean under either a Poisson or a negative binomial distribution assumption. Consequently, the MLEs $\hat{\theta} = (\hat{p}, \hat{\lambda})$ of $\theta = (p, \lambda)$ are estimates of the frequency of zeros (p) and the mean microbial count (λ). It is well known that $\hat{\theta}$ is asymptotically bivariate normal:

$$\hat{\theta} \sim N(\theta, \mathbf{I}),$$

where I is the Fisher's information matrix defined as

$$\mathbf{I} = \begin{pmatrix} I_{11} & I_{12} \\ I_{12} & I_{22} \end{pmatrix} = \begin{pmatrix} E\left(\dfrac{\partial^2 l}{\partial p^2}\right) & -E\left(\dfrac{\partial^2 l}{\partial p \partial \lambda}\right) \\ -E\left(\dfrac{\partial^2 l}{\partial p \partial \lambda}\right) & E\left(\dfrac{\partial^2 l}{\partial \lambda^2}\right) \end{pmatrix},$$

where l is the log-likelihood function of $\hat{\theta}$.

Define

$$T^2 = (\hat{\theta} - \theta)' \mathbf{I}(\hat{\theta} - \theta).$$

If θ is known, T^2 approximately follows a χ^2 distribution with 2 degrees of freedom. When θ is unknown, in order to construct the bivariate control chart for $\hat{\theta}$, the unknown parameters θ need to be estimated. This is usually accomplished by using historical data collected from the manufacturing environment deemed to be in control. Yang and Zhang (2008) outlined an estimation procedure for this purpose. Assume that the historical data consist of m sets of samples each of size n. Let $\hat{\theta}_1, \ldots, \hat{\theta}_m$ and $\hat{\mathbf{I}}_1, \ldots, \hat{\mathbf{I}}_m$ be the MLEs of θ and the Fisher's information matrix I, respectively. $\hat{\mathbf{I}}_i$ is obtained by replacing θ by $\hat{\theta}_i$. Now, let $\bar{\theta}$ and $\bar{\mathbf{I}}$ be the mean of $\hat{\theta}_i$ and $\hat{\mathbf{I}}_i$:

$$\bar{\theta} = \frac{\sum\limits_{i=1}^{m} \hat{\theta}_i}{m} \quad \text{and}$$

$$\overline{\mathbf{I}} = \frac{\sum\limits_{i=1}^{m} \hat{\mathbf{I}}_i}{m}.$$

The T^2 statistic can then be estimated as

$$\hat{T}^2 = (\hat{\boldsymbol{\theta}} - \overline{\boldsymbol{\theta}})' \overline{\mathbf{I}} (\hat{\boldsymbol{\theta}} - \overline{\boldsymbol{\theta}}). \tag{10.24}$$

The alert and action limits can be chosen to be the 95th and 99th percentiles of the χ_2^2 distribution, respectively. These limits, together with the estimate T^2 values, allow for construction of a bivariate control chart.

10.4.2.2 Example

Under the zero-inflated Poisson distribution, the probability mass function can be given by

$$\Pr(X_i = x) = \begin{cases} p + (1-p)e^{-\lambda} & \text{if } x = 0 \\ (1-p)\dfrac{\lambda^x e^{-\lambda}}{x!} & \text{else.} \end{cases} \tag{10.25}$$

10.4.2.2.1 Maximum Likelihood Estimation

The MLEs of the model parameters in the above model can be obtained through several standard statistical software packages, such as SAS (1998, 2009). They can also be calculated by the following procedure. Consider x is an observed value of X. Without loss of generality, we assume that $x_i = 0$ for $i = 1,\dots, n_1$ and $x_i > 0$ for $i = 1,\dots, n_2$, where $n_2 = n - n_1$. The likelihood function of x_i is

$$L = [p + (1-p)e^{-\lambda}]^{n_1} \prod_{i=n_1+1}^{n} [(1-p)\frac{\lambda^{x_i}}{x!}e^{-\lambda}]$$

$$= [p + (1-p)e^{-\lambda}]^{n_1} (1-p)^{n_2} \frac{\lambda^{\sum x_i}}{\prod\limits_{i=n_1+1}^{n} x_i!} e^{-\lambda n_2}.$$

Thus, the log-likelihood is

$$l = \log(L) = n_1 \log[p + (1-p)e^{-\lambda}] + n_2 \log(1-p)$$

$$+ \sum x_i \log(\lambda) - \lambda n_2 + \sum \log(x_i!).$$

The first-order partial derivatives of l with respect to parameters p and λ are given by

$$\frac{\partial l}{\partial p} = \frac{n_1(1-e^{-\lambda})}{p+(1-p)e^{-\lambda}} - \frac{n_2}{1-p}$$

$$\frac{\partial l}{\partial \lambda} = \frac{-n_1(1-p)e^{-\lambda}}{p+(1-p)e^{-\lambda}} + \frac{\sum x_i}{\lambda} - n_2.$$

Thus, the MLEs of p and λ can be obtained as the solutions to the following equations:

$$\frac{n_1(1-e^{-\lambda})}{p+(1-p)e^{-\lambda}} - \frac{n_2}{1-p} = 0 \text{ and}$$

$$\frac{-n_1(1-p)e^{-\lambda}}{p+(1-p)e^{-\lambda}} + \frac{\sum x_i}{\lambda} - n_2 = 0,$$

or, equivalently,

$$\lambda = \frac{\sum x_i}{n(1-p)} \text{ and}$$

$$e^{-\lambda} = \frac{n_1 - np}{n(1-p)}.$$

The above equations can be solved through an iterative algorithm. Because

$$I_{11} = -E\left(\frac{\partial^2 l}{\partial p^2}\right) = \frac{n_2}{(1-p)^2} - \frac{n_1(1-e^{-\lambda})^2}{[p+(1-p)e^{-\lambda}]^2}$$

$$I_{12} = -E\left(\frac{\partial^2 l}{\partial p \partial \lambda}\right) = -\frac{n_1 e^{-\lambda}}{p+(1-p)e^{-\lambda}}$$

$$I_{22} = -E\left(\frac{\partial^2 l}{\partial \lambda^2}\right) = \frac{n(1-p)}{\lambda} - \frac{n_1(1-p)e^{-\lambda}}{[p+(1-p)e^{-\lambda}]^2}, \tag{10.26}$$

an estimate of the Fisher's information matrix can be obtained by substituting the MLEs $\hat{\theta} = (\hat{p}, \hat{\lambda})$ for $\theta = (p, \lambda)$.

10.4.2.2.2 Simulation Studies

Yang (2012a) carried out several simulation studies to demonstrate the utility of the multivariate control chart. Microbial count samples were assumed to follow the zero-inflated Poisson distribution in Equation 10.25. Three simulation scenarios were used, and are described in Table 10.3.

Scenario 1 with $p = 0.8$ and $\lambda = 2$ corresponds to a case in which the environment is deemed to be in a state of control. The other two scenarios, $p = 0.7$ and $\lambda = 2$ and $p = 0.8$ and $\lambda = 3$, represent out-of-control states, with either lower frequency of zeros than what is expected or mean microbial count larger than what is considered as acceptable.

For each scenario, 5000 data sets, each containing 100 observations from the zero-inflated model Poisson model in Equation 10.25 with parameters specified in Table 10.3, were generated; thus, 5000 MLEs $(\hat{p}_i, \hat{\lambda}_i)$, $i = 1,..., 5000$, of (p, λ) were obtained. Data from the first simulation scenario were used as historical in-control data to set alert and action limits. In addition, they were also used to estimate the true values of (p, λ) and the Fisher's information matrix.

$$\bar{p} = \frac{\sum\limits_{i=1}^{5000} \hat{p}_i}{5000}$$

$$\hat{\lambda} = \frac{\sum\limits_{i=1}^{5000} \hat{\lambda}_i}{5000}$$

$$\bar{I} = \frac{\sum\limits_{i=1}^{5000} \bar{I}_i}{5000}.$$

TABLE 10.3

Simulation Scenarios

Scenario	Frequency of Zeros (p)	Mean Microbial Count (λ)	Environment in Control
1	0.8	2	Yes
2	0.7	2	No
3	0.8	3	No

For each of the 5000 data sets in each of the three scenarios, the Hotelling T^2 statistic in Equation 10.24 was calculated, thus resulting in a total of 5000 T^2 values per scenario. The corresponding control chart was obtained by plotting these estimates against the alert and action limits. The three control charts are shown in Figures 10.4 through 10.6.

As expected, for the in-control data (Figure 10.4), approximately 5% and 1% T^2 values are above the alert and action limits, respectively. For scenario 2, there are 30 T^2 values above the alert limit and 12 T^2 values above the action limit (Figure 10.5). Last, there are 69 T^2 values above the alert limit and 50 T^2 values above the action limit for scenario 3 shown in Figure 10.6.

The results of the simulation demonstrate that the multivariate control chart is an effective tool for detecting microbial excursions due to either increased frequency or magnitude of nonzero observations.

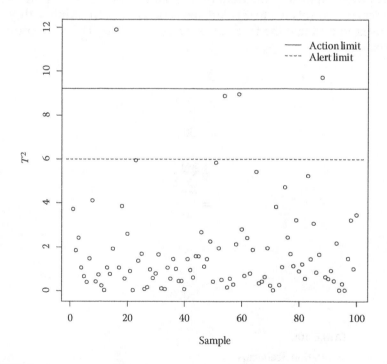

FIGURE 10.4
Plot of T^2 values with $p = 0.8$ and $\lambda = 2$ (in-control data). (From Yang, H. (2012a). Multivariate control chart for environmental monitoring. *J. Validation Technol.*, 18(4), 59–63.)

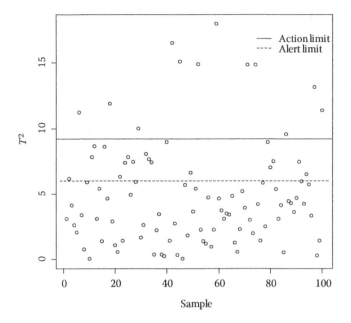

FIGURE 10.5
Plot of T^2 values with $p = 0.7$ and $\lambda = 2$ (out-of-control data). (From Yang, H. (2012a). Multivariate control chart for environmental monitoring. *J. Validation Technol.*, 18(4), 59–63.)

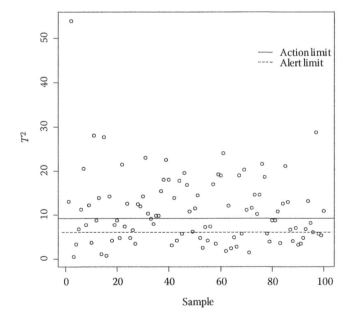

FIGURE 10.6
Plot of T^2 values with $p = 0.8$ and $\lambda = 3$ (out-of-control data). (From Yang, H. (2012a). Multivariate control chart for environmental monitoring. *J. Validation Technol.*, 18(4), 59–63.)

10.5 Concluding Remarks

EM programs, required by regulatory guidance, provide quality oversight for areas and rooms where sterile products are manufactured. Central to these programs is the establishment of alert and action limits. Because the soundness of an EM program depends heavily on the accurate determination of alert and action limits, blind application of traditional techniques, such as those based on a normal distribution, without understanding the distribution of the data may lead to inappropriate alert and action limits, causing high rate of false-positive or false-negative outcomes. Therefore, special care must be taken when selecting models to describe the data and set alert and action limits. Fortunately, the availability of statistical software packages for advanced statistical modeling makes it possible to evaluate competing models based on well-established statistical criteria. Monte Carlo simulation is also a useful tool in aiding model selection.

11

Stability Design and Analysis

11.1 Introduction

Stability of quality attributes may affect a drug product's safety and efficacy over its labeled use period (shelf life). Effective utilization of stability testing plays a critical role throughout the life cycle of a drug product. During early development, well-designed stability studies can help gain a deep understanding of the product's degradation pathways. In late phase development, stability testing provides information regarding how a variety of environmental factors such as temperature, humidity, and light affect the product quality over time. These data are also used to establish the shelf life and storage conditions of the product, in support of regulatory licensure. For marketed products, stability studies can be used to (1) update shelf life or release limit(s), if needed, to warrant product quality through a specified (shortened or extended) period; (2) provide assurance of robustness of the manufacturing process after process changes (including site, scale, formulation, storage, shipping conditions, and delivery device); and (3) aid in the evaluation and removal of non–stability-indicating tests. As the entire pharmaceutical industry is moving toward a risk-based paradigm for process and product development, full utilization of stability studies has become increasingly important not only in increasing product quality assurance but also in minimizing the risk of untoward rejection of good product lots or acceptance of compromised lots.

Stability testing is also a regulatory requirement. Since 1984, when the first stability guideline was issued by the Food and Drug Administration (FDA), several regulatory guidelines related to stability testing of new drug and biological substances and products have been published. The guidance published by the FDA in 1987 provided more specific requirements on statistical design and analysis than the original one (FDA 1987). In an effort to harmonize stability testing in different regions, a series of ICH guidelines have been developed and published since 1993 (ICH 1993, 1995b, 2003a). However, the primary focus of these guidelines is to provide recommendations on how to use stability data to propose a shelf life in a registration application. Little guidance is given to stability study design and analysis at different stages of drug development. In 2002, a working group sponsored by the World Health Organization (WHO) began to address this issue for vaccine stability testing, resulting in the publication of the WHO Guideline *Stability Evaluation of Vaccines* (WHO 2006). For the first time, a life cycle and risk-based approach to stability evaluation was recommended. Although the concept was proposed specifically for vaccines, the principles are applicable to drug and other biological products as well.

In this chapter, we describe various statistical methods used for stability study design and analysis. Specific topics include shelf life estimation and applications of stability study design and analysis to ensure product quality and regulatory compliance.

11.2 Shelf Life Estimation

11.2.1 Definitions

For all marketed pharmaceutical products, regulatory guidelines require that an expiration date or shelf life be determined and indicated on the primary container label. A formal definition of shelf life is given in ICH Q1A (R2) (ICH 2003a). It is defined as "[t]he time period during which a drug product is expected to remain within the approved shelf life specification, provided that it is stored under the conditions defined on the container label." As pointed out by Capen et al. (2012), because of the ambiguity in the term *drug product* in the shelf life definition, different interpretations may lead to different ways of collecting, analyzing, and interpreting stability data. Therefore, it is important to have a clear implementable definition of *shelf life* and *product* among all stakeholders, which would provide a common ground for developing and evaluating statistical methods for shelf life determination.

In 2006, a Stability Shelf Life Working Group under the auspices of the Product Quality Research Institute was formed and tasked with examining existing statistical methods and developing improved procedures. The effort led to a series of publications and presentations (Capen et al. 2012; Quinlan et al. 2013a,b; Stroup and Quinlan 2010). The group proposed new terminology, including *true shelf life, estimated shelf life, supported shelf life, maximum shelf life, labeled shelf life, batch,* and *product shelf life*. According to Capen et al. (2012), the *true shelf life* is the true but unknown limit on the period of storage time during which the pharmaceutical or drug product is considered fit for use and effective. It can also be referred to as the *true product shelf life*. The estimate of the *true shelf life* from stability data is called the *estimated shelf life*. The *supported shelf life* is a conservative estimate of the *true shelf life* that warrants that a large proportion of product is fit for its intended use within the estimated shelf life. The *maximum shelf life* is the maximally allowable shelf life extrapolated from data from real-time stability studies and accelerated and stressed stability testing. The *labeled shelf life* is the most conservative estimate of the *product shelf life* that is printed on the product label. It is no bigger than either the *supported shelf life* or the *maximum shelf life*. As a drug product is manufactured in batches, it is often of interest to understand the stability of a given batch. The *batch shelf life* is a characteristic of a particular batch. The Stability Shelf Life Working Group suggests that "drug product" in the ICH Q1A (R2) (ICH 2003a) is best defined as the entire collection of batches that are either produced or will be produced in the future. Using the above definitions, the group suggested that the true product shelf life be defined as a small quantile of the distribution of batch shelf life estimates. Accordingly, a random-batch model was recommended for calculating the estimated shelf life.

11.2.2 Statistical Models

In this section, several methods proposed in the literature are discussed. We first concentrate on the method recommended in ICH Q1E (2003b), which states "Regression analysis is considered an appropriate approach to evaluating the stability data for a quantitative attribute and establish a retest period or shelf life." It further suggests that at least three batches of the drug product or substance be used for estimating the shelf life. In the following, we assume that a linear model is used for describing the relationship between the stability attribute y_{ij} and time x_{ij}, $i = 1,\ldots,n; j = 1,\ldots,m$:

$$y_{ij} = \alpha + a_i + (\beta + b_i)x_{ij} + \varepsilon_{ij}, \tag{11.1}$$

where α and β are the intercept and slope parameters; a_i and b_i are deviations of the ith batch from the common intercept and slope, respectively; and ε_{ij} are measurement errors that are assumed to be independently and identically distributed (*iid*) according to a normal distribution $N(0, \sigma^2)$.

In ICH Q1E, the batch effect is considered as fixed. Depending on the outcome of batch poolability tests intended to test the hypotheses $a_i = 0$ and $b_i = 0$, each at a significance level of 0.25, shelf life is determined using one of the four regression models:

1. $y_{ij} = \alpha + \beta x_{ij} + \varepsilon_{ij}$ for common intercept and slope.
2. $y_{ij} = \alpha + (\beta + b_i)x_{ij} + \varepsilon_{ij}$ for common intercept but different slopes.
3. $y_{ij} = \alpha + a_i + \beta x_{ij} + \varepsilon_{ij}$ for different intercepts but common slope.
4. $y_{ij} = \alpha + a_i + (\beta + b_i)x_{ij} + \varepsilon_{ij}$ for different intercepts and common slope.

11.2.3 Estimation Methods

Without loss of generality, we assume that the stability attribute degrades over time, so $\beta < 0$. Let η be the lower specification limit. When the batch data can be pooled, per ICH Q1E, the labeled shelf life $\hat{\tau}_L$ is determined to be the time at which the lower 95% confidence limit $L(x)$ for the predicted mean response at time x based on the pooled model (1) intersects the lower specification limit η. Mathematically,

$$\hat{\tau}_L = \inf\{x \geq 0 : L(x) \leq \eta\},$$

where inf represents the infimum or the greatest lower bound. When the batches are not poolable, the labeled shelf life $\hat{\tau}_L$ is estimated by

$$\hat{\tau}_L = \min_{\{1 \leq i \leq n_b\}} \{\hat{\tau}_i : \hat{\tau}_i = \inf\{x \geq 0 : L_i(x) \leq \eta\}\},$$

where $L_i(x)$ is the lower limit of the 95% confidence interval for the predicted mean response of the ith batch ($i = 1,\ldots,n_b$) at time x, based on one of the above models with different slopes and intercepts.

One criticism of the ICH Q1E confidence interval method is that it provides quality assurance for the mean of all units in a batch as opposed to individual units. As a result, it may not provide adequate protection to the consumer risk (Kiermeier et al. 2004; Yang and Zhang 2012b). Since a prediction interval is used to predict the behavior of a single observation, it is naturally proposed as an alternative method (Cartensen and Nelson 1976). As pointed out by Yang and Zhang (2012b), while the prediction interval is more conservative than the confidence interval, it may not adequately address quality assurance of all units from the batch. The point can be made through the following example. Suppose that m units are randomly chosen from the batch at the end of the labeled shelf life, which was determined based on a one-sided 95% prediction interval. It can be easily verified that the probability of at least one of the m units being out of specification is $1 - (0.95)^m$, which exceeds 22% for $m \geq 5$. This may well represent an unacceptable level of consumer risk. To offset the issue, Kiermeier et al. (2004) and Komka et al. (2010) proposed to use a tolerance interval (TI) approach to shelf life estimation, with the goal of determining a shelf life that renders assurance that a high percentage of the units in a batch will be in specification. The quality assurance that a shelf life calculated in this way provides to all units in the batch is characterized by two quantities ς and $1 - \gamma$, where ς represents the percentage of units meeting the quality standard (e.g., potency being above the lower specification limit at any point before the expiration dating) and $1 - \gamma$ is the confidence level. The shelf life based on the one-sided ($\varsigma, 1 - \gamma$) tolerance interval is estimated as the time point at which the lower limit intersects the approved lower specification limit.

However, both the prediction and tolerance interval approaches are oriented toward providing assurance for consumers, while neither takes into account the producer risk. In addition, because of the lack of a common framework, it is difficult to compare these three intervals, in terms of risk and benefit. Yang and Zhang (2012b) proposed a unified risk-based approach for evaluating these three shelf life estimation methods, which relies on the demonstration that both confidence and prediction intervals can be expressed as tolerance intervals with either the same content or level of confidence. Using a realistically simulated example, they showed that although conceptually appealing, application of 95% predication and 95%/95% tolerance interval approaches may not render a reasonable balance between the consumer and producer risks. To simplify the discussion, it is assumed that lots used in the statistical analysis are poolable and the following simple regression model is used for shelf life determination:

$$y_{ij} = \alpha + \beta + x_{ij} + \varepsilon_{ij}. \tag{11.2}$$

Let $(\hat{\alpha}, \hat{\beta}, \hat{\sigma}^2)$ be the least square estimators of $(\alpha, \beta, \sigma^2)$ based on Model 11.2. The following definitions of estimated shelf life based on the confidence interval (CI), prediction interval (PI), and tolerance interval (TI) can be introduced.

11.2.3.1 Confidence Interval Method

Note that the one-sided 95% lower confidence limit for the mean value of y at time x, $\alpha + \beta x$, is given by

$$\hat{\alpha} + \hat{\beta}x - \hat{\sigma} t_{0.05, n-2} \sqrt{\left[\frac{1}{n} + \frac{(x - \bar{x})^2}{S_{xx}} \right]},$$

where $t_{0.05, n-2}$ is the 95th percentile of the t distribution with $n - 2$ degrees of freedom, and

$$\bar{x} = \frac{1}{n} \sum_{i=1}^{n} x_i \text{ and } S_{xx} = \sum_{i=1}^{n} (x_i - \bar{x})^2.$$

The estimated shelf life $\hat{\theta}_{CL}$, defined as the time at which the above one-sided 95% lower confidence limit intersects the lower specification limit, is the smaller value of the two solutions of the following equation per ICH Q1E:

$$\eta = \hat{\alpha} + \hat{\beta}x - \hat{\sigma} t_{0.05, n-2} \sqrt{\left[\frac{1}{n} + \frac{(x - \bar{x})^2}{S_{xx}} \right]}. \tag{11.3}$$

11.2.3.2 Prediction Interval Method

The shelf life $\hat{\theta}_{PL}$ based on a prediction interval is defined as the time point at which the lower limit of the one-sided 95% prediction interval for an individual observation y_{ij} intersects the lower specification limit. Therefore, it is the smaller solution to the equation

$$\eta = \hat{\alpha} + \hat{\beta}x - \hat{\sigma}\, t_{0.05,n-2}\sqrt{1 + \left[\frac{1}{n} + \frac{(x-\bar{x})^2}{S_{xx}}\right]}. \tag{11.4}$$

11.2.3.3 Tolerance Interval Method

Let $y^* = \alpha + \beta x + \varepsilon$ be the potency of a unit randomly selected from the batch at time x, described through Model 11.1. Hence, $y^* \sim N\,(\alpha + \beta x, \sigma^2)$. The lower limit of a tolerance for y^*, $g(x,\hat{\omega})$, with content ς and confidence level $1-\gamma$, with $\hat{\omega} = (\hat{\alpha}, \hat{\beta}, \hat{\sigma}^2)$, is defined as

$$P_\omega[P(y^* > g(x,\hat{\omega})\,|\,\hat{\omega}) \geq \varsigma] = 1 - \gamma. \tag{11.5}$$

The shelf life $\hat{\theta}_{TL}$ based on the TI approach is defined to be the time point at which the lower $(\varsigma, 1-\gamma)$ tolerance limit $g(x,\hat{\omega})$ intersects the lower specification limit η. That is,

$$g(x,\hat{\omega}) = \eta.$$

Two methods for determining $g(x,\hat{\omega})$ are developed. One method makes use of the generalized confidence interval (Weerahandi 1993), and the other provides a closed-form expression for $g(x,\hat{\omega})$. Details are provided in Sections 11.2.5 and 11.2.6.

11.2.4 Relationships among Three Methods

In this section, we demonstrate that the confidence limit (CL) and prediction limit (PL) discussed in the previous section can each be expressed as a tolerance limit (TL). As a result, both CL and PL contain a certain proportion of observations with certain levels of confidence. Theoretical results concerning the coverage and content of the CL and PL are derived. Theorem 11.1 shows that a PL can be expressed as a CL, which, in turn, can be expressed as a TL as shown in Theorem 11.2.

Let

$$PL(\tau) = \hat{\alpha} + \hat{\beta}x - \hat{\sigma}\, t_{n-2}(\tau)\sqrt{1 + \left[\frac{1}{n} + \frac{(x-\bar{x})^2}{S_{xx}}\right]}$$

and

$$CL(\tau) = \hat{\alpha} + \hat{\beta}x - \hat{\sigma}\, t_{n-2}(\tau)\sqrt{\left[\frac{1}{n} + \frac{(x-\bar{x})^2}{S_{xx}}\right]} \tag{11.6}$$

be the lower limit of one-sided $(1-\tau)100\%$ prediction interval of a future observation and the lower limit of one-sided $(1-\tau)100\%$ confidence interval of the mean observed value $\alpha + \beta\, x$, respectively. Here, the function $t_{n-2}(\tau)$ of τ is defined as

$$t_{n-2}(\tau) = t_{\tau,n-2}$$

to facilitate the development of the theoretical results described below.

Theorem 11.1: Relationship between CL and PL

There exists a $\tau_0 < \tau$ such that $PL(\tau) = CL(\tau_0)$, where τ_0 is the unique solution of the equation

$$t_{\tau_0,n-2} = t_{\tau,n-2}\sqrt{1 + \left[\frac{1}{n} + \frac{(x-\bar{x})^2}{S_{xx}}\right]}\Bigg/ \sqrt{\left[\frac{1}{n} + \frac{(x-\bar{x})^2}{S_{xx}}\right]}. \tag{11.7}$$

In other words, $PL(\tau)$ is the lower one-sided $(1-\tau_0)100\%$ confidence limit of $\alpha + \beta\, x$. ∎

Proof

The proof can be completed through the following simple algebraic manipulations:

$$PL(\tau) = \hat{\alpha} + \hat{\beta}x - \hat{\sigma}\, t_{n-2}(\tau)\sqrt{1 + \left[\frac{1}{n} + \frac{(x-\bar{x})^2}{S_{xx}}\right]} = \hat{\alpha} + \hat{\beta}x - \hat{\sigma}\Omega\sqrt{\left[\frac{1}{n} + \frac{(x-\bar{x})2}{Sxx}\right]},$$

where $\Omega = t_{n-2}(\tau)\sqrt{1 + \left[\frac{1}{n} + \frac{(x-\bar{x})^2}{S_{xx}}\right]}\Bigg/ \sqrt{\left[\frac{1}{n} + \frac{(x-\bar{x})^2}{S_{xx}}\right]}.$

Because $t_{n-2}(\varsigma)$ is a strictly monotonic continuous function varying over $(0, 1)$ such that $t_{n-2}(0) = -\infty$ and $t_{n-2}(1) = \infty$, by the Intermediate Value Theorem, there exists a unique $\tau_0 \in (0, 1)$ such that $t_{n-2}(\tau_0) = \Omega$. Hence,

$$PL(\tau) = \hat{\alpha} + \hat{\beta}x - \hat{\sigma}\, t_{n-2}(\tau_0)\sqrt{\left[\frac{1}{n} + \frac{(x-\bar{x})^2}{S_{xx}}\right]} = CL(\tau_0).$$

Because $t_{n-2}(\tau_0) = \Omega > t_{n-2}(\tau)$, it can be inferred that $\tau_0 < \tau$. Consequently, the PL of an observation at time x can also be thought of as a CL of the mean observation at the same time point x, but with higher level of confidence.

Theorem 11.2: Relationship between CL and TL

For a given τ and γ satisfying $0 < \tau < 1$ and $0 < \gamma < 1$, there exists ς_0 such that $CL(\tau)$ is a $(\varsigma_0, 1-\gamma)$ lower tolerance limit of $y^* = \alpha + \beta x + \varepsilon$, with $\varepsilon \sim N(0, \sigma^2)$, where ς_0 is the unique solution of the following equation for a given γ,

$$P\left(\left[Z\Delta_{CL} - \sqrt{U}\,\frac{t_{n-2}(\tau)\Delta_{CL}}{\sqrt{n-2}}\right) \le z_\varsigma\right] = 1 - \gamma \tag{11.8}$$

where $\Delta_{CL} = \sqrt{\left[\dfrac{1}{n} + \dfrac{(x-\bar{x})^2}{S_{xx}}\right]}$, $U \sim \chi^2_{n-2}$, $Z \sim N(0, 1)$ *and* z_ς *is the upper 100ςth percentile of a standard normal distribution. For a given τ and ς satisfying $0 < \tau, \varsigma < 1$, there exists γ_0 such that $CL(\tau)$ is a $(\varsigma, 1-\gamma_0)$ lower tolerance limit of $y^* = \alpha + \beta x + \varepsilon$, with γ_0 being the unique solution of Equation 11.8.* ∎

Proof

Substituting $CL(\tau)$ for $g(x, \hat{\omega})$ in $P_{\hat{\omega}}[P(y^* > g(x, \hat{\omega})|\hat{\omega}) \ge \varsigma] = 1 - \gamma$,

$$P_{\hat{\omega}}\left(P\left[y^* > \hat{\alpha} + \hat{\beta}x - \hat{\sigma}\,t_{n-2}(\tau)\sqrt{\left[\frac{1}{n} + \frac{(x-\bar{x})^2}{S_{xx}}\right]}\,\Big|\,\hat{\omega}\right] \ge \varsigma\right) = 1 - \gamma$$

$$\Leftrightarrow P_{\hat{\omega}}\left(P\left[\frac{y^* - (\alpha + \beta x)}{\sigma} > \frac{(\hat{\alpha} + \hat{\beta}x) - (\alpha + \beta x)}{\sigma} - \frac{\hat{\sigma}}{\sigma}t_{n-2}(\tau)\Delta_{CL})\,|\,\hat{\omega}\right] \ge \varsigma\right) = 1 - \gamma$$

$$\Leftrightarrow P_{\hat{\omega}}\left(\left[\frac{(\hat{\alpha} + \hat{\beta}x) - (\alpha + \beta x)}{\sigma} - \frac{\hat{\sigma}}{\sigma}t_{n-2}(\tau)\Delta_{CL})\right] \le z_\varsigma\right) = 1 - \gamma$$

$$\Leftrightarrow P_{\hat{\omega}}\left(\left[\frac{(\hat{\alpha} + \hat{\beta}x) - (\alpha + \beta x)}{\sigma\Delta_{CL}}\Delta_{CL} - \sqrt{\frac{(n-2)\hat{\sigma}^2}{\sigma^2}}\,\frac{t_{n-2}(\tau)\Delta_{CL}}{\sqrt{n-2}})\right] \le z_\varsigma\right) = 1 - \gamma$$

$$\Leftrightarrow P\left(\left[Z\Delta_{CL} - \sqrt{U}\,\frac{t_{n-2}(\tau)\Delta_{CL}}{\sqrt{n-2}})\right] \le z_\varsigma\right) = 1 - \gamma,$$

where we used the fact that both $\dfrac{y^* - (\alpha + \beta x)}{\sigma}$ and $Z = \dfrac{(\hat{\alpha} + \hat{\beta}x) - (\alpha + \beta x)}{\sigma \Delta_{CL}}$

follow the standard normal distribution, and $U = \dfrac{(n-2)\hat{\sigma}^2}{\sigma^2}$ is a random variable having a χ^2 distribution with df $= n - 2$.

Define $f(\tau, \varsigma) = P\left(\left[Z\Delta_{CL} - \sqrt{U}\,\dfrac{t_{n-2}(\tau)\Delta_{CL}}{\sqrt{n-2}})\right] \leq z_\varsigma\right)$. $f(\tau, \varsigma)$ is a strictly monotonic continuous function satisfying $f(\tau, 0) = 0$ and $f(\tau, 1) = 1$. Therefore, for fixed values of τ and γ such that $0 < \tau < 1$ and $0 < \gamma < 1$, there exists ς_0 such that

$$f(\tau, \varsigma_0) = 1 - \gamma.$$

This is equivalent to

$$P\left(\left[Z\Delta_{CL} - \sqrt{U}\,\frac{t_{n-2}(\tau)\Delta_{CL}}{\sqrt{n-2}})\right] \leq z_{\varsigma_0}\right) = 1 - \gamma.$$

Therefore, the first half of the theorem holds. The second half of the theorem can be similarly verified.

In practice, given a confidence level $1 - \tau$, either the content ς_0 or the confidence level $1 - \gamma_0$ in Theorem 11.2 can be determined, using the following method. We let

$$W = Z\Delta_{CL} - \sqrt{U}\,\frac{t_{n-2}(\tau)\Delta_{CL}}{\sqrt{n-2}}.$$

The cdf of W is

$$P(W \leq w) = \int_0^\infty \int_{-\infty}^{\frac{w}{\Delta_{CL}} + \sqrt{u}\frac{t_{n-2}(\tau)}{\sqrt{n-2}}} \varphi(z)g(u)\,dz\,du$$

$$= \int_0^\infty \Phi\left(\frac{w}{\Delta_{CL}} + \sqrt{u}\,\frac{t_{n-2}(\tau)}{\sqrt{n-2}}\right)g(u)\,du,$$

where $\varphi(.)$ and $\Phi(.)$ are the pdf and cdf of standard normal distribution, respectively, and $g(.)$ is the pdf of a χ^2 distribution with $n - 2$ degrees of freedom.

Let Q_γ denote the $100(1 - \gamma)$th percentile of distribution of W, that is,

$$P(W \leq Q\gamma) = 1 - \gamma.$$

From Equation 11.8, we have

$$z_\varsigma = Q_\gamma,$$

which implies

$$\varsigma = 1 - \Phi(Q_\gamma).$$

Therefore, the content ς can be derived from the $100(1 - \gamma)$th percentile of distribution of W, which can be obtained through either numerical integration or empirical estimation obtained by taking a large sample from the distribution of W. We have the following corollaries to Theorem 11.1 and Theorem 11.2, respectively.

Corollary to Theorem 11.1: Content Covered by CL

For a given τ such that $0 < \tau < 1$, $CL(\tau)$ is a $(50\%, 1 - \tau)$ lower tolerance limit of $y^* = \alpha + \beta x + \varepsilon$, with $\varepsilon \sim N(0, \sigma^2)$. ∎

Proof

When $\tau = \gamma$, from Equation 11.8, the content ς satisfies

$$P\left(\left[Z\Delta_{CL} - \sqrt{U}\,\frac{t_{n-2}(\tau)\Delta_{CL}}{\sqrt{n-2}}\right) \leq z_\varsigma\right) = 1 - \tau.$$

Note that

$$P\left(\left[Z\Delta_{CL} - \sqrt{U}\,\frac{t_{n-2}(\tau)\Delta_{CL}}{\sqrt{n-2}}\right) \leq z_{0.5}\right) = P\left(\left[Z\Delta_{CL} - \sqrt{U}\,\frac{t_{n-2}(\tau)\Delta_{CL}}{\sqrt{n-2}}\right) \leq 0\right)$$

$$= P\left(\left[\frac{Z}{\sqrt{\frac{U}{\sqrt{n-2}}}}\right] \leq t_{n-2}(\tau)\right) = 1 - \tau. \tag{11.9}$$

Because the function $P\left(\left[Z\Delta_{CL} - \sqrt{U}\,\frac{t_{n-2}(\tau)\Delta_{CL}}{\sqrt{n-2}}\right) \leq z_\varsigma\right)$ is strictly monotonically increasing with respect to ς, Equation 11.9 implies that $z_\varsigma = 0$; thus, $\varsigma = 0.5$.

The corollary indicates that the one-sided confidence interval $CL(\tau)$ is a one-sided tolerance interval that has 50% content with the same level of confidence. The following corollary quantifies the content of a one-sided prediction interval when viewed as a one-sided tolerance interval.

Corollary to Theorem 11.2: Content Covered by PL

For a given τ *such that* $0 < \tau < 1$, $PL(\tau)$ *is a* $(\varsigma_0, 1-\tau)$ *lower tolerance limit of* $y^* = \alpha + \beta x + \varepsilon$, *with* $\varepsilon \sim N(0, \sigma^2)$, *such that* ς_0 *is greater than or equal to 50% and a unique solution to*

$$\int_0^\infty \Phi\left(\left[\frac{z_\varsigma}{\Delta_{CL}} + \sqrt{u}\,\frac{t_{n-2}(\tau)}{\sqrt{n-2}}\sqrt{1+\frac{1}{\Delta_{CL}^2}}\right]\right)g(u)\,du = 1-\tau \tag{11.10}$$

where Φ, z_ς, *and* $g(u)$ *are the cdf of the standard normal distribution, the* (100ς)*th percentile of the standard normal distribution, and the density function of a* χ^2 *distribution with* $df = n-2$, *respectively.* ∎

Proof

Replacing $g(x, \hat{\omega})$ in Equation 11.5 by $PL(\tau)$, we obtain

$$P_{\hat{\omega}}\left(P\left[y^* > \hat{\alpha} + \hat{\beta}x - \hat{\sigma}t_{n-2}(\tau)\sqrt{1+\frac{1}{n}+\frac{(x-\bar{x})^2}{S_{xx}}}\,\Big|\,\hat{\omega}\right] \geq \varsigma\right) = 1-\tau.$$

The above equality can be rewritten as

$$P\left(\left[Z\Delta_{CL} - \sqrt{u}\,\frac{t_{n-2}(\tau)\sqrt{1+\Delta_{CL}^2}}{\sqrt{n-2}}\right) \leq z_\varsigma\right] = 1-\tau$$

$$\Leftrightarrow P\left(\left[Z \leq \frac{z_\varsigma}{\Delta_{CL}^2} + \sqrt{u}\,\frac{t_{n-2}(\tau)\sqrt{1+1/\Delta_{CL}^2}}{\sqrt{n-2}}\right)\right] = 1-\tau$$

$$\Leftrightarrow E\left\langle P\left(\left[Z \leq \frac{z_\varsigma}{\Delta_{CL}} + \sqrt{u}\,\frac{t_{n-2}(\tau)}{\sqrt{n-2}}\sqrt{1+\frac{1}{\Delta_{CL}^2}}\,\Big|u\right]\right)\right\rangle = 1-\tau$$

$$\Leftrightarrow E\left\langle \Phi\left(\left[\frac{z_\varsigma}{\Delta_{CL}} + \sqrt{u}\,\frac{t_{n-2}(\tau)}{\sqrt{n-2}}\sqrt{1+\frac{1}{\Delta_{CL}^2}}\right]\right)\right\rangle = 1-\tau$$

$$\Leftrightarrow \int_0^\infty \Phi\left(\left[\frac{z_\varsigma}{\Delta_{CL}} + \sqrt{u}\,\frac{t_{n-2}(\tau)}{\sqrt{n-2}}\sqrt{1+\frac{1}{\Delta_{CL}^2}}\right]\right)g(u)\,du = 1-\tau.$$

Let $g(\varsigma) = \int_0^\infty \Phi\left(\left[\frac{z_\varsigma}{\Delta_{CL}} + \sqrt{u}\,\frac{t_{n-2}(\tau)}{\sqrt{n-2}}\sqrt{1+\frac{1}{\Delta_{CL}^2}}\right]\right)g(u)\,du$. It can be verified that $g(\varsigma)$ is continuous and strictly monotonic over $[0, 1]$, with $g(0) = 0$ and $g(1) = 1$.

By the Intermediate Value Theorem, there exists ς_0 such that $g(\varsigma_0) = 1-\tau$, where $0 < 1-\tau < 1$. In addition, the claim that $\varsigma_0 \geq 50\%$ can be proved by contradiction. Suppose that $\varsigma_0 < 50\%$. Then, $z_{\varsigma_0} > z_{0.5} = 0$. Note that

$$\left((Z,U) : \left[Z\Delta_{CL} - \sqrt{U}\,\frac{t_{n-2}(\tau)\Delta_{CL}}{\sqrt{n-2}} \right) \leq z_{0.5} \right)$$

$$\subset \left((Z,U) : \left[Z\Delta_{CL} - \sqrt{U}\,\frac{t_{n-2}(\tau)\sqrt{1+\Delta_{CL}^2}}{\sqrt{n-2}} \right) \leq z_{\varsigma_0} \right).$$

It becomes evident that

$$1-\tau = P\left(\left[Z\Delta_{CL} - \sqrt{U}\,\frac{t_{n-2}(\tau)\sqrt{1+\Delta_{CL}^2}}{\sqrt{n-2}} \right) \leq z_{\varsigma} \right)$$

$$< 1-\tau = P\left(\left[Z\Delta_{CL} - \sqrt{U}\,\frac{t_{n-2}(\tau)\sqrt{1+\Delta_{CL}^2}}{\sqrt{n-2}} \right) \leq z_{\varsigma} \right) = 1-\tau,$$

which is a contradiction. Therefore, it can be concluded that ς_0 has to be no smaller than 50%.

The results in Theorems 11.1 and 11.2 show that the CL, PL, and TL can be interpreted interchangeably and converted to one another. Therefore, they can all be interpreted in the same context of coverage for the mean, a single observation, or content. The result in Corollary 11.1 shows that a $(1-\tau)$ 100% one-sided confidence limit always has 50% content with the same level of confidence; Corollary 2 indicates that a PL has content greater than or equal to that of a CL. It is of interest to establish an upper bound for the content of a PL. Since content ς in Equation 11.10 is an implicit function of the quantity $\Delta_{CL} = \sqrt{\left[\dfrac{1}{n} + \dfrac{(x-\bar{x})^2}{S_{xx}} \right]}$, we empirically explore the relationship by calculating ς for a wide range of values of Δ_{CL} (which is bounded by $1/\sqrt{n}$, with n being the sample size of the stability study). The results for $n = 21$ are displayed in Figure 11.1. It appears that ς is monotonically decreasing with respect to Δ_{CL} and achieves its maximum at $1/\sqrt{n}$. If a stability study is conducted using the stability design suggested in ICH guidelines, with $x_i = 0, 3, 6, 9, 12, 18,$ and 24 months, and three replicates at each x_i, this upper bound of the content covered by the 95% PI is estimated to be 88%. Thus, the shelf life estimated based on the PI method might not provide enough quality assurance to all units in the batch.

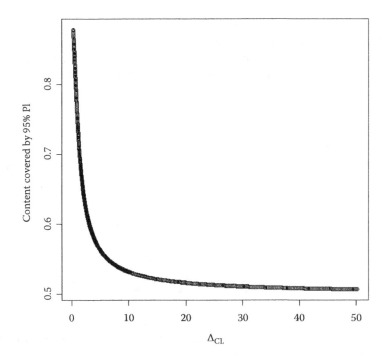

FIGURE 11.1
Relationship between content of a PI (ς) and Δ_{CL}.

11.2.5 Generalized Confidence Interval Approach to Tolerance Interval

The application of the tolerance interval method to estimate shelf life requires calculation of the tolerance limit $g(x, \hat{\omega})$ in Equation 11.5. For a given x, let $h(\hat{\omega}, t; x)$ be a $(1-\gamma)100\%$ lower confidence limit for $P(y^* > t)$ That is,

$$P_{\hat{\omega}}[P(y^* > t) \geq h(\hat{\omega}, t; x)] = 1 - \gamma.$$

If we solve the equation

$$h(\hat{\omega}, t; x) = \varsigma, \tag{11.11}$$

then the solution $t = g(x, \hat{\omega})$ satisfies Equation 11.5 and is a (ς, $1-\gamma$) lower tolerance limit for y^*.
Because

$$h(\hat{\omega}, -\infty; x) = 1 \text{ and } h(\hat{\omega}, \infty; x) = 0,$$

and $h(\hat{\omega}, t; x)$ is monotonically increasing with t, by the Intermediate Value Theorem (Silverman 1989), the solution to Equation 11.11 exists and is unique. A method based on the generalized confidence interval approach (Weerahandi 1993) to determine $h(\hat{\omega}, t; x)$ is presented below.

Let $Y = (Y_1, \ldots, Y_n)$ be random observations at time point x_i, $i = 1, \ldots, n$, and $y = (y_1, \ldots, y_n)$ be observed values of Y. It can be readily seen that

$$P(y^* > t) = \Phi\left(\frac{\alpha + \beta x - t}{\sigma}\right). \tag{11.12}$$

A generalized pivotal quantity (GPQ) of $P(y^* > t)$ in Equation 11.12 is given by

$$\Phi\left(\frac{\hat{\alpha} + \hat{\beta} x - t}{\sigma \hat{\sigma}_{yy}/\sigma_{YY}} - \frac{\hat{A} + \hat{B} x - t - (\alpha + \beta x - t)}{\sigma}\right)$$

$$= \Phi\left(\frac{\hat{\alpha} + \hat{\beta} x - t}{\sigma \hat{\sigma}_{yy}\sqrt{n-2/U}} - Z\sqrt{\frac{1}{n} + \frac{(x-x)^2}{S_{xx}}}\right) \equiv h(U, Z)$$

where $(\hat{\alpha}, \hat{\beta}, \hat{\sigma}_{yy})$ and $(\hat{A}, \hat{B}, \hat{\sigma}_{YY})$ are least square estimators of (α, β, σ), based on $(y_1, \ldots, y_n)$ and $(Y_1, \ldots, Y_n)$, respectively, and

$$U = \frac{(n-2)\hat{\sigma}_{YY}^2}{\sigma^2} \sim \chi_{n-2}^2, \quad Z = \frac{\hat{A} + \hat{B} x - t - (\alpha + \beta x - t)}{\sigma\sqrt{\frac{1}{n} + \frac{(x-\bar{x})^2}{S_{xx}}}} \sim N(0, 1).$$

Then, $h(U, Z)$ is free of parameters. When the random vector $Y = (Y_1, \ldots, Y_n)$ is replaced by its observed value $y = (y_1, \ldots, y_n)$, $h(U, Z)$ is equal to $P(y^* > t)$. Therefore, it satisfies the requirements for being a GPQ for $P(y^* > t)$ (see Weerahandi 1993), and a one-sided lower $(1-\gamma)100\%$ confidence limit for $P(y^* > t)$ is given by (h_γ, ∞), where h_γ is the γ100th percentile of the distribution of $h(U, Z)$. This percentile h_γ can be estimated through the following Monte Carlo algorithm: (1) Simulate U and Z m times from their respective distributions, to generate (u_i, z_i), $i = 1, \ldots, m$. (2) Rank the values $h(u_i, z_i)$ and denote them as $h^{(1)}, \ldots, h^{(m)}$. (3) Determine the γ100th percentile of the ranked values, which is an estimate of h_γ. Refer to Zhang et al. (2010) for further details.

11.2.6 Interpretation of Shelf Life Estimates

In Section 11.2.4, the relationships among the confidence, prediction, and tolerance intervals was established. These enable comparison of the three interval approaches in terms of either their content at some fixed confidence level or confidence level for a given content. In this section, we show that the shelf life estimates based on the three interval methods are lower confidence limits of the theoretical mean shelf life $\theta = \dfrac{\eta - \alpha}{\beta}$ with varying confidence levels. We continue to use $\hat{\theta}_{CL}$, $\hat{\theta}_{PL}$, and $\hat{\theta}_{TL}$ to denote the shelf life estimates, based on confidence, prediction, and tolerance intervals, respectively. The relationships among these three shelf life estimates are summarized in Theorem 11.3.

Theorem 11.3

Assume that the shelf life estimates $\hat{\theta}_{CL}$, $\hat{\theta}_{PL}$, and $\hat{\theta}_{TL}$ are obtained based on $(1-\alpha) \times 100\%$ confidence interval, a $(1-\alpha) \times 100\%$ prediction interval, and tolerance interval that has ς content with $(1-\alpha) \times 100\%$ confidence, respectively. Under this assumption, $\hat{\theta}_{CL}$, $\hat{\theta}_{PL}$, and $\hat{\theta}_{TL}$ are the lower confidence limits of the mean shelf life θ at confidence levels of $(1-\alpha) \times 100\%$, $(1-\tau_0) \times 100\%$ and $(1-\tau_1) \times 100\%$, respectively, where τ_0 is a solution of Equation 11.7 and τ_1 is a solution of Equation 11.8 with $(\tau, \varsigma, \gamma)$ in Equation 11.8 being replaced by (α, τ_1, α). ∎

Proof

The proof that $\hat{\theta}_{CL}$ is a lower $(1-\alpha) \times 100\%$ confidence limit of θ was given by Shao and Chow (2001) and is described briefly below:

Let $CL(x) = \hat{\alpha} + \hat{\beta}x - \hat{\sigma} t_{n-2}(\alpha) \sqrt{\left[\dfrac{1}{n} + \dfrac{(x-\bar{x})^2}{S_{xx}} \right]}$ be the $(1-\alpha) \times 100\%$ confi-

dence limit of $\alpha + \beta x$. Thus, $\hat{\theta}_{CL} = \inf\{x \geq 0 : CL(x) \leq \eta\}$. By definition, $\hat{\theta}_{CL} > \theta$ implies $\eta = CL(\hat{\theta}_{CL}) < CL(\theta)$, where $CL(\theta)$ is the lower $(1-\alpha) \times 100\%$ confidence limit of $\alpha + \beta\theta = \eta$. Consequently,

$$P[\hat{\theta}_{CL} > \theta] \leq P[\eta < CL(\theta)] = \alpha.$$

Therefore, $P[\hat{\theta}_{CL} \geq \theta] \geq 1 - \alpha$. In other words, $\hat{\theta}_{CL}$ is the lower $(1-\alpha) \times 100\%$ confidence limit of the mean shelf life θ. Following the above steps and using Theorems 11.1 and 11.2, the remainder of the theorem can be easily verified.

One immediate benefit of the above theorem is that the performance of the three shelf life estimates can be quantified through their coverage probabilities for the theoretical mean shelf life θ.

11.2.7 Shelf Life Estimation Method Comparisons

In the previous sections, a unified perspective of shelf life estimation based on confidence, prediction, and tolerance intervals was developed. As a result, confidence and prediction approaches can both be perceived as tolerance interval methods. The shelf life estimates from each method provides a certain level of assurance regarding units in the batch, in terms of the percentage of units that remain within specification with a certain level of statistical confidence during the shelf life of the product. In this section, through simulation, we quantify the level of quality assurance provided by the shelf life estimates, based on the ICH Q1E recommended one-sided 95% CI method and one-sided 95% prediction interval. We also evaluate the impact of degradation rate and assay variability on the level of quality assurance provided by the CI and PI methods. As discussed in Section 11.1, the quality assurance that a shelf life estimate provides to the units is characterized by two quantities ς and $1-\gamma$, where ς represents the percentage of units with potency greater than the lower specification limit before the expiration date, and $1-\gamma$ is the confidence level. Since the CI and PI can be perceived as tolerance intervals either having the same content with different levels of confidence or having different contents with the same level of confidence, a comparison between the two methods is feasible. A second simulation study was also conducted to evaluate the risks and benefits of using one interval approach versus the other.

11.2.7.1 Simulation Study I

Data were simulated from Model 11.2 in Section 11.2.3, using the ICH Q1E stability design with testing time points $x_i = 0, 3, 6, 9, 12, 18$, and 24 months, with three replicates at each x_i. The model parameter α and the lower specification limit η were chosen to be 105 and 90, respectively, two values of β (-0.25 and -0.5) were used, and σ ranged from 0.1 to 2.0 (same parameters were used in the simulations by Shao and Chow 2001).

11.2.7.1.1 Results of Simulation Study I

The simulated data were fit to Model 11.2, giving rise to estimates of the model parameters. One-sided 95% confidence and prediction limits were calculated along with shelf life estimates $\hat{\theta}_{CL}$ and $\hat{\theta}_{PL}$. Treating the CIs and PIs as tolerance intervals with a fixed 95% confidence level, their corresponding contents are calculated, based on Corollaries 11.1 and 11.2. The results are presented in Table 11.1. As expected, regardless of the variability and

TABLE 11.1

Content of Confidence and Prediction Intervals (95% Confidence)

Degradation Slope β	Variability α	95% CI Shelf Life	95% CI Content	95% PI Shelf Life	95% PI Content
−0.5	0.1	29.75	0.500	29.55	0.812
	0.5	29.02	0.500	28.05	0.819
	2.0	26.63	0.500	22.66	0.845
−0.25	0.1	58.98	0.500	58.76	0.697
	0.5	55.81	0.499	54.72	0.708
	2.0	47.07	0.500	42.64	0.752

degradation rate, the 95% confidence interval always contains 50% of the units. When the degradation rate $\beta = -0.5$, the prediction interval contains over 81%–85% of the units, which represents more than a 31% increase in content when compared to the 95% confidence interval. For example, when $\sigma = 0.1$, the prediction interval contains 81.2% of the distribution. In other words, at $\hat{\theta}_{PL}$, the potency of 81.2% of the units will be above the lower limit of 90, with 95% confidence, compared to 50% of the units at $\hat{\theta}_{CL}$ with the same confidence. The content of the PI is smaller when the degradation rate $\beta = -0.5$ compared to when it is -0.5. It also decreases as the variability σ increases from 0.1 to 2.0. Overall, the PI is a more conservative approach than the CI approach, as it contains a larger content with the same confidence. Unlike the CI, the content of the PI is affected by both the degradation rate and the variability in the data.

A second comparison between the CI and PI methods was also performed. This time, we treated both the CI and PI as tolerance intervals with a fixed content of 80% and calculated the confidence levels with which they have 80% content. The results are displayed in Table 11.2. It can be seen that when $\beta = -0.5$, the one-sided nominal 95% confidence interval has 80% content with an estimated confidence level decreasing from 61.1% to 51.7% as the variability increases from 0.1 to 2.0. When $\beta = -0.25$, the CI has the same content but with higher estimated confidence (decreasing from 85.4% to 80.9%, as the variability increases 0.1 to 2.0). By comparison, the 95% PI has 80% content with confidence of 95% and 92% for $\beta = -0.5$ and $\beta = -0.25$, respectively. The confidence level of the PI is only slightly affected by the variability over the range studied ($\sigma = 0.1$ to 2.0). The difference in confidence level between CI and PI is more pronounced for $\beta = -0.5$ than for $\beta = -0.25$. In any case, the PI exhibits a higher confidence level for 80% content than does the CI.

11.2.7.1.2 Discussion of Simulation Study I

From this unified perspective, it is seen that the ICH-recommended method for estimating shelf life provides only assurance that 50% of potency values of units in a batch will remain within specification limits at the estimated expiration date. Depending on the drug and its intended use, this

TABLE 11.2

Estimated Confidence Levels of Confidence and Prediction Intervals with 80% Content

β	σ	Nominal 95% CI		Nominal 95% PI	
		Shelf Life	Confidence Level	Shelf Life	Confidence Level
−0.5	0.1	29.75	0.601	29.55	0.957
	0.5	28.97	0.582	28.00	0.961
	2.0	26.68	0.517	22.67	0.978
−0.25	0.1	59.00	0.854	58.78	0.922
	0.5	55.69	0.844	54.60	0.923
	2.0	47.22	0.809	42.75	0.931

level of quality assurance might or might not be acceptable. For example, if the drug is a vaccine intended to be used in a large healthy population, a shelf life that only warrants 50% of units in a batch having potency within the therapeutic limits right before the expiration date does not seem to be acceptable to either public health authorities or vaccine recipients. However, for an oncology drug product, the risk for patients to take a drug with a high chance to fall outside specifications outweighs the risk for them not to take the drug at all; thus, the use of FDA-recommended methods might be appropriate. There are other circumstances in which it might be perfectly fine to determine shelf life based on the 95% one-sided confidence interval approach. During early clinical development of a drug candidate, clinical trial materials are formulated on a small scale in a laboratory setting. The manufacturing process is far from optimized, and the final product specifications are not available. In such cases, it makes sense to release clinical trial materials if the sponsor has some confidence that the materials would provide some clinical benefit. Similar remarks can be made about prediction interval approach. It is reasonable to argue that depending on the intended use of a drug, the FDA-recommended method or other interval approaches suggested in the literature may or may not be stringent. The unified view of the interval approaches makes it possible to evaluate the appropriateness of choosing one method over the other in the shelf life estimation.

The results of the first simulation study indicate that the actual confidence levels of the CI and PI, and the content of the PI, when viewed as tolerance intervals, are dependent on the degradation rate of the drug. The unified method proposed in this chapter allows for prediction of the level of quality assurance that a given shelf life estimate might provide, based on available knowledge about the degradation rate, before long-term stability data of the commercial product become available. The estimation can be accomplished by using stability data generated during the clinical development stage. This preliminary estimate of quality assurance is especially useful both for fine-tuning formulation of the drug before late phase clinical trials take place and for negotiating the product labeling with regulatory authorities when the drug is being reviewed for marketing approval. The early assessment of the level of quality assurance a given shelf life estimate would provide maximizes the manufacturer's chance of success for developing a stable formulation and getting regulatory approval for the final product. It is very much in line with the philosophy of quality by design.

The interval approaches can be compared "vertically" in terms of either content at some fixed confidence level, or confidence level with fixed content. They can also be assessed "horizontally" with respect to the coverage probabilities they provide for the theoretical mean shelf life $\theta = \dfrac{\eta - \alpha}{\beta}$. Using the lower 95% confidence and prediction limits results in shelf life estimates $\hat{\theta}_{CL}$ and $\hat{\theta}_{PL}$, respectively. As discussed previously, $\hat{\theta}_{CL}$ covers θ with 95% confidence (Shao and Chow 2001). By Theorem 11.1, the $1 - \tau_0$ confidence level of

$\hat{\theta}_{PL}$ satisfies Equation 11.7 and is clearly greater than 95% but <100%. Since the prediction interval produces an estimate of the theoretical shelf life with no more than 5% added confidence when compared to that derived from the FDA-recommended CI method, the gain does not seem to be so great. From the standpoint of direct estimation of the theoretical shelf life, the FDA method does not appear to be unduly less stringent.

11.2.7.2 Simulation Study II

A second simulation study was carried out by Yang and Zhang (2012b) to assess the risks and benefits of each of the three interval approaches. Once again, Model 11.2 was used to simulate data, with $x_i = 0, 3, 6, 9, 12, 18,$ and 24 months, and three replicates at each x_i. The model parameters α and β and the lower specification limit η were 105, −0.5, and 90, respectively, as used in the previous simulation. However, four values (0.01, 0.5, 2.0, and 5.0) were used for σ, representing extremely low, very low, low, and moderate variability, respectively.

11.2.7.2.1 Results of Simulation Study II

The model parameters were estimated by fitting the simulated data to Model 11.2. Fixing the confidence level at 95%, both the contents and shelf life estimates based on the three intervals were determined and are shown in Table 11.3. As expected, the 95% confidence interval has a content of 50% and, as before, the prediction interval content ranges from 81% to 88%. In addition, the content increases as the overall variability increases. The content of the 95%/95% TI remains constant; it is 95% regardless of the variability. The TI has the largest content (95%), which represents 45% more content than CI. From the point of view of consumer risk, the TI approach is most desirable. However, this gain might only be obtained at a greater expense to the producer, particularly when the overall variability is high. From Table 11.3, when the variability is extremely low ($\sigma = 0.01$), all three methods resulted

TABLE 11.3

Contents of Confidence and Prediction Intervals with 95% Confidence

	95% CI		95% PI		95% TI	
σ	**Shelf Life**	**Content**	**Shelf Life**	**Content**	**Shelf Life**	**Content**
0.01	30.1	50.0%	30.1	81.1%	30.1	95.0%
0.5	29.0	50.0%	29.6	81.2%	27.3	95.0%
2.0	26.7	50.0%	22.8	84.4%	19.7	95.0%
5.0	23.5	50.0%	12.7	87.6%	6.1	95.0%

Source: Yang, H. and Zhang, L. (2012b). Evaluation of statistical methods for estimating shelf life of drug products: a unified and risk-based approach. *J. Validation Technol.*, http://www.ivtnetwork.com/sites/default/files/IVTJVT0512_067-074_Yang-%7B1237440%7D.pdf (accessed on April 16, 2016).

in the same estimate of shelf life, 30.1 months. However, the variability has a much more pronounced effect on the shelf life estimates based on prediction and tolerance intervals than those based on the confidence interval. For example, with moderate variability ($\sigma = 5$ or 5% total CV), the shelf life estimates based on prediction and tolerance intervals are reduced to 12.7 and 6.1 months, respectively. When compared to 23.5 months based on the confidence interval approach, these two estimates represent 46% and 74% reductions in shelf life. A shelf life of only 6 months can easily make a product commercially nonviable, thus greatly discouraging a producer from marketing the product.

11.2.7.2.2 Discussion of Simulation Study II

The results of the second simulation study show that the prediction and tolerance interval approaches are too conservative. For example, when the total process and assay variability is 5.0, the shelf life estimates are 12.7 and 6.1 months, respectively, based on the PI and TI. In reality, a 6-month shelf life is too short to make a product commercially viable. It is also true that when the total variability is extremely low or very low, there are only marginal differences in shelf life among the three interval methods. The results suggest that improvement in manufacturing consistency and assay variability would give rise to comparable shelf life estimates and level of protection to both consumer and producer risks.

Last, for simplicity, batch-to-batch variability is not included in the current model, and therefore inference is only pertinent to the mean or individual units from the batch or batches under study. In order to determine a shelf life that provides quality assurance for all future batches, a random effects model that accounts for batch variability is needed.

11.3 Random-Batch Modeling

As previously discussed, per ICH Q1E, the purpose of a stability study is to establish a shelf life during which a quantitative attribute remains within acceptance criteria for all future batches manufactured, packaged, and stored under similar (labeled) conditions. However, as noted by many researchers (Capen et al. 2012), the ICH-recommended regression method is incompatible with this intent, as are the alternative methods discussed so far. This incompatibility is caused by treating batches as a fixed effect. In order to extrapolate the shelf life estimated from the batches used in the regression analyses to all future batches, the batch should be viewed as a random effect (Capen et al. 2012; Chow 2007; Lin 1994; Quinlan et al. 2013a,b). Understanding that there are more sources of variability than measurement error, Kiermeier et al. (2004) considered tablet-to-tablet variability and suggested a tolerance interval method to estimate true product shelf life of a batch, which is defined as a small quantile of the distribution of the measure stability characteristic. Komka et al. (2010) attempted to generalize the method to multiple batches, in which the batch is viewed as a random effect. However, their investigation was restricted to a single batch. Only more recently was an analysis strategy assuming a random-batch effect thoroughly investigated by the Stability Shelf Life Working Group (Capen et al. 2012; Quinlan et al. 2013a,b). Hereafter, we refer to the group as the Working Group. In the following sections, we primarily focus on discussing the advantages and disadvantages of this new strategy.

11.3.1 Methods Based on Random Batch

The random-batch model takes the same form as the model in Equation 11.1 but assumes that the deviation of intercept and slope for a given batch is random. Let $Y_i = (y_{i1},...,y_{im})$, $Y = (Y_1',...,Y_n')'$, $b = (\alpha,\beta)^T$, $X_i = \begin{pmatrix} 1 & ... & 1 \\ x_i & ... & x_i \end{pmatrix}'_{m \times 2}$,

$X = (X_1',...,X_n')'$, $e_i = (\varepsilon_{i1},...,\varepsilon_{im})^T$, and $e = (e_1',...,e_n')'$. Let $u = (u_0, u_1)$ be deviations of a batch from the mean intercept and slope. It is assumed that $u = (u_0, u_1)$ follows a bivariate normal distribution, $u \sim MVN(0, D)$, with

$$D = \begin{pmatrix} \sigma_\alpha^2 & 0 \\ 0 & \sigma_\beta^2 \end{pmatrix}.$$

Hence, Model 11.1 can be expressed as

$$Y = Xb + Zu + e, \tag{11.13}$$

with $Y \sim MVN(Xb, V)$, $V = X'DX + \sigma_e^2 I_{(mn) \times (mn)}$. Three shelf life estimation methods were suggested by Quinlan et al. (2013a,b) and are described below.

11.3.1.1 Random-Batch Shelf Life Estimation Method I

Let $\hat{\beta}$ and $\hat{V}$ be the estimates of β and the variance of $\hat{\beta}$, respectively. The $(1-\alpha) \times 100\%$ confidence interval for the mean response y measured at time t is given by

$$CI_L(t), CI_U(t) = \hat{\alpha} + \hat{\beta}t \pm t_{1-\alpha/2, df, \delta} \sqrt{x(X'\hat{V}^{-1}X)^- x'}, \tag{11.14}$$

where $t_{1-\alpha/2, n-p^*}$ is the $(1-\alpha/2)$th quantile of the noncentral t distribution with $n - p^*$ degrees of freedom, p^* is the rank of X, $x = (1, t)$, and $(X'\hat{V}^{-1}X)^-$ is a generalized inverse of $X'\hat{V}^{-1}X$.

The estimated shelf life is

$$\hat{\tau}_{TI} = \min\{\inf\{t \ge 0 : TI_L(t) < \eta\}, \inf\{t \ge 0 : TI_U(t) > \lambda\},$$

where η and λ are the lower and upper specification limits, respectively.

When the stability attribute is known to be either decreasing or increasing over time, only a one-sided tolerance interval is needed to determine the shelf life. Under such circumstances, the critical value $t_{1-\alpha/2,df,\delta}$ should be replaced by $t_{1-\alpha,df,\delta}$. This method is referred to as the reflection method (Quinlan et al. 2013a).

11.3.1.2 Random-Batch Shelf Life Estimation Method II

From Model 11.1, a point estimate of the batch shelf life can be obtained as

$$\hat{\tau}(\hat{\alpha}, \hat{\beta}) = \frac{\eta - \hat{\alpha}}{\hat{\beta}}. \tag{11.15}$$

Because $\hat{\tau}(\hat{\alpha}, \hat{\beta})$ approximately follows a normal distribution $N(\tau(\alpha, \beta), h(X'V^{-1}X)^- h'$ with

$$h = \left[\frac{\partial \tau(\alpha, \beta)}{\partial \alpha}, \frac{\partial \tau(\alpha, \beta)}{\partial \beta} \right],$$

the estimated (labeled) shelf life, defined as the lower confidence limit of the mean shelf life $\frac{\eta - \alpha}{\beta}$, is given by

$$\hat{\tau}(\hat{\alpha}, \hat{\beta}) - t_{1-\alpha, n-p*} \sqrt{\hat{h}(X'\hat{V}^{-1}X)^- \hat{h}'}, \tag{11.16}$$

where p^* is the rank of X and $\hat{h}$ is h evaluated at $\beta = \hat{\beta}$.

11.3.1.3 Random-Batch Shelf Life Estimation Method III

Lastly, Quinlan et al. (2013a) suggest shelf life t_c be determined such that it is the minimum among all possible values satisfying

$$|x_c\beta - \eta| \le t_{1-\alpha, n-p*} \sqrt{x_c X'\hat{V}^{-1}X)^- x_c'}, \tag{11.17}$$

where $x_c = (1, t_c)$.

11.3.2 Random-Batch Shelf Life Estimation Method Evaluations

Quinlan et al. (2013a,b) investigated the performance of the random-batch estimation methods they proposed, along with the ICH-recommended method, through several simulation studies for the number of batches to be equal to 3, 6, 9, and 12. In the ICH method, the batch effect is treated as fixed, and a poolability test is conducted. Mean shelf life estimates based on the above four methods are compared separately for data sets for which batches were poolable ($P > 0.25$), those for which the batches were not poolable ($P \leq 0.25$), and all data sets combined. Data were simulated from Model 11.13 with the assumptions that $\mathbf{b} = (100, -0.15)$, $\eta = 95$, $\mathbf{u} \sim MVN(\mathbf{0}, \mathbf{D})$, with

$$\mathbf{D} = \begin{pmatrix} 0.15 & 0 \\ 0 & 0.00005 \end{pmatrix},$$

and measurement variance $\sigma_e^2 = 1$. Within each batch, results were simulated at time points 0, 3, 6, 9, 12, 18, 24, and 36 months. For each batch number, a total of 1000 data sets were generated. The simulation was repeated five times. The results are presented in Tables 11.4 and 11.5.

TABLE 11.4

Mean and Ranges of Shelf Life Estimates Based on Three Batches and Five Simulations Each Having 1000 Iterations

Method	All	Poolable Data	Nonpoolable
ICH	25.2 (25.1–25.4)	28.6 (28.4–28.8)	23.5 (23.4–23.7)
I	25.3 (25.1–25.5)	26.9 (26.7–27.0)	24.5 (24.3–24.7)
II	22.8 (22.7–23.0)	25.0 (24.9–25.1)	21.7 (21.5–21.9)
III	25.5 (25.3–25.7)	27.1 (26.9–27.2)	24.7 (24.4–24.9)

Source: Quinlan, M., Stroup, W., Schwenke, J., and Christopher, D. (2013b). Evaluating the performance of the ICH guidelines for shelf life estimation. *J. Biopharm. Stat.*, 23, 881–896.

TABLE 11.5

Mean and Ranges of Shelf Life Estimates Based on Six Batches and Five Simulations Each Having 1000 Iterations

Method	All	Poolable Data	Nonpoolable
ICH	24.1 (24.0–24.1)	29.8 (29.7–29.9)	22.7 (22.6–22.8)
I	29.0 (28.9–29.0)	28.6 (29.5–29.7)	28.8 (28.7–28.9)
II	28.4 (28.4–28.5)	29.2 (29.1–29.3)	28.2 (28.1–28.3)
III	29.2 (29.1–29.2)	29.8 (29.7–29.9)	29.0 (28.9–29.0)

Source: Quinlan, M., Stroup, W., Schwenke, J., and Christopher, D. (2013b). Evaluating the performance of the ICH guidelines for shelf life estimation. *J. Biopharm. Stat.*, 23, 881–896.

Note that the true shelf life is $(100 - 95)/0.15 = 33.3$ months. From Table 11.4, it can be seen that for the data consisting of three batches, the ICH method provides a more accurate shelf life estimate than the other three methods when the batches are poolable, whereas it provides a slightly more conservative estimate than Procedures I and III otherwise. Procedure II appears to have the worst performance. Using all the data, the ICH method is comparable to Procedures I and III and estimates a longer mean shelf life than Procedure II. When data were simulated based on six batches, the ICH method produced comparable mean shelf life estimates to Procedure III and gives a slightly more accurate result than Procedures I and II when the batches are poolable. However, when batches are not poolable, the ICH method uniformly does worse (i.e., estimates a shorter shelf life) than the other three methods. This is expected since as more batches are used in the analysis, the minimum shelf life estimate of all the batches is farther away from the true shelf life than if the batches are pooled.

Quinlan et al. (2013a) also conducted additional simulations to compare the performance of the ICH method to that of Procedure I for 9 and 12 batches. It was found that as the number of batches increases, the ICH method becomes more conservative, giving a risk of even smaller shelf life estimates compared to any of the random-batch methods.

11.3.3 Mixed Model Tolerance Interval

Let $\hat{\boldsymbol{\beta}}$ and $\hat{\mathbf{V}}$ be the estimates of $\boldsymbol{\beta}$ and the variance of $\hat{\boldsymbol{\beta}}$, respectively. Again, to simplify our discussion, we assume that the measured quality attribute decreases over time. By extending Hahn's work (1970), Quinlan et al. (2013a) derived the confidence interval of the qth quantile of the mean response y measured at time t:

$$\text{TI}_L(t), \text{TI}_U(t) = \hat{\alpha} + \hat{\beta} t \pm t_{1-\alpha/2, df, \delta} \sqrt{\mathbf{x}(\mathbf{X}'\hat{\mathbf{V}}^{-1}\mathbf{X})^-\mathbf{x}'}, \tag{11.18}$$

where $t_{1-\alpha/2, df, \delta}$ is the $(1 - \alpha/2) \times 100$th quantile of the noncentral t distribution with df and noncentrality parameter $\delta = -\Phi^{-1}(q)\sqrt{n_b}$, with $\Phi(\cdot)$ being the cdf of the standard normal distribution, n_b being the number of batches used in the stability study, $\mathbf{x} = (1, t)$, and $(\mathbf{X}'\hat{\mathbf{V}}^{-1}\mathbf{X})^-$ being a generalized inverse of $\mathbf{X}'\hat{\mathbf{V}}^{-1}\mathbf{X}$.

The estimated shelf life is

$$\hat{\tau}_{TI} = \min\{\inf\{t \geq 0 : \text{TI}_L(t) < \eta\}, \inf\{t \geq 0 : \text{TI}_U(t) > \lambda\}, \tag{11.19}$$

where η and λ are the lower and upper specifications.

A relationship between a given percentile, say, the 5th percentile, of the distribution of the estimated shelf life $\hat{\tau}(\hat{\alpha},\hat{\beta}) = \dfrac{\eta - \hat{\alpha}}{\hat{\beta}}$ and a quantile of the mean response y is measured (Quinlan et al. 2013a). However, this relationship is dependent on the unknown variability of intercept and slope in Model 11.13. Therefore, it cannot be used to guide the selection of a percentile of the y response, which corresponds to a preselected percentile of the distribution of $\hat{\tau}(\hat{\alpha},\hat{\beta}) = \dfrac{\eta - \hat{\alpha}}{\hat{\beta}}$, so as to allow for determining a shelf life based on the above TI method. Consequently, the method is of little practical use.

11.4 Shelf Life Based on Piecewise Regression

The shelf life of a pharmaceutical product is often determined based on a linear regression analysis recommended in the ICH guidelines. A linear model has been broadly used to describe product stability. However, since product stability is influenced not only by known factors such as storage temperature but also by unknown variables, the rate of product degradation may change over time. For example, for a vaccine product we developed, potency degradation appears to occur in phases, where there are distinctly different rates of degradation associated with different phases of storage. During the initial phase, the degradation rate is relatively high. In the second phase, the drop in potency seems to occur at a lower rate than before. Although the precise time at which the degradation rate changes is unknown, it is roughly in the vicinity of 8 weeks after product release. This time point is often referred to as a *breakpoint* in the literature. It is of great interest to objectively determine the breakpoint so that the product shelf life can be properly estimated based on data collected from the breakpoint onward. Figure 11.2 depicts the stability profile of potency for a lot that has a biphasic nature, with a breakpoint at day 25.

In this section, we use a piecewise regression model to estimate the shelf life of a product that degrades in two phases. The model fits linear segments to data collected before and after the breakpoint, although other nonlinear curves may be used. The breakpoint is formally defined as the time where the two linear segments intersect each other. It is formulated as a parameter in the model and can be estimated using the traditional least squares method, along with other model parameters. The goodness of fit of the model is evaluated by testing the hypothesis that the reduction in the sum of squares for error due to fitting the piecewise model is insignificant when compared to a single linear model.

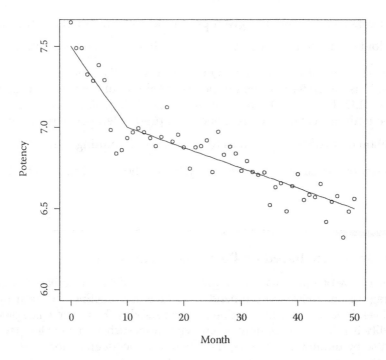

FIGURE 11.2
Biphasic stability profile of a vaccine lot.

11.4.1 Piecewise Regression Model

We use y and x to represent measured potency and time, respectively. Suppose a stability study consists of n time points x_i, $i = 1, \ldots, n$, with corresponding measured potency values y_i. For simplicity, we assume that there is only one replicate of stability sample tested per time point. The relationship between the potency and time may be described through the linear model given in Equation 11.2:

$$y_i = \alpha + \beta x_i + \varepsilon_i, \tag{11.20}$$

where α and β are the intercept and slope parameters and ε_i are measurement errors that are assumed to be *iid* according to a normal distribution $N(0, \sigma^2)$. However, when the product stability is biphasic in nature, a single linear or nonlinear model may not adequately describe the product's stability profile. Under such circumstances, the following piecewise model may be used:

$$y_i = \alpha_1 + \beta_1 x_i + \varepsilon_i \quad \text{for} \quad x_i \le c \text{ and}$$

$$y_i = \alpha_2 + \beta_2 x_i + \varepsilon_i \quad \text{for} \quad x_i > c, \tag{11.21}$$

where c is an unknown breakpoint such that

$$\alpha_1 + \beta_1 c = \alpha_2 + \beta_2 c. \tag{11.22}$$

In other words, c is the time point at which the two line segments intersect each other. Model 11.22 can be reparameterized as

$$y_i = \alpha_1 + \beta_1 x_i + \varepsilon_i \quad \text{for} \quad x_i \leq c \text{ and}$$

$$y_i = \alpha_1 + \beta_1 x_i + \beta(x_i - c) + \varepsilon_i \quad \text{for} \quad x_i > c, \tag{11.23}$$

with

$$\beta = \beta_2 - \beta_1, \tag{11.24}$$

which is the difference between the slopes of the two line segments. Potency y, described through Equation 11.21, can be viewed as a nonlinear function of time x. Let $\theta = (\alpha_1, \beta_1, \beta, c, \sigma^2)$ be the unknown parameters in Model 11.21 and $\hat{\theta} = (\hat{\alpha}_1, \hat{\beta}_1, \hat{\beta}, \hat{c}, \hat{\sigma}^2)$ be its least square estimates (LSE), and let $\hat{y}$ be the predicted mean potency value at time x. Similarly, we let $\tilde{\theta} = (\tilde{\alpha}_1, \tilde{\beta}_1, \tilde{\sigma}^2)$ be the LSE of $\theta_0 = (\alpha_1, \beta_1, \sigma^2)$ and $\tilde{y}$ be the predicted mean potency at time x, based on Model 11.20. Then, the sums of squared errors due to Models 11.20 and 11.21, which we refer to as reduced (R) and full (F) models, are given by

$$SSE(R) = \sum_{i=1}^{n} (y_i - \tilde{y}_i)^2 \sim \sigma^2 \chi^2 (n-3) \text{ and}$$

$$SSE(F) = \sum_{i=1}^{n} (y_i - \hat{y}_i)^2 \sim \sigma^2 \chi^2 (n-5).$$

Therefore, the following hypotheses concerning the necessity of using Model 11.21

$$H_0: \beta = 0 \quad \text{versus} \quad H_1: \beta \neq 0, \tag{11.25}$$

where β is given in Equation 11.24, can be tested using an extra sums of squares test suggested by Neter (1990):

$$F^* = \frac{[SSE(R) - SSE(F)]/2}{SSE(F)/(n-5)} \sim F_{2,n-5}.$$

Hypothesis H_0 is rejected at the 5% significance level if $F^* > F_{0.95;2,\,n-5}$, where $F_{0.95;2,\,n-5}$ is the 95th percentile of the central F distribution with degrees of freedom of 2 and $n-5$. If H_0 is rejected, the piecewise model (Equation 11.21) is deemed more appropriate for describing the product stability profile than a single linear model and is thus suitable for shelf life estimation.

11.4.2 Shelf Life Estimation Using Piecewise Regression

When the piecewise regression model is considered appropriate for shelf life estimation, the shelf life can be estimated as time at which the one-sided lower 95% confidence interval of the predicted mean value based on the linear model in the second phase intersects the lower specification limit η. Using the δ method, we could estimate the variance of $\hat{y} = \hat{\alpha}_1 + \hat{\beta}_1 x + \hat{\beta}(x - \hat{c})$ such that (assuming all co-variances are zero)

$$\sigma_{\hat{y}}^2 = \text{var}[\hat{\alpha}_1] + \text{var}[\hat{\beta}_1]x^2 + \text{var}[\hat{\beta}](x - \hat{c})^2 + \hat{\beta}^2 \, \text{var}[\hat{c}].$$

Thus, an approximate one-sided 95% lower confidence limit for the mean value of $\hat{y}$ at time x is given by

$$\hat{\alpha}_1 + \hat{\beta}_1 x + \hat{\beta}(x - \hat{c}) - 1.645\sigma_{\hat{y}}.$$

Then, the shelf life is the smaller root of the following equation with respect to x,

$$\hat{\alpha}_1 + \hat{\beta}_1 x + \hat{\beta}(x - \hat{c}) - 1.645\sigma_{\hat{y}} = \eta. \tag{11.26}$$

11.5 Other Applications of Stability Studies

11.5.1 Design Space of Storage Temperature

It is a regulatory requirement that a drug product be stored under the conditions specified in the product label insert to ensure its quality. As the product may be shipped to different regions, excursions outside of the approved temperature range may occur. In this circumstance, an investigation must be conducted to assess the impact of the excursion. The manufacturer is also required to file a product deviation report with the regulatory authority. The investigation not only costs resources but also may delay the release of the product. Applying the design space concept, Yang (2012b) proposed establishing a design space (DS) for storage temperature based on Arrhenius modeling (Silberberg 2006). The design space is defined as a range of temperatures for which the degradation rate of the product is bounded by an acceptable limit, with a certain level of confidence. The method was illustrated through a vaccine example. Historical data suggested that a degradation rate is considered acceptable if it does not exceed 0.122 $\log_{10}$ titer/month over the labeled shelf life. The DS for storage temperature in this case is the range of temperatures for which the one-sided upper 95% confidence limit for the degradation rate is no more than 0.122 $\log_{10}$ titer/month.

An accelerated stability study was simulated, using temperatures $T = 20°C$, $30°C$, $40°C$, and $50°C$, which are outside of the normal range of storage temperature ($5°C \pm 3°C$). Potency data were generated at months 0, 3, and 6, in accordance with recommendations of ICH Q1A (R2) (2003). For each temperature, the data were fit to the linear model in Equation 11.1 to obtain an estimate $\hat{k}_T$ of the degradation rate k_T at that temperature T. The estimates $\hat{k}_T$ were further fit to the Arrhenius model $k_T = Ae^{-\frac{\Delta H}{RT}}$, with temperature T in Kelvin ($K = °C + 273.15$), R being the universal gas constant (8.314), and ΔH being activation energy; after log-transformation,

$$\ln(\hat{k}_T) = \ln(k_T) + \varepsilon = \alpha + \beta \frac{1}{T} + \varepsilon, \qquad (11.27)$$

where ε is variability of the estimate of $\ln(\hat{k}_T)$ and is assumed to follow a normal distribution with mean 0 and variance σ_k^2.

Let $\hat{\alpha}$, $\hat{\beta}$, and $\hat{\sigma}_k$ be the least squares estimates of α, β, and σ_k, respectively. Thus, the log degradation rate at temperature T can be predicted through the following equation:

$$\ln(\tilde{k}_T) = \hat{\alpha} + \hat{\beta} \frac{1}{T},$$

along with its one-sided upper 95% confidence limit. An example was given by Yang (2012b) and is described here. The $\hat{\alpha}$, $\hat{\beta}$, and $\hat{\sigma}_k$ were calculated to be 15.467, −5300.4, and 0.2337, respectively, for the model parameters α, β, and σ_k. Therefore, the estimated regression line is given by

$$\ln(\tilde{k}_T) = 15.467 - 5300.4 \frac{1}{T}.$$

An approximate one-sided upper 95% confidence limit for k_T is calculated as

$$e^{\ln(\tilde{k}_T) + t_2(0.05)\hat{\sigma}\sqrt{1/4 + (T^{-1} - \bar{T}^{-1})^2 / \sum_{i=1}^{4}(T_i^{-1} - \bar{T}^{-1})^2}},$$

where $t_2(0.05)$ is the 95th percentile of the t distribution with 2 *df* and $\bar{T} = \sum_{i=1}^{4} T_i^{-1}/4$. Finally, the DS is determined by

$$DS = \left\{ T : e^{15.467-5300.4/T+t_2(0.05)\hat{\sigma}\sqrt{1/4+(T-\bar{T})^2/\sum_{i=1}^{4}(T_i-\bar{T})^2}} \leq 0.122 \right\}. \qquad (11.28)$$

Solving the inequality in Equation 11.28 for T results in

$$T \leq 17.9°C.$$

Note that the labeled storage temperature is 5°C ± 3°C. The actual design space is determined to be 2°C to 17.9°C.

11.5.2 Evaluation of Stability Design Using Simulation

The shelf life of a drug product is determined from data generated from stability studies designed in accordance with regulatory guidelines (ICH 1993, 1995b, 1998, 2003a,b). For this purpose, typically three lots, representative of the final commercially packaged product, are tested at time points of 0, 3, 6, 9, 12, 18, and 24 months (see Table 11.6). Multiple lots are used to account for lot-to-lot variability, thus allowing for extrapolation of findings from the current study to future lots.

Since stability studies are usually costly, it is desirable to reduce the amount of testing. Several alternative designs such as matrixing and bracketing designs have been suggested (Barron 1994; Chow 2007; ICH 2002; Lin and Fairweather 1997; Nordbrock and Valvani 1995). However, while reducing the overall cost of stability testing, the reduced designs may also decrease the reliability of model parameter estimation, thus incurring the risk of providing an unreliable estimate of shelf life. It is in the manufacturer's best interest to evaluate this risk before adopting a reduced stability program. The risk assessment can be performed using statistical simulations. Yang (2012b) evaluated two alternate designs listed in Tables 11.7 and 11.8 against that in Table 11.5.

TABLE 11.6

Stability Design with Three Lots

Time (Month)	0	3	6	9	12	18	24
Lot 1	Δ	Δ	Δ	Δ	Δ	Δ	Δ
Lot 2	Δ	Δ	Δ	Δ	Δ	Δ	Δ
Lot 3	Δ	Δ	Δ	Δ	Δ	Δ	Δ

Source: Yang, H. (2012b). Ensure product quality and regulatory compliance through novel stability design and analysis. *J. Validation Technol.*, 18(3), 52–59.

Note: Δ, Time point where potency value is measured.

TABLE 11.7

Reduced Stability Design I

Time (Month)	0	3	6	9	12	18	24
Lot 1	Δ	Δ			Δ	Δ	Δ
Lot 2	Δ		Δ	Δ	Δ		Δ
Lot 3	Δ			Δ	Δ	Δ	Δ

Source: Yang, H. (2012b). Ensure product quality and regulatory compliance through novel stability design and analysis. *J. Validation Technol.*, 18(3), 52–59.

Note: Δ, Time point where potency value is measured.

TABLE 11.8

Reduced Stability Design II

Time (Month)	0	3	6	9	12	18	24
Lot 1	Δ	Δ			Δ	Δ	Δ
Lot 2	Δ		Δ		Δ		Δ
Lot 3	Δ			Δ	Δ		Δ
Lot 4	Δ				Δ	Δ	Δ

Source: Yang, H. (2012b). Ensure product quality and regulatory compliance through novel stability design and analysis. *J. Validation Technol.*, 18(3), 52–59.

Note: Δ, Time point where potency value is measured.

In the context of stability design evaluation, stability data sets under different designs can be repeatedly simulated based on a degradation model such as Equation 11.1 and input parameters α, β, and σ, which are usually estimated from development data. For each round of simulation, shelf life can be estimated for each of the designs under evaluation. The repeated simulations generate large sets of shelf life estimates, making it possible to calculate accuracy and precision of the shelf life estimate based on each design and assess the appropriateness of using reduced designs for the stability study in support of product licensure.

Tables 11.7 and 11.8 list two reduced designs of interest, one specified in ICH Q1E and the other similar to what is suggested by Schofield (2009), assuming that four lots of product are available for stability testing.

Suppose that the stability characteristic under evaluation is potency, with a specification range of 6.5 to −7.0 $\log_{10}$ titer. For each of the three designs above, 1000 random samples were simulated from the model

$$y = 7.0 + 0.025x + \varepsilon, \tag{11.29}$$

where $\varepsilon \sim N(0, 0.01^2)$. The mean shelf life is equal to $(7.0 - 6.5)/0.025 = 20$ months.

For each design and each simulation i, $1 \le i \le 1000$, the above model was fit to the data, and the shelf life $\hat{\theta}_i$ was determined from Equation 11.29 using the ICH Q1E method. To determine the performance of each design, the mean estimated shelf life, its range, accuracy, and precision were calculated and presented in Table 11.9:

$$\bar{\theta} = \frac{1}{1000} \sum_{i=1}^{1000} \hat{\theta}_i,$$

$$\text{Range} = [\min(\hat{\theta}_i), \max(\hat{\theta}_i)],$$

$$\text{Accuracy} = |\bar{\theta} - 20|,$$

$$\text{Precision} = \frac{1}{999} \sum_{i=1}^{n} (\hat{\theta}_i - \bar{\theta})^2.$$

As seen from the table, all three designs render comparable estimates of shelf life, although each underestimates the true shelf life of 20 months by approximately 1 month. The underestimation is expected because the shelf life based on ICH Q1E method is a biased underestimate of the true shelf life (Chow 2007). Furthermore, the estimate from the full design is slightly more accurate than the two reduced designs due to having more data. However, the second reduced design, consisting of four lots, is most precise, as evidenced by a narrower range of shelf life estimates (15.81–22.41) and smaller SD (1.05) than either of the others. This design has 51 test results compared to 81 in the full design. Therefore, it results in approximately 37% [(81 − 51)/81] savings in total testing. In light of these findings, design II (Table 11.8) is a good alternative to the full design.

This example is intended to illustrate the use of Monte Carlo simulation to identify reduced designs that provide a fine balance between efficiency and risk. The outcomes may be influenced by assay and process variability. For

TABLE 11.9

Results of Simulation Comparing Performance of Three Stability Designs in Estimating the Shelf Life (Months)

Design	Estimated Mean	Range (Min–Max)	Accuracy	Precision
Full	19.16	15.62–23.52	0.84	1.19
Reduced I	18.94	14.40–23.29	1.06	1.24
Reduced II	19.02	15.81–22.41	0.92	1.05

Source: Yang, H. (2012b). Ensure product quality and regulatory compliance through novel stability design and analysis. *J. Validation Technol.*, 18(3), 52–59.

a real product, alternate models may be used, incorporating other sources of variation. Nevertheless, the simulation procedure remains similar to what was shown above.

11.5.3 Bayesian Stability Analysis

Yang (2012b) described an example demonstrating the utility of Bayesian stability analysis to predict the outcome of an annual stability study. The annual stability study is a regulatory requirement. For each annual manufacturing campaign, one lot of product is required to be selected for real-time stability monitoring, with the intention of verifying the product's shelf life. It is of interest to predict the outcome of the stability study when partial data become available. This ongoing update allows for a timely response to any unexpected results. It is assumed for the purposes of discussion that the key stability indicator is the degradation rate. The acceptance criterion is that the rate of decrease is no more than $0.025 \log_{10}$ titer/month, which confirms a 20-month shelf life when the lot is released at an acceptable potency level of $7.0 \log_{10}$ titer. Potency measurements are taken at 0, 3, 6, 9, 12, 18, and 24 months. Let $Y_m = (y_1, \ldots, y_m)$ denote the potency data collected up to time point $x_m (<24)$, and $\hat{\beta}$ be the estimate of slope based on Y_m. The posterior probability

$$p = \Pr[\beta \geq -0.025 | \hat{\beta}] \tag{11.30}$$

provides a level of confidence that the stability of the lot behaves as expected. It is assumed that the slope β of commercial lots has a normal distribution $N(\beta_0, \sigma_0^2)$. Because $\hat{\beta}$ also follows a normal distribution with mean β and variance $\sigma_\beta^2 = \sigma^2 / S_{xx}(m)$, where $S_{xx}(m) = \sum_{i=1}^m [x_i - \bar{x}(m)]^2$, with $\bar{x}(m) = \frac{1}{m} \sum_{i=1}^m x_i$ (20), it can be easily verified that the posterior distribution of b is

$$\beta | \hat{\beta} \sim N\left(\frac{\sigma_\beta^2}{\sigma_\beta^2 + \sigma_0^2} \beta_0 + \frac{\sigma_0^2}{\sigma_\beta^2 + \sigma_0^2} \hat{\beta}, \frac{\sigma_\beta^2 \sigma_0^2}{\sigma_\beta^2 + \sigma_0^2} \right).$$

Consequently,

$$\Pr[\beta \geq -0.025 | \hat{\beta}] = 1 - \Phi\left(\left[-0.025 - \frac{\sigma_\beta^2}{\sigma_\beta^2 + \sigma_0^2} \beta_0 - \frac{\sigma_0^2}{\sigma_\beta^2 + \sigma_0^2} \hat{\beta} \right] \Big/ \sqrt{\frac{\sigma_\beta^2 \sigma_0^2}{\sigma_\beta^2 + \sigma_0^2}} \right),$$

where Φ is the cdf of the standard normal distribution.

As an illustration, suppose that $\hat{\beta} = -0.027$ and $S_{xx}(9) = 45$ based on data collected up to 9 months. It is further assumed that the mean and variance

β_0 and σ_0^2 in the prior distribution are -0.01 and 0.01^2, respectively, implying a very stable product. Under these assumptions and an assay variability of $\sigma^2 = 0.04$, it can be calculated that

$$\Pr[\beta \geq -0.025 | \hat{\beta}] = 91.2\%.$$

Therefore, there is a 91% probability that the product will have a desirable stability profile, even though the partial data seemingly suggest a faster degradation rate.

11.6 Concluding Remarks

Stability testing, as an integral part of drug product development, plays a very important role in every aspect of drug product development. If effectively utilized, it not only enables the manufacturer to build efficiency in the product development but also ensures compliance to regulatory standards. Since stability testing is usually costly and time-consuming, the application of novel statistical methods in stability study design and analysis can result in robust study designs with reduced cost.

12

Investigation of Out-of-Specification and Out-of-Trend Results

12.1 Introduction

Out-of-specification (OOS) and out-of-trend (OOT) results may be observed during substance or drug product release or stability testing, which may significantly affect the results of a statistical analysis and of the disposition of a drug substance or product lot. Therefore, when an OOS or OOT result occurs, it is critical to conduct a thorough investigation to identify the root cause(s) so that the results can be appropriately addressed. Over the past decades, many violations of current good manufacturing practice (cGMP) concerning OOS/OOT resulted in legal proceedings, drug recalls, and disruption of supply chain. Despite heightened regulatory oversight, failure to properly investigate OOS results continues to be a significant part of Food and Drug Administration (FDA) Form 483 findings. Although FDA guidance outlines steps for OOS investigation (FDA 2006), it does not provide guidelines for using statistical methods to assist OOS investigations. Numerous working practices and various degrees of understanding of current expectations in this area have led to many different statistical approaches to investigating OOS results. In this chapter, statistical methods for OOS investigation that represent good science and conform to current regulatory guidelines are presented. In addition, various statistical methods for identifying OOT results are also included in the chapter.

12.2 Background

12.2.1 FDA versus Barr Laboratories

From August 1989 to September 1991, FDA conducted several general inspections of two plants of Barr Laboratories, Inc., a generic drug manufacturer headquartered in New Jersey. The inspections resulted in a list of objectionable findings, including routinely retesting, resampling, and reprocessing without adequate investigation and documentation of OOS results (Madsen 1994). For example, when there was an OOS result, Barr Laboratories would test two more samples and use the best two to determine if the batch met quality standards. However, Barr disagreed that their practices were not compliant with the GMPs, and as the argument intensified, eventually in April 1992, Barr sued FDA for "ad hoc" drug regulation and FDA asked the court to order Barr to stop shipments of its product in question, on the grounds that Barr products were adulterated (Longwell 2016). Judge Alfred Wolin of the US District Court for the District of New Jersey heard the cases and handed down a ruling on February 4, 1993. Among the findings was a decision regarding OOS investigation. It was stated that (1) Any OOS results requires a failure investigation. The extent of the investigation may vary, depending on the type of error; (2) Barr's handling of lots with an initial OOS result by testing twice more and releasing the lot if 2 out 3 results, and the average of the 3 results pass the specification is inappropriate; and (3) FDA's claim that a single OOS result invalidates a lot was rejected.

12.2.2 Impacts of Barr Ruling

The Barr Decision highlighted the lack of clarity in the current regulations regarding OOS results. For example, in his ruling, Judge Wolin noted, "Thus, the CGMP regulations provide the yardstick with which FDA investigators, and the Court in the instant action, measure firm behavior. Ironically, the regulations themselves, whose broad and sometimes vague instructions allow conflicting, but plausible, views of the precise requirements, transform what might be a routine evaluation into an arduous task." In addition, he also ruled that outlier tests could not be used for chemical analysis data because they were not suggested in the United States Pharmacopoeia (USP) chapters.

The Barr ruling spawned many regulatory efforts to address potential loopholes in regulations and unintended omissions in USP chapters. In 1994, soon after the Barr ruling, a draft guidance entitled "Investigating Out-of-Specification Test Results for Pharmaceutical Production" was developed and issued by the FDA, and was finalized in 2006. The guidance requires that an investigation be conducted in the event of an OOS test result. The investigation should be conducted in a phased manner, and each step of the investigation should be fully documented. It also specifies circumstances in which statistical methods for detection and removal of outliers may be used. Recognizing that the lack of guidance for chemical measurements has impeded proper application of statistical methods and procedures, a General USP Chapter <1010> Analytical Data—Interpretation and Treatment was developed and published (USP 2005), which addresses the use of statistical principles and methods, along with other good laboratory practices, for the analysis and interpretation of data obtained from chemical and other analyses.

12.3 FDA OOS Guidance

The purposes of laboratory testing are (1) to confirm that components, containers and closures, in-process materials, and finished products conform to specifications, including stability specifications, and (2) to support analytical and process validation. Laboratory testing is required by cGMP, and so is the investigation of OOS results. In 2004, the FDA published guidance on the investigation of OOS results for pharmaceutical production, which provides the agency's current thinking on how OOS test results should be evaluated. It discusses at length the responsibilities of laboratory personnel in OOS investigation, stepwise laboratory investigation, additional testing that may be necessary, when to expand the investigation outside the laboratory, and the final evaluation of all test results. The primary purpose of an OOS investigation is to determine the root cause of the OOS results, regardless of whether or not the OOS result leads to acceptance or rejection of the batch. The guidance suggests that the investigation be carried out in a timely, unbiased, well-documented, and scientifically sound manner, starting with a preliminary assessment of laboratory error. An obvious error that occurred during the testing may be identified, in which case, no formal investigation is needed. Otherwise, a formal stepwise laboratory assessment, consisting of three phases, should be carried out, with the aim of finding an assignable cause for the OOS.

12.3.1 Phase I Investigation

The investigation in this phase is to determine if the OOS result can be assigned to an error in the testing laboratory. Limited testing may be done using the same test preparations as generated by the OOS to aid the OOS investigation. In the event that an assignable cause is identified, the original sample is tested again and evaluated for its compliance to the acceptance criteria. If it is confirmed that the OOS was due to a laboratory error, the investigation is closed after the root cause is documented, and the effect of this assignable cause on other test results is assessed and corrective actions are taken.

12.3.2 Phase II Investigation

If an assignable laboratory cause for the OOS result cannot be identified in the first phase of investigation, a full-scale investigation should be conducted. This may include both production process review and additional laboratory testing. However, such an investigation should be planned in advance according to a written SOP. The FDA guidance states "Part of the investigation may involve *retesting* of a portion of the original sample. The sample used for the retesting should be taken from the same homogeneous material that was originally collected from the lot, tested, and yielded the OOS results." In addition, additional tests based on resampling may be warranted. Unlike retesting that analyzes the original, homogeneous sample material, *resampling* refers to any additional units collected as part of the original sampling procedure or from a new sample collected from the batch.

12.3.3 Phase III Investigation

The purpose of this final phase of investigation is to summarize the cause of the OOS result, document the OOS investigation, and note any corrective actions and preventive measures. The decision concerning acceptance or rejection of the batch is made, and the rationale is documented. There is no limit on further testing to determine the OOS cause and allow for a corrective action to be taken. Should the root cause of the OOS result be related to the laboratory, additional equipment maintenance and training may be warranted.

12.4 Statistical Methods for OOS Investigation

In this section, we discuss various statistical methods that can be applied to assist OOS investigations. Chief among these are outlier tests, retesting, and resampling.

12.4.1 Graphical Tools

An outlier is often referred to as a value that is markedly different from others in the data set. There are many causes of outlying observations such as deviation from prescribed analytical test procedures and inherent variability of samples being tested. Outliers may significantly affect conclusions. A variety of graphical tools can be used to identify outliers. For example, boxplots and normal probability plots, also called Q–Q plots, are useful for identifying outliers. Individual value plots with added symbols denoting the mean, median, quartiles, and other percentiles are also useful. The primary underlying assumption of these graphical methods is that the data are a random sample and are clustered together except for the outliers.

12.4.1.1 Boxplot

A boxplot is a graphical tool that describes data based on specific quantiles estimated from the data. As shown in Figure 12.1, the bottom and top of the

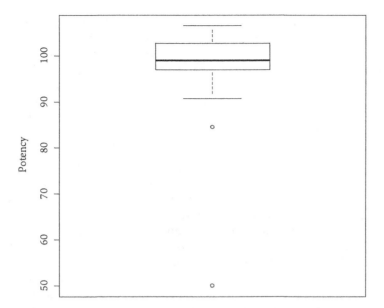

FIGURE 12.1
Example of a boxplot to detect outliers.

box correspond to the 25th (Q_1) and 75th (Q_3) quantiles, respectively, and the line within the box is the median (Q_2). The variability of the data is described through the two vertical lines extending from the box. Data points beyond the range covered by the two lines are deemed to be outliers and are plotted as individual points. In addition to potential use for outlier detection, a boxplot also conveys other useful information such as spread and skewness of the data. As it is very convenient to construct a boxplot, it should be used as part of any OOS investigation. The boxplot uses a specific definition of an outlier as a point more than $1.5 \times$ IQR, where IQR = interquartile range = $Q_3 - Q_1$.

12.4.1.2 Normal Probability (Q–Q) Plot

A normal probability (Q–Q) plot is obtained by plotting ordered observations against the corresponding quantiles of the normal distribution from which the data were assumed to be generated (Wilk and Gnanadesikan 1968). A Q–Q plot can be used to evaluate distributional assumptions. Suppose that $X = (X_1, \ldots, X_n)$ are the observed data. The random observations $X_1, \ldots, X_n$ are ordered from the smallest to the largest, to give rise to the ordered observations $X^{(1)} < X^{(2)} < \ldots X^{(n)}$. The ith ordered observation is paired with its percentile z_{p_i} of the standard normal distribution, where $p_i = (i - 0.5)/n$. The paired points $\left(X^{(i)}, z_{p_i}\right)$ are plotted. In statistics, if a random variable y follows a normal distribution with mean μ and variable σ^2, it can be expressed as $y = \mu + \sigma x$, where x is a random variable having the standard normal distribution. In other words, there is a linear relationship between the two variables. Consequently, if the sampling distribution of the observed data is normal, the data will lie on approximately a straight line. A Q–Q plot is displayed in Figure 12.2. The data appear to be normally distributed. Thus, it is reasonable to assume that there is no outlier in the data.

The boxplot and the Q–Q plot are tools that provide descriptive summaries of the data. However, a formal statistical analysis can assess how significant the outliers are in reference to a distribution or a well-established model. The detection of outliers relies on the distribution of the reference sample. An outlier based on a normal distribution assumption might not be an outlier if the normal assumption is untrue. Therefore, it is important to evaluate whether or not the data come from a certain distribution before an outlier test is performed. Various statistical techniques in the literature can be used to test the normality assumption. In the event that the normality assumption does not hold, a proper transformation of the data may be carried out to ensure the assumption is met. In such cases, outlier testing needs to be performed on the transformed data.

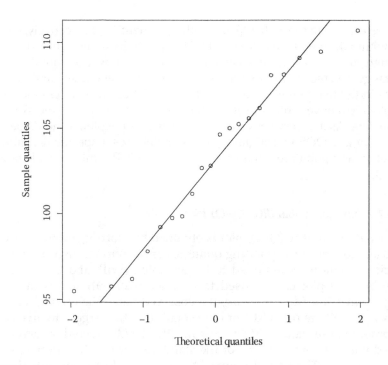

FIGURE 12.2
Q–Q plot of empirical quantiles against quantiles of the standard normal distribution.

12.4.2 Univariate Outlier Tests

12.4.2.1 Grubb's Test

Several outlier tests are available. Most frequently used is a method called Grubb's test (Grubb 1950), which uses the maximum deviation from the sample mean

$$G = \frac{\max_{\{1 \le i \le n\}} |X_i - \bar{X}|}{s} \tag{12.1}$$

and compares it to the cutoff value $\dfrac{n}{\sqrt{n-1}} \sqrt{\dfrac{t_{\alpha/(2n)}^2 (n-2)}{n-2+t_{\alpha/(2n)}^2 (n-2)}}$. If G exceeds the cutoff, the value that is most distant from the sample mean is an outlier. The test can be repeated after the outlier is removed. In practice, a table such as Table 12.1 listing cutoff values for a range of n values is used.

Now, we assume that a random sample consisting of 10 vials from a lot is tested, resulting in these potency values: 102.0, 100.1, 101.3, 100.0, 99.6, 99.9, 100.2, 99.5, 100.0, and 95.7. Then, $\bar{X} = 99.83$, $s = 1.65$, and $G = 2.51$, which is larger than the critical value 2.29. Therefore, the value 95.7 is an outlier.

As a word of caution, although the Grubb's test can be applied iteratively to remove multiple outliers, it is not appropriate to use when the sample size is less than 7 because the test identifies most observations as outliers.

12.4.2.2 Dixon's Test

Dixon's Q test is another method for outlier detection (Dean and Dixon 1951). If the smallest value is suspected to be an outlier, calculate the ratio of the difference between the smallest and second smallest value to the difference between the smallest and largest values. The ratio is calculated as the difference between the largest value and second largest value and the difference between the smallest and largest values if the largest value is suspected to be an outlier. Mathematically,

$$r = \frac{X_{(2)} - X_{(1)}}{X_{(n)} - X_{(1)}} \quad \text{or} \quad \frac{X_{(n)} - X_{(n-1)}}{X_{(n)} - X_{(1)}}, \tag{12.2}$$

where $X_{(1)} \le X_{(2)} \le \dots \le X_{(n-1)} \le X_{(n)}$ are ordered values of the original observations $X_1, X_2, \dots, X_{(n-1)} \le X_{(n)}$.

TABLE 12.1

Critical Values of Grubb's Outlier Test

n	3	4	5	6	7	8	9	10
Critical value	1.15	1.48	1.71	1.89	2.02	2.13	2.21	2.29

TABLE 12.2

Critical Values of Dixon's Q Test

n	Significance Level		
	90%	95%	99%
3	0.941	0.97	0.994
4	0.765	0.829	0.926
5	0.642	0.71	0.821
6	0.56	0.625	0.74
7	0.507	0.568	0.68
8	0.468	0.526	0.634
9	0.437	0.493	0.598
10	0.412	0.466	0.568

The statistic r is compared to the critical value corresponding to N in Table 12.2 for a prespecified significance level. An outlier is confirmed if r exceeds the critical value. For the above example, $r = (99.5 - 95.7)/(102.0 - 95.7) = 0.559 > 0.526$. Thus, Dixon's test also concludes that the value 95.7 is an outlier at the 95% significance level.

12.4.2.3 Hampel's Test

Hampel's outlier test is based on the median and median absolute deviation (MAD) (Hampel 1974). It is presumably a more reliable outlier test that detects all potential outliers at once. The method first calculates the median of the data $m = \text{median}_{\{1 \le i \le n\}}\{X_i\}$ and $\text{MAD} = 1.483 \times \text{median}_{\{1 \le i \le n\}}|X_i - m|$, which is a normalization factor

$$H_i = \frac{|X_i - m|}{\text{MAD}}, i = 1, \ldots, n. \tag{12.3}$$

Observations with H greater than 3.5 are deemed as outliers. After removing these outliers, the test can be repeated for the reduced data set.

We performed Hampel's test on the previous data set. The median = 100 and MAD = 0.22, and 11 observations have H values less than 3.5 but not the value 95.7, whose H value is 19.33. This observation was declared to be an outlier. After removing this value, the test was reapplied to the remaining data, and there were no more outliers identified.

12.4.2.4 Prediction Interval

A prediction interval is also useful for an OOS investigation where the behavior of suspected outlying individual observations is of primary concern. If the OOS result is far beyond the range predicted based on data generated under normal manufacturing conditions, it is likely a real outlier. A prediction interval provides a range for a randomly selected future observation from the population to fall in, with a prespecified level of confidence (Hahn and Meeker 1991). When the distribution of the population is normal with mean μ and variance σ^2, construction of the prediction interval is relatively straightforward. Let X_{n+1} be a future observation and $X = (X_1, ..., X_n)$ be the current data obtained by testing a random sample from the population. Because the statistic $T_{n+1} = \dfrac{X_{n+1} - \bar{X}}{s/\sqrt{1+1/n}}$ follows a t distribution with $n-1$ degrees of freedom,

$$P\left[\left|\frac{X_{n+1} - \bar{X}}{s/\sqrt{1+1/n}}\right| < t_{1-\alpha/2}(n-1)\right]$$

$$= P[\bar{X} - t_{1-\alpha/2}(n-1)s/\sqrt{1+1/n} < X_{n+1} < \bar{X} + t_{1-\alpha/2}(n-1)s/\sqrt{1+1/n} \qquad (12.4)$$

$$= 1 - \alpha.$$

Thus, the interval

$$\left(\bar{X} - t_{1-\alpha/2}(n-1)s/\sqrt{1+1/n}, \bar{X} + t_{1-\alpha/2}(n-1)s/\sqrt{1+1/n}\right) \qquad (12.5)$$

is the $100(1-\alpha)\%$ prediction interval for a future observation X_{n+1}.

Now, we assume that the potency specification limits are (90, 110). Suppose that a test of a sample from a new batch yields a potency of 85, which is an OOS result. Is this observation an outlier? To answer the question, we use the data described in the previous section to calculate the 95% prediction interval:

$$\left(100.1 - 2.262 \times 4.38/\sqrt{1+1/9},\ 100.1 + 2.262 \times 4.38/\sqrt{1+1/9}\right) = (89.7, 110.5).$$

Since 85 is not within the prediction interval, it is likely that something else other than random variation has caused this outlying result.

Last, the above prediction interval for a single future observation can be generalized to construct prediction intervals for all of m future observations, or the average of these m observations. For a detailed discussion, please refer to Hahn and Meeker (1991).

12.4.2.5 Bayesian Method

The 1993 legal ruling in *United States v. Barr Laboratories* stated that the history of the product must be considered when evaluating analytical results and deciding on the disposition of the batch under evaluation. Bayesian principles provide a framework for the incorporation of historical data in an OOS investigation, in the form of a prior distribution. In addition, a Bayesian approach also facilitates a probabilistic statement of how likely an OOS result is to be a true outlier. For the purposes of illustration, we assume that X_{n+1} is a suspected outlier, and that $X_i, i = 1,...n$, are data collected from the analytical testing laboratory where the suspected OOS result X_{n+1} is observed. It is further assumed that

$$X_i \sim N(\mu, \sigma^2),$$

where both the mean μ and variance σ^2 are unknown.

12.4.2.5.1 Informative Prior

Castillo and Colosimo (2007) used the following conjugate priors to derive the predictive posterior distribution of a new observation $\tilde{X}$:

$$\mu | \sigma^2 \sim N(\mu_0, \sigma^2/\kappa_0)$$

$$\sigma^2 \sim \mathrm{Inv} - \chi^2\left(v_0, \sigma_0^2\right),$$

where the hyperparameters $\mu_0, \kappa_0, v_0,$ and σ_0^2 are assumed to be either known or estimated.

It can be easily verified that both the joint prior distribution of (μ, σ^2) and the joint posterior distribution $(\mu, \sigma^2) | \bar{X}, s^2$ are Normal – Inverse – χ^2:

$$(\mu, \sigma^2) \sim N - \mathrm{Inv} - \chi^2\left(\mu_0, \sigma_0^2 / \kappa_0; v_0, \sigma_0^2\right), \text{ and}$$

$$(\mu, \sigma^2) | \bar{X}, s^2 \sim N - \mathrm{Inv} - \chi^2\left(\mu_n, \sigma_n^2; v_n, \sigma_n^2\right),$$

where

$$\mu_n = \frac{\kappa_0}{\kappa_0 + n} \mu_0 + \frac{n}{\kappa_0 + n} \bar{X},$$

$$\kappa_n = \kappa_0 + n,$$

$$v_n = v_0 + n, \text{ and}$$

$$v_n \sigma_n^2 = v_0 \sigma_0^2 + (n-1)s^2 + \frac{\kappa_0}{\kappa_0 + n}(\bar{X} - \mu_0)^2.$$

It can be further shown that marginal posterior distributions are

$$\sigma^2 | \overline{X}, s^2 \sim \text{Inv} - \chi^2 \left(v_n, \sigma_n^2 \right) \text{ and } \mu | \overline{X}, s^2 \sim t_{v_n} \left(\mu_n, \sigma_n^2 / \kappa_n \right).$$

Therefore, the predictive posterior distribution of $\tilde{X}$ can be obtained through the following integration:

$$p(\tilde{X}|X) = \iint p(\tilde{X}|\mu, \sigma^2) | \overline{X}, X) p(\mu, \sigma^2 | X) d\mu d\sigma^2,$$

which yields

$$\tilde{X} | X \sim t_{v_n} \left(\mu_n, \frac{\sigma_n^2 (\kappa_n + 1)}{\kappa_n} \right). \tag{12.6}$$

Assume that an observed OOS result X_{OOS} exceeds the upper specification limit. X_{OOS} is a confirmed outlier if $P(\tilde{X} \geq X_{\text{OOS}} | X) < p_0$, where p_0 is a predetermined small number such as 1%. If X_{OOS} is below the lower specification limit, it is a confirmed outlier if $P(\tilde{X} \leq X_{\text{OOS}} | X) < p_0$. This probability can be obtained through a procedure modified from that by Castillo and Colosimo (2007), as follows:

1. Simulate σ_*^2 from $\text{Inv} - \chi^2 \left(v_n, \sigma_n^2 \right)$.
2. Simulate $\mu_* \sim t_{v_n} \left(\mu_n, \sigma_*^2 / \kappa_n \right)$.
3. Simulate $\tilde{X} \sim N \left(\mu_*, \sigma_*^2 \right)$.
4. Repeat Steps 1–3 m times.
5. Estimate $P(\tilde{X} \leq X_{\text{OOS}} | X)$ as the proportion of m times that $\tilde{X} \leq X_{\text{OOS}}$.

12.4.2.5.2 *Noninformative Prior*

When there are little historical data available to construct the prior distributions, one may use Jeffreys' noninformative priors (Castillo and Colosimo 2007):

$$p(\mu) \propto \text{constant}$$

$$p(\sigma^2) \propto \frac{1}{\sigma^2}.$$

Following similar derivation steps (see Castillo and Colosimo 2007 for details), we have

$$\sigma^2 | \mathbf{X} \sim \text{Inv} - \chi^2(n - 1, s^2)$$

$$\mu | \mathbf{X} \sim t_{n-1}(\bar{X}, s^2/n),$$

$$\tilde{X} | \mathbf{X} \sim t_{n-1}\left(\bar{X}, \left(1 + \frac{1}{n}s^2\right)\right). \tag{12.7}$$

Similar to the informative prior example above, the outlier assessment for the OOS investigation can be carried out through simulation, to estimate $P(\tilde{X} \leq X_{\text{OOS}} | \mathbf{X})$.

12.4.3 Multivariate Outlier Methods

In the event that there are OOS results from multiple tests of the same samples for multiple attributes, the univariate methods described in the previous sections may be applied separately to each attribute to assist the investigation of root cause. However, not accounting for the correlation among the test results for related attributes may fail to detect true outliers. Methods for multivariate control charts described in Section 8.4 can be used to detect outliers based on multivariate data.

12.4.4 Model-Based Methods

Statistical analysis of analytical data often involves fitting a model to describe the relationship between the measured response, such as potency and independent variable, and another factor such as drug concentration. Unlike identifying outliers in relation to the "center" of the data, the detection of outliers can be carried out by utilizing the relationship between the response and independent variables.

12.4.4.1 Method Based on Studentized Residuals

Although both linear and nonlinear models are commonly used to characterize analytical data, in the following discussion, we assume that the data can be adequately described through a linear model. To further simplify the discussion of the outlier detection method in the context of linear regression, we also assume that the analytical data follow the following simple linear model:

$$y_i = \alpha + \beta x_i + \varepsilon_i, \tag{12.8}$$

where y_i ($1 \leq i \leq n$) is an individual test result; x_i is the value of the ith covariate; α and β are the intercept and slope parameters, respectively; and ε_i is the ith measurement error; the ε_i values are assumed to be independently and identically distributed according to $N(0, \sigma^2)$.

In a vector–matrix format, Model 12.8 can be written as

$$\mathbf{Y} = \mathbf{Xb} + \mathbf{e},$$

where $\mathbf{Y} = (y_1,...,y_n)'$, $\mathbf{b} = (\alpha, \beta)^T$, $\mathbf{X} = \begin{pmatrix} 1 & \cdots & 1 \\ x_1 & \cdots & x_n \end{pmatrix}'_{n \times 2}$ $\mathbf{e}_i = (\varepsilon_1,..., \varepsilon_n)^T$, and $\mathbf{e} = \left(e'_1,...,e'_n\right)'$.

Let

$$\mathbf{H} = (h_{ii}) = \mathbf{X}(\mathbf{X}'\mathbf{X})^{-1}\mathbf{X}'. \tag{12.9}$$

The fitted response values are

$$\hat{\mathbf{y}} = \mathbf{Hy}. \tag{12.10}$$

The residuals are

$$\hat{\mathbf{e}} = \hat{\mathbf{y}} - \mathbf{y}, \tag{12.11}$$

with $\mathrm{var}[\hat{\mathbf{e}}] = (\mathbf{I}_n - \mathbf{H})\sigma^2$. Since $\mathrm{var}[\hat{e}_i] = (1 - h_{ii})\sigma^2$ do not have a constant variance, a large residual does not necessarily imply an outlier, and a true outlier may not have a large residual. However, this difficulty can be overcome through the following procedure. To assess the impact of a suspected outlier y_i on the regression model, a new fitted value $\hat{y}_i(i)$ is obtained from fitting Model 12.8 to a subset of data that contain all observations but y_i. It can be shown that (Iglewicz and Hoaglin 1993)

$$y_i - \hat{y}_i(i) = \frac{\hat{e}_i}{1 - h_{ii}}, \tag{12.12}$$

where the left-hand side of Equation 12.12 can be calculated from the estimates obtained from fitting all data to Model 12.8. Let s^2 and $s^2(i)$ be the residual mean squares from the regression with and without observation y_i, respectively. It can be shown that (Iglewicz and Hoaglin 1993)

$$(n-3)s^2(i) = (n-2)s^2 - \frac{\hat{e}_i^2}{1 - h_{ii}},$$

with

$$s^2 = \sum_{i=1}^{n} \hat{e}_i^2 / (n-2).$$

It can be verified that the studentized residual

$$\tilde{e}_i = \frac{\hat{e}_i}{s(i)\sqrt{1-h_{ii}}}$$

follows the Student t distribution with $n - 3$ degrees of freedom. An outlier detection method can be naturally devised by identifying observations that give rise to studentized residuals exceeding the limits $\pm t_{1-\alpha/2, n-3}$.

The studentized residual method discussed in this section can be extended to cases where either there is more than one covariate or the model is nonlinear. It is also worth pointing out that application of the linear regression model requires that the observations are independent of each other. There are situations in which multiple samples from the same preparation are tested at the same time or over time. Therefore, the measured responses are correlated. To account for the correlation structure among the observed responses, more sophisticated models are needed to describe the data and develop outlier detection methods. Tse and Xiang (2009) proposed a method based on a generalized linear mixed model. For details, please refer to their paper.

12.5 Retesting and Resampling

During the full-scale OOS investigation, additional testing of either a portion of the original sample or of different units from the same lot may be performed. However, to prevent the practice of "testing into compliance," the FDA OOS guidance (2006) clearly requires a predefined retest plan, which includes the maximum number of retests to be performed, stopping rules for retesting, and acceptance criteria for the retest results. The results from both initial testing and retesting/resampling will be used in making the decision concerning the disposition of the batch. In essence, a double-sampling plan should be defined beforehand. The plan should be designed in such a way that both the rate of falsely accepting a batch when it does not meet quality standards (consumer risk) and the rate of falsely rejecting a batch when it meets quality standards (producer risk) are minimized. In the following sections, we address the issue of how to develop a double-sampling plan for

OOS investigation. Since a double-sampling plan is an extension of a single-sampling plan, we first discuss how to develop a single-sampling plan.

12.5.1 Single-Sampling Plan

A single-sampling plan is a test scheme in which a decision concerning the disposition of a drug substance or product batch is made based on testing n units from the batch. A simple sampling plan is defined by the sample size n and a prespecified cutoff number c. The batch is accepted if there is no more than c defective units in the sample; otherwise, the batch is rejected. Whether or not a unit is defective is judged by an acceptance criterion; for example, an OOS result can be deemed defective. The two numbers n and c of a single-sampling plan are chosen such that both consumer risk (CR) and producer risk (PR) are bounded by prespecified limits. The smaller the number c is, the lower the consumer risk. For example, when c is equal to zero, the batch is accepted only if the test results of all n units are within specifications, which renders greater assurance of the batch quality than any other single-sampling plan with the same sample size. It is important to note that the probability that a batch contains units that do not meet the quality standard can never be zero. Therefore, there must be a level of defectives that is considered acceptable. This level is commonly called the acceptable quality level (AQL). By contrast, the quality level that is deemed to be unacceptable by the consumer is called consumer's quality level (CQL). In order to develop an acceptance sampling plan, both of these two numbers need to be defined in advance. It is also necessary that the AQL is smaller than the CQL; otherwise, most of the batches would not be able to pass acceptance testing. Let p_p and p_c denote the AQL and CQL, respectively. The PR and CR are defined as

$$PR = \Pr(\text{Reject the lot, given the true proportion}$$
$$\text{of defects in the lot is AQL}) = 1 - \Pr(x \le c \mid p_p)$$

$$CR = \Pr(\text{Accept the lot, given the true proportion}$$
$$\text{of defects in the lot is CQL}) = \Pr(x \le c \mid p_c).$$

To calculate the above probabilities, statistical assumptions about the sampling distributions need to be made. Suppose that the batch size is N and there are d units in the batch that are defective. Under these assumptions, the number of defectives x in a sample of size n can be described through a hypergeometric distribution:

$$\Pr(x;d,N,n) = \binom{d}{x}\binom{N-d}{n-x} \Big/ \binom{N}{n}. \tag{12.13}$$

Thus, PR and CR are obtained as

$$PR = 1 - \sum_{i=0}^{c} \Pr(i; d_p, N, n)$$

$$= 1 - \sum_{i=0}^{c} \binom{d_p}{i} \binom{N - d_p}{n - i} \Big/ \binom{N}{n}, \tag{12.14}$$

$$CR = \sum_{i=0}^{c} \Pr(i; d_c, N, n)$$

$$= \sum_{i=0}^{c} \binom{d_c}{i} \binom{N - d_c}{n - i} \Big/ \binom{N}{n}, \tag{12.15}$$

where $d_p = Np_p$ and $d_c = Np_c$ are expected numbers of defectives from the batch when its quality level is AQL or CQL, respectively.

For a large batch size N, the hypergeometric distribution can be approximated by a binomial distribution. Thus, PR and CR are obtained as

$$PR = 1 - \sum_{i=0}^{c} \binom{n}{i} p_p^i (1 - p_p)^{n-i}$$

$$CR = \sum_{i=0}^{c} \binom{n}{i} p_c^i (1 - p_c)^{n-i}. \tag{12.16}$$

12.5.2 Double-Sampling Plan

A double-sampling plan provides a questionable batch another chance if the test results of the first sample are inclusive. A decision concerning disposition of the batch can be reached either after testing the first sample or at the end of the second testing. Initially, a sample of size n_1 is taken randomly from the batch and the number of defectives x_1 is counted. If $x_1 \leq c_1$, the first acceptance number, the batch is accepted. If $x_1 > r_1$, the rejection number, the batch is rejected. Otherwise, if $c_1 < x \leq r_1$, a second sample of size n_2 is taken and the total number of defectives $x_T = x_1 + x_2$ is determined. The batch is accepted if $x_T \leq c_2$, the acceptance number for the combined samples; otherwise, the batch is rejected. The sample sizes n_1 and n_2 and the acceptance numbers c_1

and c_2 are chosen to ensure that PR and CR are within prespecified limits. We assume that the number of defectives follows a binomial distribution. The PR and CR can be readily calculated:

$$PR = P(\text{Reject the lot, given the lot has an acceptable } p_p)$$

$$= 1 - P(\text{Accept the lot, given the lot has an acceptable } p_p)$$

$$= 1 - [P(x_1 \le c_1) + P(x_1 = c_1 + 1)P(x_2 \le c_2 - x_1) + \ldots + P(x_1 = r_1)P(x_2 \le c_2 - x_1)]$$

$$= 1 - \left\{ \sum_{i=0}^{c_1} \binom{n_1}{i} p_p^i (1-p_p)^{n_1-i} + \sum_{j=c_1+1}^{r_1} \binom{n_1}{j} p_p^j (1-p_p)^{n_1-j} \sum_{k=0}^{c_2-j} \binom{n_2}{k} p_p^k (1-p_p)^{n_2-k} \right\}.$$

Similarly,

$$CR = P(\text{Accept the lot, given the lot has an acceptable } p_c)$$

$$= P(x_1 \le c_1) + P(x_1 = c_1 + 1)P(x_2 \le c_2 - x_1) + \ldots$$

$$+ P(x_1 = r_1)P(x_2 \le c_2 - x_1)]$$

$$= \sum_{i=0}^{c_1} \binom{n_1}{i} p_c^i (1-p_c)^{n_1-i} + \sum_{j=c_1+1}^{r_1} \binom{n_1}{j} p_c^j (1-p_c)^{n_1-j} \sum_{k=0}^{c_2-j} \binom{n_2}{k} p_c^k (1-p_c)^{n_2-}.$$

(12.17)

By properly choosing the sample size and decision rules, double-sampling plans can provide the same levels of protection to the consumer and producer risks as a single-sampling plan. In addition, on average, it also has a smaller average sample size than a single-sampling plan with the same AQL and RQL. However, it is logistically more complicated to implement than a single-sampling plan.

12.5.3 Retesting and Resampling Plans

A full-scale OOS investigation may include either retesting a portion of the original sample or resampling from the batch in question (FDA 2006). Retesting refers to testing these additional samples from the same homogeneous material for which the OOS results were observed, while resampling consists of analyzing additional units collected as part of the original sampling procedure or from a new sample from the same batch. In either situation, the purpose of retesting is to assess whether the additional results help explain the initial OOS result(s) so that the batch can be properly disposed. The double-sampling plan discussed in the previous section can be used to lend statistical vision to the OOS investigation.

12.6 Investigation of OOT Results

The issue of OOT results is often raised in the context of stability testing of a drug product, which is known to degrade over time. There has not been a consensus on the definition of an OOT result. Per the PhRMA CMC Statistics and Expert Teams, consisting of representatives from PhRMA member companies (hereafter, we refer to the group as Stability Teams) (2005), an OOT result is a stability result that does not follow the expected trend, either in comparison with other stability batches or with respect to previous results from the batch collected during a stability study. We refer to the former as a batch OOT and the latter as a single-value OOT. Figures 12.3 and 12.4 show examples of these two types of OOT results.

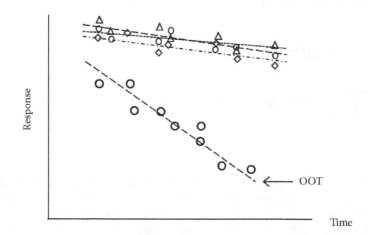

FIGURE 12.3
A batch appears to be out of trend when compared to results of other batches.

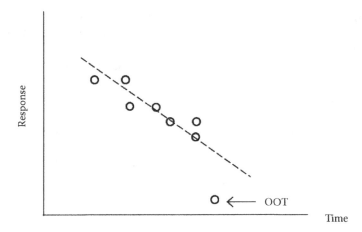

FIGURE 12.4
A single value does not appear to trend well with data collected from the same study.

As noted by the Stability Teams (2005), the identification of OOT results has increasingly become a regulatory issue for commercial drug products. Although the legal and regulatory basis to mandate OOT result investigations does not exist, an OOT result may eventually lead to an OOS result. Therefore, the identification of OOT results is a good industry practice. However, despite the importance of identifying OOT results and their root cause, how to conduct effective OOT investigations has not been fully addressed in scientific literature or regulatory guidance. An attempt was made by the Stability Teams to tackle OOT-related issues, review current practices, and summarize potential solutions, which led to a publication (2005). This chapter presents four statistical methods discussed in that publication that can be potentially used to address OOT issues. They include the (1) regression control chart method, (2) by time point method, (3) slope control chart method, and (4) Z-score method. Each method is briefly described below.

12.6.1 Regression Control Chart Method

This approach is used to confirm a suspected OOT result, based on data from the same stability study. It is assumed that the data can be described through a linear or nonlinear model. For the sake of illustration, a linear model (Equation 12.8) is assumed to be appropriate for describing the data. Let $(\hat{\alpha}, \hat{\beta}, \hat{\sigma}^2)$ be the least square estimators of $(\alpha, \beta, \sigma^2)$. Regression control limits can be obtained as

$$\hat{\alpha} + \hat{\beta}x \pm k\hat{\sigma}, \tag{12.18}$$

where the multiplier k is chosen to provide expected level of confidence. As discussed in Chapter 11, k can be selected such that the limits in Equation

12.18 can be interpreted as confidence, prediction, or tolerance limits. Since the goal here is to confirm a suspected value as a real OOT or not OOT, it may be appropriate to establish the limits in Equation 12.18 as prediction limits. A result is considered OOT if it is outside of the control limits.

12.6.2 By Time Point Method

When data from other batches are available, the behavior of a batch can be assessed based on a cross section of historical data collected at each stability time point. The limits at a given time point t are expressed as

$$\bar{X}_t \pm ks_t, \tag{12.19}$$

where $\bar{X}_t$ and s_t are mean and sample standard deviation at time t.

The Stability Teams (2005) suggested choosing k in Equation 12.19 so that the limits form a tolerance interval. However, because there is variability attributed to both batch and analytical method, the tolerance interval at each time point cannot be simply obtained by a proper choice of the multiplier k in Equation 12.19. Assuming a balanced design in which the number of observations from each batch is the same across all batches at a given time point, two alternative methods can be used to obtain the tolerance interval. The first method was proposed by Hoffman and Kringle (2005). The second approach was suggested by Krishnamoorthy and Mathew (2009) based on GPQ analysis. See Chapter 2 for detailed discussions of the two methods.

12.6.3 Slope Control Chart Method

A third approach suggested by the Stability Teams (2005) is to detect single-value OOT results by comparing the slope at the time point with the suspected OOT result(s) to the range of expected slope calculated from historical batches. At each time point, a linear regression analysis is performed and the slope is estimated for each batch. Assuming normality of measurement errors, the least squares estimate of slope follows a normal distribution. Therefore, the expected range of slopes can be calculated as a tolerance interval, based on the slope estimates at each time point.

12.7 Concluding Remarks

Inadequate OOS investigations comprise a major cause of FDA warning letters. Although the FDA issued guidance on investigating OOS test results in pharmaceutical production, little detail is offered on statistical methods for this purpose. Different interpretations of the guidance are likely to lead to the adoption of inconsistent approaches for OOS investigations. In addition, there is a growing concern among regulators and scientists involved in pharmaceutical manufacturing regarding how OOT results are identified. Despite the potentially serious consequences of OOT results, there are a limited number of publications on the subject. In this chapter, various statistical methods were discussed for OOS result investigations and OOT result identification. Since there is no consensus on the methods or statistical evaluations of the performance of these methods, further research into OOS and OOT issues is definitely warranted.

References

Adley, C. et al. (2015). Bioburden and biofilm management in pharmaceutical drug substance manufacturing. PDA Technical Report No. 69.

Agresti, A. (1990). *Categorical Data Analysis*. John Wiley & Sons, New York.

Akers, J. (2008). Microbiological considerations in selection and validation of filter sterilization. In *Filtration and Purification in the Pharmaceutical Industry*, ed by Jornitz, M.W. and Melzer, T.H., Informa Healthcare Inc.

Allen, P.V., Dukes, G.R., and Gerger, M.E. (1991). Determination of release limits: A general methodology. *Pharm. Res.* 9(9), 1210–1213.

Ahmed, M., Aqqar, B., Gu, F., and Ball, D. (2012). Fault Detection and Diagnosis Using Principal Component Analysis of Vibration Data from a Reciprocating Compressor. *2012 UKACC International Conference on Control*, Cardiff, UK. https://www.researchgate.net/publication/261147617_Fault_detection_and _diagnosis_using_Principal_Component_Analysis_of_vibration_data_from_a _reciprocating_compressor.

Anscombe, F.J. (1973). Graphs in statistical analysis. *Am Stat.*, 27(1), 17–21.

Arfaj, A.S.A., Chowdhary, A.R., Khalil, N., and Ali, R. (2007). Immunogenicity of singlet oxygen modified human DNA: Implications for anti-DNA antibodies in systemic lupus erythematosus. *Clin. Immunol*, 124, 83–89.

Baltimore, D. (1970). RNA-dependent DNA polymerase in virions of RNA tumour viruses. *Nature*, 226, 1209–1211.

Banerjee, S. and Roy, A. (2014). *Linear Algebra and Matrix Analysis for Statistics, Texts in Statistical Science*. 1st ed., Chapman and Hall/CRC.

Barron, A.M. (1994). Use of fractional factorial (or matrix) designs in stability analysis. *Proceedings of Biopharmaceutical Section of American Statistical Association*. Alexandria, VA.

Berger, R.L. (1982). Multiparameter hypothesis testing and acceptance sampling. *Technometrics*, 24, 295–300.

Berger, R.L. and Hsu, J.C. (1996). Bioequivalence trials, intersection-union tests, and equivalence confidence sets. *Stat. Sci.* 11, 283–319.

Billingsley, P. (1986). *Probability and Measure*. John Wiley & Sons.

Bissell, A.F. (1990). How reliable is your capability index? *Applied Stat.*, 39(3), 331–340.

Borman, P., Nethercote, P., Chaftield, M., Thompson, D., and Truman, K. (2007). The application of quality by design to analytical methods. *Pharm. Technol.*, 31(10), 142–152.

Boulanger, B., Chiap, P., Dewe, W. et al. (2003). An analysis of the SFSTP guide on validation of chromatographic bioanalytical methods: Progresses and limitations. *J. Pharm. Biomed. Anal.* 32, 753–765.

Boulanger, B., Devanaryan, V., Dewe, W., and Smith, W. (2007a). Statistical considerations in analytical method validation. In *Pharmaceutical Statistics Using SAS: A Practical Guide,* ed by Dmitrienko, A., Chuang-Stein, C., and D'Agostino, R., SAS Publishing.

Boulanger, B., Dewe, W., Gibert, A., Govaerts, B., and Maumy-Bertrand, M. (2007b). Risk management for analytical methods based on the total error concept: Concilating the objectives of the pre-study and in-study validation phases. *Chemom. Intell. Lab. Syst.*, 86, 198–207.

Boyd, S. and Vandenberghe, L. (2004). *Convex Optimization.* Cambridge University Press.

Brüggemann, L., Wolfang, Q., and Wennrich, R. (2006). Test for non-linearity concerning linear calibrated chemical measurements. *Accred. Qual. Assur.*, 11, 625–631.

Bryder, M., Etling, H., Fleming, J., Hu, Y., and Levy, P. (2015). Topic 1—Stage 2 process validation: Determining and justifying the number of process qualification batches, ISPE discussion paper: PV stage 2, number of batches (version 2). https://www.pharmamedtechbi.com/~/media/Supporting%20Documents /The%20Gold%20Sheet/47/2/stage2processvalidation1.pdf.

Burdick, R.K., LeBlond, D., Sandell, D., and Yang, H. (2013). Statistical methods for validation of procedure accuracy and precision. *Pharmacopeial Forum*, 39(3).

Callahan, J.D. and Sajjadi, N.C. (2003). Testing the null hypothesis for a specified difference—The right way to test for parallelism. *BioProcess. J.*, Mar/Apr 1–6.

Capen, C., Christopher, D., Forenzo, P., Ireland, C., Liu, O., Lyapustina, S., O'Neill, J., Patterson, N., Quinlan, M., Sandell, D., Schwenke, J., Stroup, W., and Tougas, T. (2012). On the shelf life of pharmaceutical products. *AAPS Pharm. Sci. Technol.*, 13(3), 911–918.

Caputo, R.A. and Huffman, A. (2004). Environmental monitoring: Data trending using a frequency model. *PDA J. Pharm. Sci. Technol.*, 58(5), 254–260.

Cartensen, J.T. and Nelson, E. (1976). Terminology regarding labeled and contained amounts in dosage forms. *J. Pharm. Sci.*, 65(2), 311–312.

Casella, G. and Berger, R.L. (1990). *Statistical Inference.* Duxbury Press, Belmont, CA.

Cassella, G. and Berger, R. (2002). *Statistical Inference.* Duxbury.

Castillo, E.D. and Colosimo, B.M. (2007). An introduction to Bayesian inference in process monitoring, control and optimization. In *Bayesian Process Monitoring, Control and Optimization*, ed by Colosimo, B.M. and Castillo, E.D., Chapman & Hall/CRC.

Chow, S.-C. (2007). *Statistical Design and Analysis of Stability Studies.* Chapman & Hall/CRC.

Chow, S.-C. and Liu, J.-P. (1992). *Design and Analysis of Bioavailability and Bioequivalence Studies.* Marcel Dekker, Inc., New York, Basel, Hong Kong.

Chow, S.-C. and Liu, J.-P. (2008). *Design and Analysis of Bioavailability and Bioequivalence Studies.* Chapman and Hall/CRC.

Christensen, A., Melgaard, H., and Iwersen, J. (2003). Environmental monitoring based on a hierarchical Poisson–Gamma model. *J. Qual. Technol.*, 35(3), 275–285.

Clinical Laboratory Standard Institute (CLSI) (2003). Evaluation of the Linearity of Quantitative Measurement Procedures: A Statistical Approach; Approved Guideline. http://www.clsi.org/source/orders/free/ep6-a.pdf.

Clopper, C.J. and Pearson, E.S. (1934). The use of confidence or fiducial limits illustrated in the case of the binomial. *Biometrika*, 26(4), 404–413.

CMC Biotech Working Group (2009). A-Mab: A Case Study in Bioprocess Development. www.casss.org/associations/9165/.../A-Mab_Case_Study_Version_2-1.pdf (accessed on April 15, 2016).

CMC Vaccine Working Group (2012). A-VAX: Applying Quality by Design to Vaccines. www.ispe.org (accessed on April 15, 2016).

Colgan, C., Hanna-Brown, M., Pellett, J., Wrisley, L., Sluggett, G., Morgado, J., Harrington, B., Szucs, R., Barnett, K., Graul, T., and Steeno, G. (2014). Using quality by design to develop robust chromatographic methods. *Pharm. Technol.*, 38(8), http://www.pharmtech.com/using-quality-design-develop-robust-chromatographic-methods (accessed on April 14, 2016).

Conover, W.J. (1999). *Practical Nonparametric Statistics*. 3rd ed. Wiley, New York.

Cook, J. (2009). Note on negative binomial distribution. http://www.johndcook.com/negative binomial.pdf (accessed on April 16, 2016).

Daniel, C. (1985). Patterns in residuals from a line through five points. Presented to the Northern New Jersey Chapter of the American Statistical Association. May 6, 1985.

Darling, A.J. (2000). Design and interpretation of viral clerance studies for biopharmaceutical products. In *Methods in Biotechnology, Vol. 9: Downstream Processing of Proteins: Methods and Protocols*, ed by Desai. M.A., Humana Press Inc., Totowa, NJ.

Darling, A.J., Boose, J.A., and Spaltro, J. (1998). Virus assay methods: Accuracy and validation. *Biologicals*, 26, 105–110.

Dean, R.B. and Dixon, W.J. (1951). Simplified statistics for small numbers of observations. *Anal. Chem.*, 23(4), 636–638.

DeGroot, M.H. (1986). *Probability and Statistics*. 2nd ed., Addison–Wesley.

DeSilva, B., Smith, W., Weiner, R. et al. (2003). Recommendations for the bioanalytical method validation of ligand-binding assays to support pharmacokinetic assessments of macromolecules. *Pharm. Res.*, 20, 1885–1900.

DeVor, R.E., Chang, T.H., and Sutherland, J.W. (1992). *Statistical Quality Design and Control*. Macmillan Publishing Company.

Dortant, P.M., Claaaswn, I.J., van Kreyl, C.F., van Steenis, G., and Wester, P.W. (1997). Risk assessment on the carcinogenic potential of hybridoma cell DNA: Implications for residual contaminating cellular DNA in biological products. *Biologicals*, 25(4), 381–390.

Drezner, Z. and Wesolowsky, G.O. (1989). On the computation of the bivariate normal integral. *Journal of Statist. Comput. Simul.*, 35, 101–107.

EFPIA/PhRMa (2010). Pharmaceutical Research and Manufacturers of America Analytical Technical Group and European Federation of Pharmaceutical Industries and Associations (EFPIA) Analytical Design Space Topic Team. Implications and opportunities of applying QbD principles to analytical measurements. *Pharm. Technol.*, 34(2), 52–59.

Elliott, P., Billingham, S., Bi, J., and Zhang, H. (2013). Quality by design for biopharmaceuticals: A historical review and guide for implementation. *Pharm. Bioprocess.*, 1(1), 105–122.

EMA (1995). ICH Topic Q2 (R1) Validation of Analytical Procedures: Text and Methodology. http://www.ema.europa.eu/docs/en_GB/document_library/Scientific_guideline/2009/09/WC500002662.pdf (accessed on April 17, 2016).

EMA (1996). CPMP Note for Guidance on Manufacture of Finished Dosage Form.

EMA (1997). ICH Topic Q5A (R1) Quality of Biotechnological Products: Viral Safety Evaluation of Biotechnology Products Derived from Cell Lines of Human or Animal Origin. CPMP/ICH/295/95. Canary Wharf, London. http://www.ema.europa.eu/docs/en_GB/document_library/Scientific_guideline/2009/09/WC500002801.pdf (accessed on April 17, 2016).

EMA (2001). Note for Guidance on Plasma-Derived Medicinal Products.

EMA (2006). Guideline on Virus Safety Evaluation of Biotechnological Investigational Medicinal Products.

EMA (2012). EMA Guideline on the Requirements for Quality Documentation Concerning Biological Investigational Medicinal Products in Clinical Trials.

Erdman, D., Jackson, L., and Sinko, A. (2008). Zero-inflated Poisson and zero-inflated negative binomial models using the COUNTREG procedure. *SAS Global Forum*, 2008.

Ermer, J. and Nethercote, P. (2015). *Method Validation in Pharmaceutical Analysis*. Wiley-VCH, Verlag GmbH & Co. KGaA.

European Biopharmaceutical Enterprise (EBE) (2013). EBE Concept Paper: Considerations in setting specification. http://www.ebe-biopharma.eu/documents/47/25/Considerations-in-Setting-Specifications.

European Directorate for the Quality of Medicines (2004). *European Pharmacopoeia*, Chapter 5.3, Statistical Analysis. EDQM, Strasburg, France; 473–507.

Faddy, M.J. and Smith, D.M. (2008). Extended Poisson process modelling of dilution series data. *Applied Stats.*, 57(4), 461–471.

Fay, M.P. (2010). Two-sided exact tests and matching confidence intervals for discrete data. *The R Journal*, 2(1), 53–58.

FDA (1987). Guideline for Submitting Documentation for the Stability of Human Drugs and Biologics. Center for Drugs and Biologics, Office of Drug Research and Review, Food and Drug Administration, Rockville, MD.

FDA (1993). Points to Consider in the Characeterization of Cell Lines Used to Produce Biologicals. FDA, Bethesda, MD.

FDA (1997). Points to Consider in the Manufacture and Testing of Monocloncal Antibody Products for Human Use.

FDA (2000). Guidance for Industry (Draft): Analytical Procedures and Methods Validation. http://www.fda.gov/cder/guidance.

FDA (2001a). Guidance for Industry: Statistical Approaches to Establishing Bioequivalence. U.S. Department of Health and Human Services, Food and Drug Administration, Center for Drug Evaluation and Research (CDER), January 2001.

FDA (2001b). Guidance for Industry: Bioanalytical Methods Validation.

FDA (2004a). Pharmaceutical cGMPs for the 21st Century: A Risk-Based Approach: Final Report.

FDA (2004b). Guidance for Industry: PAT—A Framework for Innovative Pharmaceutical Development, Manufacturing and Quality Assurance.

FDA (2004c). FDA Guidance for Industry: Sterile Drug Products Produced by Aseptic Processing—Current Good Manufacturing Practice.

FDA (2006). Guidance for Industry: Investigating Out-of-Specification (OOS) Test Results for Pharmaceutical Production.

FDA (2010). Guidance for Industry: Characterization and Qualification of Cell Substrates and Other Biological Materials Used in the Production of Viral Vaccines for Infectious Disease Indications. U.S. Department of Health and Human Services, Food and Drug Administration Center for Biologics Evaluation and Research.

FDA (2011). Guidance for Industry on Process Validation: General Principles and Practices.

FDA (2015). Guidance for Industry: Analytical Procedures and Methods Validation for Drugs and Biologics. http://www.fda.gov/downloads/drugs/guidance complianceregulatoryinformation/guidances/ucm386366.pdf (accessed on April 17, 2016).

Fieller, E.C. (1944). A fundamental formula in the statistics of biological assay and some applications. *J. Pharm. Pharmacol.*, 17, 117–123.

Findlay, J.W.A., Smith, W.C., Lee, J.W. et al. (2000). Validation of immunoassays for bioanalysis: A pharmaceutical industry perspective. *J. Pharm. Biomed. Anal.*, 21, 1249–1273.

Finney, D.J. (1938). The distribution of the ratio of the estimates of the two variances in a sample from a bivariate normal population. *Biometrika*, 30, 190–192.

Finney, D.J. (1978). *Statistical Method in Biological Assay.* 3rd ed., Charles Griffin & Co., London and High Wycombe.

Gelman, A., Carlin, J., Stern, H., and Rubin, D. (2004). *Bayesian Data Analysis.* 2nd ed., New York, Chapman & Hall.

Gottschalk, P.J. and Dunn, J.R. (2005). Measuring parallelism, linearity, and relative potency in bioassay and immunoassay data. *J. Biopharm. Stat.*, 15(3), 437–463.

Govaerts, B., Dewe, W., Maumy, M. and Boulanger, B. (2008). Pre-study analytical method validation: Comparison of four alternative approaches based on quality-level estimation and tolerance intervals. *Qual. Reliab. Eng. Int.*, 24, 557–680.

Graybill, F.A. and Wang, C.M. (1980). Confidence intervals on nonnegative linear combinations of variances. *J. Am. Stat. Assoc.*, 75, 869–873.

Greenwood, P.E. and Nikulin, M.S. (1996). *A Guide to Chi-squared Testing.* Wiley, New York.

Gronemeyer, P., Ditz, R., and Strube, J. (2014). Trends in upstream and downstream process development for antibody manufacturing. *Bioengineering*, 1, 188–212.

Grubb, F.E. (1950). Sample criteria for testing outlying observations. *Ann. Math. Stat.*, 21(1): 27–58.

Guenther, W. (1972). Simple approximation to the negative binomial (and regular binomial). *Technometrics*, 14, 385–398.

Haaland, P. (1989). *Experimental Design in Biotechnology.* CRC Press.

Hahn, G.J. (1970). Statistical intervals for a normal population, Part 4, Formulas, assumptions, some derivations. *J. Qual. Technol.*, 2, 195–206.

Hahn, G.J. and Meeker, W.Q. (1991). *Statistical Interval: A Guide for Practitioners.* Wiley.

Hahn G.J. and Nelson, W. (1973). A survey of prediction intervals and their applications. *J. Qual. Technol.*, 5(4), 178–188.

Haight, F.A. (1967). *Handbook of the Poisson Distribution.* John Wiley & Sons, New York.

Hampel, F.R. (1974). The influence curve and its role in robust estimation. *J. Am. Stat. Assoc.*, 69, 382–393.

Hanley, J.A. (1989). Receiver operating characteristic (ROC) methodology: The state of the art. *Crit. Rev. Diagn. Imaging*, 29, 307–335.

Hauck, W.W., Capen, R.C., Callahan, J.D., Muth, J.E.D., Hsu, H., Lansky, D., Sajjadi, N.C., Seaver, S.S., Singer, R.R. and Weisman, D. (2005). Assessing parallelism prior to determining relative potency. *PDA J. Pharm. Sci. Technol.*, 59, 127–137.

Hazewinkel, M. (2001). Trapezium formula. In *Encyclopedia of Mathematics.* Springer.

Hilbe, J.M. (2007). *Negative Binomial Regression.* Cambridge University Press, Cambridge, UK.

Hinkley, D.V. (1969). On the ratio of two correlated normal random variables. *Biometrika*, 56, 635–639.

Hofer, D. (2009). Discussion. *J. Qual. Technol.*, 41(2), 137–139.

Hoffman, D. (2004). Negative binomial control limits for count data with extra-Poisson variation. *Pharm. Stat.*, 2, 127–132.

Hoffman, D. and Kringle, R. (2005). Two-sided tolerance intervals for balanced and unbalanced random effects models. *J. Biopharm. Stat.*, 15(2) 283–293.

Hoffman, D. and Kringle, R. (2007). A total error approach for the validation of quantitative analytical methods. *Pharm. Res.*, 24, 1157–1164.

Hotelling, H. (1947). Multivariate quality control illustrated by the air testing of sample bombsights. In *Techniques of Statistical Analysis*, ed by Eisenhart, C., Hastay, M.W., and Wallis, W.A., McGraw-Hill, New York.

Hotelling, H. (1951). A generalized *t* test and measure of multivariate dispersion. *Proceedings of the Second Berkeley Symposium on Mathematical Statistics and Probability*. University of California Press, Los Angeles and Berkeley, 23–42.

Hsieh, E., Hsiao, C.-F., and Liu J.-P. (2009). Statistical methods for evaluating the linearity in assay validation. *J. Chemom.*, 23, 56–63.

Hsieh, E. and Liu, J.-P. (2008). On statistical evaluation of the linearity in assay validation. *J. Biopharm. Stat.*, 18, 677–690.

Hubert, Ph., Nguyen-Huu, J.J., Boulanger B. et al. (2004). Harmonization of strategies for the validation of quantitative analytical procedures: A SFSTP proposal—Part I. *J. Pharm. Biomed. Anal.*, 36, 579–586.

Hubert, Ph., Nguyen-Huu, J.J., Boulanger B. et al. (2007a). Harmonization of strategies for the validation of quantitative analytical procedures: A SFSTP proposal—Part II. *J. Pharm. Biomed. Anal.*, 45, 70–81.

Hubert, Ph., Nguyen-Huu, J.J., Boulanger B. et al. (2007b). Harmonization of strategies for the validation of quantitative analytical procedures: A SFSTP proposal—Part III. *J. Pharm. Biomed. Anal.*, 45, 82–96.

ICH (1993). Q1A Stability Testing of New Drug Substances and Products.

ICH (1995a). Q2A Validation of Analytical Methods: Definitions and Terminology. http://www.pharma.gally.ch/ich/q2a038195en.pdf (accessed on April 17, 2016).

ICH (1995b). Q5C Quality of Biotechnological Products: Stability Testing of Biotechnological/Biological Products.

ICH (1996). Q2 Validation of Analytical Procedures: Methodology. http://www.fda.gov/downloads/drugs/guidancecomplianceregulatoryinformation/guidances/ucm073384.pdf.

ICH (1998). Q1B Photostability Testing of New Active Substances and Medicinal Products.

ICH (1999a). ICH Q6A Specifications: Test Procedures and Acceptance Criteria for New Drug Substances and New Drug Products: Chemical Substances.

ICH (1999b). ICH Q6B Specifications: Test Procedures and Acceptance Criteria for Biotechnological/Biological Product. EMEA, September.

ICH (2002). Q1D Bracketing & Matrixing Designs for Stability Testing of New Drug Substances and Drug Products.

ICH (2003a). Q1A (R2) Stability Testing of New Drug Substances and Products.

ICH (2003b). Q1E Evaluation of Stability Data.

ICH (2005). Q2 (R1) Validation of Analytical Procedures: Text and Methodology—International Conference on Harmonization of Technical Requirements for Registration of Pharmaceuticals for Human Use. http://www.ich.org/fileadmin/Public_Web_Site/ICH_Products/Guidelines/Quality/Q2_R1/Step4/Q2_R1__Guideline.pdf.

ICH (2006). Q8 (R2) Pharmaceutical Development. http://www.fda.gov/downloads/Drugs/.../Guidances/ucm073507.pdf.

ICH (2007a). Q9 Quality Risk Management. http://www.ich.org/fileadmin/Public_Web_Site/ICH_Products/Guidelines/Quality/Q9/Step4/Q9_Guideline.pdf.

ICH (2007b). Q10 Pharmaceutical Quality Systems. http://www.fda.gov/downloads /Drugs/.../Guidances/ucm073517.pdf.

ICH (2011). Q11 Concept Paper. http://www.ema.europa.eu/docs/en_GB/document _library/Scientific_guideline/2011/06/WC500107128.pdf.

Iglewicz, B. and Hoaglin, D. (1993). Volume 16: How to Detect and Handle Outliers. In *The ASQ Basic References in Quality Control: Statistical Techniques*, ed by Mykytka, E.F., American Society for Quality (ASQ).

Ishii, K.J., Gursel, I., Gursel, M., and Klinman, D.M. (2004). Immunotherapeutic utility of stimulatory and suppressive oligodeoxynucleotides. *Curr. Opin. Mol. Ther.*, 6, 166–174.

Ishikawa, K. (1968). *Guide to Quality Control*. JUSE, Tokyo.

Jackson, J.E. (1956). Quality control methods for two related variables. *Industrial Quality Control*, XII, 7, 4–8.

Jackson, J.E. (1959). Quality control methods for several related variables. *Technometrics*, 1(4), 359–377.

Jackson, J.E. and Bradley, R.A. (1959). Multivariate sequential procedures for testing means. The Development of Statistical Methods for Experimental Design in Quality Control and Surveillance Testing, Tech. Report No. 10, Virginia Polytechnic Institute.

Jackson, J.E. and Bradley, R.A. (1961a). Sequential x2 and T2 tests and their application to an acceptance sampling problem. *Technometrics*, 3, 519–534.

Jackson, J.E. and Bradley, R.A. (1961b). Sequential x2 and T2 Tests. *Ann. Math. Stat.*, 32, 1063–1077.

Jenkins, G.I. (1967). Multivariate methods applied to product testing and specifications. *J. R. Stat. Soc., Ser. D*, 17(2), 141–155.

Johnson, N.L., Kemp, A.W., and Kotz, S. (2005). *Univariate Discrete Distributions*. 3rd ed., Wiley.

Jonkman, J. and Sidik, K. (2009). Equivalence testing for parallelism in the four-parameter logistic model. *J. Biopharm. Stat.*, 19(5), 818–837.

Jornitz, M.W., Akers, J.E., Agalloco, J.P., Madsen, R.E., and Melzer, T.H. (2003). Considerations in sterile filtration. Part II: The sterilizing filter and its organism challenge: A critique of regulatory standards. *PDA J. Pharm. Sci. Technol.*, 57(2), 88–96.

Kiermeier, A., Jarrett, R.G., and Verbyla, A.P. (2004). A new approach to estimating shelf-life. *Pharm. Stat.*, 3:3–11.

Klinman, D.M., Xie, H., and Ivins, B.E. (2006). CpG oligonucleotides improve the protective immune response induced by the licensed anthrax vaccine. *Ann. N. Y. Acad. Sci.*, 1082, 137–150.

Klinman, D.M., Yamshchikov, G., and Ishigatsubo, Y. (1997). Contribution of CpG motifs to the immunogenicity of DNA vaccines. *J. Immunol.*, 158, 3635–3639.

Kojima, Y., Xin, K.-Q., Ooki, T., Hamajima, K., Oikawa, T., Shinoda, K., Ozaki, T., Hoshino, Y., Jounai, N., Nakazawa, M., Kinman, D., and Okuda, K. (2002). Adjuvant effect of multi-CpG motifs on an HIV-1 DNA vaccine. *Vaccine*, 20, 2857–2865.

Komka, K., Kemeny, S., and Banfai, B. (2010). Novel tolerance interval model for the estimation of the shelf life of pharmaceutical products. *J. Chemom.*, 24(3–4), 131–139.

Kourti, T. and MacGregor, J.F. (1995). Process analysis, monitoring and diagnosis, using multivariate projection methods. *Chemom. Intell. Lab. Syst.*, 28, 3–21.

Kozlowski, S. and Swann, P. (2009). Considerations for biotechnology product quality by design. In *Quality by Design for Biopharmaceuticals: Principles and Case Studies*, ed by Rathore, A.S. and Mhatre, R., Wiley & Sons, Inc.

Krause, P.R. and Lewis, Jr., A.M. (1998). Safety of viral DNA in biological products. *Biologicals*, 36(3), 184–197.

Kringle, R.O. and Khan-Malek, R.C. (1994). A statistical assessment of the recommendations from a conference on analytical methods validation in bioavailability, bioequivalence, and pharmacokinetic studies. *Proceedings of the Biopharmaceutical Section of the American Statistical Association*. Alexandria, VA, 510–514.

Krishnamoorthy, K. and Mathew, T. (2004). One-sided tolerance limits in balanced and unbalanced one-way random models based on generalized confidence limits. *Technometrics*, 46, 44–52.

Krishnamoorthy, K. and Mathew, T. (2009). *Statistical Tolerance Regions: Theory, Applications, and Computation*. Wiley.

Kroll, M.H., Præstgaard, J., Michaliszyn, E., and Styer, P.E. (2000). Evaluation of the extent of nonlinearity in reportable range studies. *Arch. Pathol. Lab. Med.*, 124, 1331–1338.

Krouwer, J. and Schlain, B. (1993). A method to quantify deviations from assay linearity. *Clin. Chem.*, 39(8), 1689–1693.

Kushler, R.H. and Hurley, P. (1992). Confidence bounds for capability indices. *J. Qual. Technol.*, 24(4), 188–195.

Lambert, D. (1992). Zero-inflated Poisson regression models with an application to defects in manufacturing. *Technometrics*, 34, 1–14.

LeBlond, D., Tan, C., and Yang, H. (2013). Confirmation of analytical method calibration linearity. *Pharmacopeial Forum*, May–June Issue, 39(3).

LeBrun, P. (2012). Bayesian design space applied to pharmaceutical. Unpublished dissertation. University de Liege https://www.google.com/url?sa=t&rct=j&q=&esrc=s&frm=1&source=web&cd=3&ved=0ahUKEwijkrXoq8HKAhXI1x4KHXjoDEYQFggoMAI&url=https%3A%2F%2Forbi.ulg.ac.be%2Fbitstream%2F2268%2F126503%2F1%2Fthesis.pdf&usg=AFQjCNG-IxFztbhvUfL_3qMwMqKXH4LvZw&bvm=bv.112454388,d.dmo.

Lee, J., Devanarayan, V., Barrett, Y., Weiner, R., Allinson, J., Fountain, S., Keller, S., Weinryb, I., Green, M., Duan, L., Rogers, J., Millham, R., O'Brien, P., Sailstad, J., Khan, M., Ray, C., and Wagner, J. (2006). Fit-for-purpose method development and validation for successful biomarker measurement. *Pharm. Res.*, 23(2), 312–328.

Lehmann, E.L. and Romano, J.R. (2005). *Testing Statistical Hypothesis*. Springer.

Lewis, Jr., A.M., Krause, P., and Peden, K. (2001). A defined-risks approach to the regulatory assessment of the use of neoplastic cells as substrates for viral vaccine manufacture. *Dev. Biol. (Basel)*, 106, 513–535.

Li, N. and Yang, H. (2012). Statistical evaluations of viral clearance studies for biological products. *Biologicals*, 40(6), 439–444.

Liao, C.T., Lin, T.Y., and Iyer, H.K. (2005). One- and two-sided tolerance intervals for general balanced mixed models and unbalanced one-way random models. *Technometrics*, 47, 323–335.

Liao, J.J.Z., Tian, Y., and Capen, R.C. (2011). Assessing the similarity of bioanalytical methods. *PDA J. Pharm. Sci. Technol.*, 65(1), 55–62.

Lin, T.Y.D. (1994). Applicability of matrix and bracket approach to stability design. *Proceedings of the Biopharmaceutical Section of the American Statistical Association.* Alexandria, VA, 142–147.

Lin, T.Y.D. and Fairweather, W.R. (1997). Statistical design (bracketing and matrixing) and analysis of stability data for the US market. *Proceedings of IBC.*

Liu, J. and Hsieh, E. (2010). Evaluation of linearity in assay validation. In *Encyclopedia of Biopharmaceutical Statistics.* 2nd ed., Informa Healthcare, 467–474.

Longwell, A. (2016). United States of American v. Barr Labs, Inc. 812 F. Supp. 458, GMP lessons from a federal Judge. http://fdclaw.com/cases/gmp/ (accessed on April 20, 2016).

Madsen, Jr., R.E. (1994). US vs Barr Laboratories: A technical perspective. *PDA J. Pharm. Sci. Technol.*, 48(4), 176–179.

Manola, A. (2012). Assessing Release Limits and Manufacturing Risk from a Bayesian Perspective. Mid-West Biopharmaceutical Statistics Workshop, May 2012, Muncie, ID.

Martin, G.P., Barnett, K.L., Burgess, C., Curry, P.D., Ermer, J., Gratzl, G.S., Hammond, J.P., Herrmann, J., Kovacs, E., LeBlond, D.J., LoBrutto, R., McCasland-Keller, A.K., McGregor, P.L., Nethercote, P., Templeton, A.C., Thomas, D.P., and Weitzel, J. (2013). Stimuli to the revision process: Lifecycle management of analytical procedures: Method development, procedure performance quantification, and procedure performance verification. *Phamacopeial Forum*, 39(5). http:/www.usp.org/uspnf /stimuli-article-lifecycle-management-analytical-procedures-posted-comment.

Massart, D.L., Vandeginste, B.G.M., Buydens, L.M.C., De Jong, S., Lewi, P.J., Smeyers-Verbeke, J. (1997). *Handbook of Chemometrics and Qualimetrics: Part A.* Elsevier, Amsterdam.

MCR Biostatistics Unit (2016). http://www.mrc-bsu.cam.ac.uk/software/bugs/.

Mee, R. (1984). β-expectation and β-content tolerance limits for balanced one-way ANOVA random model. *Technometrics*, 26, 251–254.

Mee, R. (1988). Estimation of the percentage of a normal distribution lying outside a specified interval. *Commun. Stat. Theory Methods*, 17(5), 1465–1479.

Metz, C.E. (1978). Basic principles of ROC curve analysis. *Semin. Nucl. Med.*, 8, 283–298.

Miller, K., Bowsher, R., Celniker, A. et al. (2001). Workshop on bioanalytical methods validation for macromolecules: Summary report. *Pharm. Res.*, 18, 1373–1383.

Montgomery, D.C. (2009). *Introduction to Statistical Quality Control.* 6th ed., John Wiley & Sons, New York.

Narula, S. (1979). Orthogonal polynomial regression. *Int. Stat. Rev.*, 47(1), 31–36.

NCCLS (1986). NCCLS proposed guideline EP6-P. Evaluation of the Linearity of Quantitative Method. Villanova, PA.

Neter, J. (1990). *Applied Linear Statistical Models.* 3rd ed., CRC Press.

Nethercote, P. and Ermer, J. (2012). Quality by design for analytical methods: Implications for method validation and transfer. *Pharm. Technol.*, 36(10), 74–79.

Nethrcote, P., Borman, P., Bennett, T., Martin, G., and McGregor, P. (2010). QbD for better method validation and transfer. *Pharm. Manuf.*, http://www.pharma manufacturing.com/articles/2010/060/ (accessed on April 17, 2016).

Nijhuis, M. and Van den Heuvel, E.R. (2007). Closed-form confidence intervals on measures of precision for an 728 interlaboratory study. *J Biopharm Stat.*, 17(1), 123–142.

Nordbrock, E. and Valvani, S. (1995). PhRMA Stability Working Group. In *Guidelines for Matrix Designs of Drug Product Stability Protocols.*

Novick, S. and Yang, H. (2013). Directly testing the linearity assumption for assay validation. *J. Chemom.*, 27(5), 117–123.

Novick, S., Yang, H., and Peterson, J. (2012). A Bayesian approach to parallelism testing *Stat. Biopharm. Res.*, 4(4), 357–374.

O'Connell, M.A., Belanger, B.A., and Haaland, P.D. (1993). Calibration and assay development using the four-parameter logistic model. *Chemom. Intell. Lab. Syst.*, 20, 97–114.

PDA (2015). PDA Technical Report No. 69 Bioburden and Biofilm Management in Pharmaceutical Manufacturing Operations. https://store.pda.org/TableOf Contents/TR69_TOC.pdf.

Peden, K., Sheng, L., Pal, A., and Lewis, A. (2006). Biological activity of residual cell substrate DNA. *Dev. Biol. (Basel)*, 123, 45–56, discussion 55–73. *In Vitro Cellular and Development Biology. Monograph No. 6: Abnormal Cells, New Products, and Risks,* ed by Hopps, H.E., and Petricciani, J.C., Tissue Culture Association, Gaithersburg, MD, 1985.

Peltzman, S. (1973). An evaluation of consumer protection legislation: The 1962 drug amendments. *J. Polit. Econ.*, 81(5), 1051.

Pepe, M.S., Gu, J.W., and Morris, D.E. (2010). The potential of genes and other markers to inform about risk. *Cancer Epidemiol Biomarkers Prev.*, 19(3), 655–665.

Peterson, J.J. (2004). A posterior predictive approach to multiple response surface optimization. *J. Qual. Technol.*, 36, 139–153.

Peterson, J.J. (2007). A review of Bayesian reliability approaches to multiple response surface optimization. In *Bayesian Statistics for Process Monitoring, Control, and Optimization,* ed by Colosimo, B.M. and del Castillo, E., Chapman and Hall/CRC Press, Inc.

Peterson, J.J. (2008). A Bayesian approach to the ICH Q8 definition of design space. *J. Biopharm. Stat.*, 18, 959–975.

Peterson, J.J. (2009). What your ICH Q8 design space needs: A multivariate predictive distribution. *Pharm. Manuf.*, 8(10), 23–28.

Peterson, J.J. and Lief, K. (2010). The ICH Q8 definition of design space: A comparison of the overlapping means and the Bayesian predictive approaches. *Stat. Biopharm. Res.*, 2, 249–259.

Peterson, J.J. and Yahyah, M. (2009). A Bayesian design space approach to robustness and system suitability for pharmaceutical assays and other processes. *Stat. Biopharm. Res.*, 1(4), 441–449.

Peterson, J.J., Miró-Quesada, G., and del Castillo, E. (2009a). A Bayesian reliability approach to multiple response optimization with seemingly unrelated regression models. *Qual. Technol. Qual. Manage.*, 6(4), 353–369.

Peterson, J.J., Snee, R.D., McAllister, P.R., Schoefield, T.L., and Carella, A.J. (2009b). Statistics in pharmaceutical development and manufacturing (with discussion). *J. Qual. Technol.*, 111–134.

Petricciani, J. and Loewer, J. (2001). An overview of cell DNA issues. *Dev. Biol. (Basel)*, 106, 275–782, discussion 317–329.

PhRMA CMC Statistics, Stability Expert Teams (2005). Identification of out-of-trend stability results, part II, *Pharm. Technol.*, October 2005, http://www.pharmtech .com/identification-out-trend-stability-results-part-ii-phrma-cmc-statistics-sta bility-expert-teams (accessed on April 15, 2016).

Press, S.J. (1972). *Applied Multivariate Analysis: Using Bayesian and Frequentist Methods of Inference*. R.E. Krieger Pub. Co.

Quinlan, M., Stroup, W., Christopher, D., and Schwenke, J. (2013a). On the distribution of batch shelf lives. *J. Biopharm. Stat.*, 23, 897–920.

Quinlan, M., Stroup, W., Schwenke, J., and Christopher, D. (2013b). Evaluating the performance of the ICH guidelines for shelf life estimation. *J. Biopharm. Stat.*, 23, 881–896.

Rathore, A. and Mhatre, R. (2009). *Quality by Design for Biopharmaceuticals: Principles and Case Studies*. Wiley & Sons, Inc.

Robert, C. and Casella, G. (2004). *Monte Carlo Statistical Methods*. 2nd ed., Springer.

Roberts, S.W. (1959). Control chart tests based on geometric moving averages. *Technometrics*, 1, 239–250.

Robson, D.S. (1959). A simple method for constructing orthogonal polynomials when the independent variable is unequally spaced. *Biometrics*, 15(2), 187–191.

Rothenfusser, S., Tuma, E., Wagner, M., Endres, S., and Hartmann, G. (2003). Recent advance in immunostimulatory CpG oligonucleotides. *Curr. Opin. Mol. Ther.*, 5, 98–106.

Rozet, E., Govaerts, B., Lebrun, P., Michail, K., Ziemons, E., Wintersteigerc, R., Rudaz, S., Boulanger, B., and Hubert, P. (2011). Evaluating the reliability of analytical results using a probability criterion: A Bayesian perspective. *Anal. Chim. Acta*, 705, 193–206.

Saffaj, T. and Ihssane, B. (2012). A Bayesian approach for application to method validation and measurement uncertainty. *Talanta*, 92, 15–25.

SAS (1998). *SAS User's Guide*. SAS, Inc.

SAS (2009). *SAS/STAT User's Guide, Version 9*. SAS Institute, Cary, NC.

Satterthwaite, F.W. (1946). An approximate distribution of estimates of variance component. *Biometric Bull.*, 2, 110–114.

Schenerman, M.A., Axley, M.J., Oliver, C.N., Ram, K., and Wasserman, G.F. (2009). Using a risk assessment process to determine criticality of product quality attributes. In *Quality by Design for Biopharmaceutical: Principles and Case Studies*, ed by Rathore, A.S. and Mhatre, R., Wiley.

Schilling, E.G. (1982). *Acceptance Sampling in Quality Control*. Marcel Dekker, Inc., New York and Basel, Milwaukee.

Schofield, T. (2009). Product stability study design and analysis to support product licensure. *Biologicals*, 37: 387–396.

Schuirmann, D.J. (1987). A comparison of the two one-sided tests procedure and the power approach for assessing the equivalence of average bioavailability. *J. Pharmacokinet. Biopharm.*, 15, 657–680.

Shakun, M. (1965). Multivariate acceptance procedures for general specification ellipsoids. *J. Am. Stat. Assoc.*, 60(311), 905–913.

Shao, J. and Chow, S.-C. (1991). Constructing release targets for drug products: A Bayesian decision theory approach. *Appl. Stat.*, 40(3), 381–391.

Shao, J. and Chow, S.-C. (2001). Drug shelf life estimation. *Stat. Sin.*, 11, 737–745.

Sheng, L., Cai, F., Zhu, Y., Pal, A., Athanasiou, M., Orrison, B., Blair, D.G., Hughes, S.H., Coffin, J.M., Lewis, A.M., and Peden, K. (2008). Oncogenicity of DNA in vivo: Tumor induction with expression plasmids for activated H-ras and c-myc. *Biologicals*, 36(3), 184–197.

Sheng-Fowler, L., Cai, F., Fu, H., Zhu, Y., Orrison, B., Foseh, G., Blair, D.G., Hughes, S.H., Coffin, J.M., Lewis, Jr., A.M., and Peden, K. (2010). Tumors induced in mice by direct inoculation of plasmid DNA expressing both activated H-*ras* and c-*myc*. *Int. J. Biol. Sci.*, 6, 151–162.

Sheng-Fowler, L., Lewis, Jr., A.M., and Peden, K. (2009a). Issues associated with residual cell-substrate DNA in viral vaccines. *Biologicals*, 37, 190–195.

Sheng-Fowler, L., Lewis, Jr., A.M., and Peden, K. (2009b). Quantitative determination of the infectivity of the proviral DNA of a retrovirus in vitro: Evaluation of methods for DNA inactivation. *Biologicals*, 37, 259–269.

Silberberg, M.S. (2006). *Chemistry*. 4th ed., McGraw-Hill, New York.

Silverman, R.A. (1989). *Essential Calculus with Applications*. Dover Publications, Inc., New York.

Sondag, P., Joei, R., and Yang, H. (2015). Confidence interval on ratios of parameters of two four parameters logistic curves. *PDA J. Pharm. Sci. Technol.*, 69(4), 467–470.

Spiegelhalter, D.J., Abrams, K.R., and Myles, J.P. (2004). *Bayesian Approaches to Clinical Trials and Health-Care Evaluation*. Wiley, Hoboken, NJ.

Stockdale, G. and Cheng, A. (2009). Finding design space and a reliable operating region using a multivariate bayesian approach with experimental design. *Qual. Technol. Quant. Manage.*, 6(4), 391–408.

Strang, G. (2005). *Linear Algebra and Its Applications*. 4th ed, Cengage Learning, Stamford, CT.

Stroup, W. and Quinlan, M. (2010). Alternative shelf life estimation methodologies. *Proceedings of 2010 Joint Statistical Meeting, American Statistical Association*, Alexandria, VA, 2056–2066.

Swets, J. and Pickett, R.M. (1982). *Evaluation of Diagnostic Systems: Methods from Signal Detection Theory*. Academic Press, New York.

Tague, T.R. (2004). Seven basic quality tools. In *The Quality Toolbox*. American Society for Quality, Milwaukee, Wisconsin.

Thyregod, P. (1998). *En Introduktion Til Statistik*. Bind S. Institute for Mathematical Modelling, Technical University of Denmark, Lyngby.

Tse, S.K. and Xiang, L. (2009). Outlier detection in clinical research. In *Encyclopedia of Biopharmaceutical Statistics*, ed by Chow, S.C., Marcel Dekker.

Tsong, Y., Hammerstrom, T., Sathe, P., and Shah, V.P. (1996). Statistical assessment of mean differences between two dissolution data sets. *Drug Inf. J.*, 30, 1105–1112.

USP (1989). General Information <1225> Validation of Compendial Methods. *United States Pharmacopeia XXVI*, 2439–2442.

USP (1997). USP <1231> Water for Pharmaceutical Purposes. *Pharmacopeial Forum*, 30(5), 1744.

USP (2000). USP <111> Design and Analysis of Biological Assays. In *United States Pharmacopeia 24*/National Formulary, 19, 1842–1844.

USP (2003). General Information Chapter <1111> Microbiological Quality of Non-Sterile Pharmaceutical Products. *Pharmacopeial Forum*, 29(5), 1733–1735.

USP (2004a). General Chapter <61> Microbial Limit Tests. 27-NF 22, 2152–2157.

USP (2004b). USP <62> Microbiological Examination of Non-Sterile Products: Tests for Specified Microorganisms.

USP (2005). General Chapter <1010> Analytical Data—Interpretation and Treatment. 36-*NF* 31, 452–464.

USP (2010a). In-Process Revision <1032> Development and Design of Bioassays [NEW] (USP34-NF29 2S). *Pharmacopoeial Forum* 36(3.4).

USP (2010b). In-Process Revision <1034> Analysis of Biological Assays [NEW] (USP34-NF29 2S). *Pharmacopoeial Forum* 36(3.4).

USP (2013). General Information <1210> Statistical Tools for Analytical Procedure Validation. *Pharmacopeial Forum*, 40(5).

van Loco, J., Elskens, M., Croux, C., and Beernaert, H. (2002). Linearity of calibration curves: Use and misuse of the correlation coefficient. *Accred. Qual. Assur.*, 7, 281–285.

Weerahandi, S. (1993). Generalized confidence intervals. *J. Am. Stat. Assoc.*, 88, 899–905.

Weerahandi, S. (1995a). *Exact Statistical Methods for Data Analysis*. Springer-Verlag, New York.

Weerahandi, S. (1995b). Generalized confidence intervals. *J. Am. Stat. Assoc.*, 88, 899–905.

Weerahandi, S. (2004). *Generalized Inference in Repeated Measures: Exact Methods in MANOVA and Mixed Model*. Wiley, Hoboken, NJ.

Wei, G.C.G. (1998). Simple methods for determination of the release limits for drug products. *J. Biopharm. Stat.*, 8(1), 103–114.

Wei, G.C.G. (2003). Release targets. In *Encyclopedia of Biopharmaceutical Statistics*, ed by Chow, S.-C., Marcel Dekker, 833–837.

WHO (2006). WHO Guidelines on Stability Evaluation of Vaccines. http://www .who.int/biologicals/publications/trs/areas/vaccines/stability/Microsoft%20 Word%20-%20BS%202049.Stability.final.09_Nov_06.pdf (accessed on April 16, 2016).

WHO (2007). Meeting Report—WHO Study Group on Cell Substrates for Production of Biologicals. June 11 and 12, 2007, 1–30. http://www.who.int/biologicals /publications/meetings/areas/vaccines/cells/Cells.FINAL.MtgRep.IK.26 _Sep_07.pdf (accessed on April 15, 2016).

Wilk, M.B. and Gnanadesikan, R. (1968). Probability plotting methods for the analysis of data. *Biometrika (Biometrika Trust)*, 55(1), 1–17.

Wilson, J.D. (1997). Setting alert and action limits for environmental monitoring. *PDA J. Pharm. Sci. Technol.*, 51(4), 161–162.

Wolfinger, R.D. (1998). Tolerance intervals for variance component models using Bayesian simulation. *J Qual. Technol.*, 3018–3032.

Wood, E.E. (1946). The theory of certain analytical procedures with particular reference to micro-biological assays. *Analyst*, 71, 1–14.

Woodcock, J. (2012). Reliable drug quality: An unresolved problem. *PDA J. Pharm. Sci. Technol.*, 66, 270–272.

Yang, H. (2012a). Multivariate control chart for environmental monitoring. *J. Validation Technol.*, 18(4), 59–63.

Yang, H. (2012b). Ensure product quality and regulatory compliance through novel stability design and analysis. *J. Validation Technol.*, 18(3), 52–59.

Yang, H. (2013a). Setting specifications of correlated quality attributes. *PDA J. Pharm. Sci. Technol.*, 67, 533–543.

Yang, H. (2013b). Establishing acceptable limits of residual DNA (2013). *PDA J. Pharm. Sci. Technol.*, March–April Issue, 67, 155–163.

Yang, H. (2013c). How many batches are needed for process validation under the new FDA guidance? *PDA J. Pharm. Sci. Technol.*, 67, 53–62.

Yang, H. (2013d). Setting specifications of correlated quality attributes *PDA J. Pharm. Sci. Technol.*, 67, 533–543.

Yang, H. and Zhang, L. (2008). Multivariate control chart for environmental monitoring. *Proceedings of 2008 JSM*.

Yang, H. and Zhang, L. (2012a). Evaluations of parallelism testing methods using ROC analysis. *Stat. Biopharm. Res.*, 2(12), 67–74.

Yang, H. and Zhang, L. (2012b). Evaluation of statistical methods for estimating shelf life of drug products: A unified and risk-based approach. *J. Validation Technol.*, http://www.ivtnetwork.com/sites/default/files/IVTJVT0512_067-074_Yang -%7B1237440%7D.pdf (accessed on April 16, 2016).

Yang, H. and Zhang, J. (2015). A generalized pivotal quantity approach to analytical method validation based on total error. *PDA J. Pharm. Sci. Technol.*, 69, 725–735.

Yang, H. and Zhang, J. (2016). A Bayesian approach to residual host cell DNA safety assessment. *PDA J. Pharm. Sci. Technol.*, 70, 157–162.

Yang, H., Kim, J., Zhang, L., Strouse, R., Schenerman, M., and Jiang, X. (2012). Parallelism testing of 4-parameter logistic curves for bioassay. *PDA J. Pharm. Sci. Technol.*, May–June Issue, 262–269.

Yang, H., Li, N., and Chang, S. (2013a). A risk-based approach to setting sterile filtration bioburden limits. *PDA J. Pharm. Sci. Technol.*, 67, 601–609.

Yang, H., Novick, S., and LeBlond, D. (2015a). Testing analytical method linearity within a pre-specified range. *J. Biopharm. Stat.*, 25(2), 334–350.

Yang, H., Wei, Z., and Schenerman, M. (2015b). A statistical approach to determining criticality of residual host cell DNA. *J. Biopharm. Stat.*, 25(2), 234–246.

Yang, H., Zhang, L., and Galinski, M. (2010). A probabilistic model for risk assessment of residual host cell DNA in biological products. *Vaccine*, 28(19), 3308–3311.

Yang, H., Zhang, J., Yu, B., and Zhao, W. (2015c). *Statistical Methods for Immunogenicity Risk Assessment*. Chapman & Hall/CRC.

Yang, H., Zhao, W., O'Day, T., and Fleming, W. (2013b). Environmental monitoring: Setting alert and action limits based on a zero-inflated model. *PDA J. Pharm. Sci. Technol.*, 67(1), 1–9.

Yu, L.X. (2008). Pharmaceutical quality by design: Product and process development, understanding, and control. *Pharm. Res.*, 25(4), 781–791.

Yu, L.X., Amidon, G., Khan, M.A., Hoag, S.W., Polli, J., Raju, J.K., and Woodcock, J. (2014). Understanding pharmaceutical quality by design. *AAPS J.*, 16(4), 771–783.

Zhang, L., Matthew, T., Yang, H., Krishnamoorthy, K., and Cho, I. (2010). Tolerance limits for a ratio of two correlated normal variables. *J. Biopharm. Stat.*, 20, 172–184.

Zhao, W. and Yang, H. (2015). *Statistical Methods for Drug Combination Study Design and Analysis*. Chapman & Hall/CRC.

Zhou, S.S. (2011). Biopharmaceutical process evaluated for viral clearance. https:// www.united.com/ual/en/gb/flight-search/book-a-flight/results/rev?f=LHR&t =IAD&d=2016-01-21&tt=1&sc=7&px=1&taxng=1.

Index

Page numbers with f and t refer to figures and tables, respectively.